Caregiver Patient Communications

Readings

Brent D. Ruben
Nurit Guttman
Rutgers University - New Brunswick

KENDALL/HUNT PUBLISHING COMPANY
2460 Kerper Boulevard P.O. Box 539 Dubuque, Iowa 52004-0539

ISBN 0-8403-8368-1

Printed in the United States of America
10 9 8 7 6 5 4 3 2 1

Table of Contents

Models of Caregiver-Patient Relationship

Dimensions of Caregiving

Caregiver-Patient Interaction: Empirical Research and Implications

The Issue of "Patient Compliance"

Patient Satisfaction and Quality of Care

Enhancing Communication Competencies and Patient Rights

Medicine, Society and Culture: Alternative Perspectives on the Context of Caregiving

Preface

Communication between caregivers and patients is an area of increasing interest and concern in medical, academic and popular literature. As patients, our most vivid recollections of a medical encounter more often relate to how or what the caregiver said or did not say to us, and to how we were treated interpersonally rather than to other facets of the medical treatment (Ruben, 1990, 1992, and in this volume).

The readings in this book have been chosen to provide the reader with an overview of some of the major issues related to caregiver-patient communication and their implications. The book begins with three essays that discuss theoretical perspectives or models of the caregiver-patient relationship. These essays underscore the importance of identifying the assumptions and expectations that underlie relationships between health care providers and lay persons, and their implications for lay and professional perceptions of health, illness, and medical treatment (e.g. see Calnan, 1987; Kaplan, 1987; Lau et al., 1989). There are numerous perspectives regarding the responsibilities and roles of both caregivers and patients, and different assumptions by the parties involved can be a source of conflict and misunderstanding (Brickman et al., 1982; Northouse & Northouse, 1985).

The multitude of approaches suggests that the relationship between caregivers and patients is a very complex one, and one that cannot be taken for granted by either party. The first essay presents what has become a classic typology of three basic models. Szasz and Hollander, in an article originally published in 1956 in *Archives of Internal Medicine*, suggest that different types of relationships between practitioners and their patients emerge, related to technical procedures and social settings. In the first two models the meaning of diagnosis and treatment is controlled by the physician. In the third, the model of "mutual participation," evaluation of the therapeutic result and the notions of disease and health are essentially negotiated between the physician and patient as equal partners.

Engel, by adopting a general systems approach, further develops the latter perspective. Engel outlines a model which he calls "biopsychosocial" that incorporates biomedical aspects, as well as psychological and social aspects that are seen as important contributors to the definition and treatment of illness. Engel suggests that by focusing solely on biomedical factors and on the role of the physician, health caregiving ignores other factors that are important in the patient's life or other caregivers who could be working in collaboration rather than as adversaries. Engel emphasizes collaboration across professional affiliation and inclusion of the "patient's voice" or criteria. The latter, according to this model, should be accepted as equally important and legitimate. These models and more recent formulations are reviewed and discussed by Perry. Though differing in many respects, these perspectives suggest that an exclusively biomedical view of medical care is too restrictive, and they emphasize the importance of communication in medical encounters.

The essays in the second section amplify the psychosocial dimensions of caring. Barlund, Cousins, and Suchman and Mathews argue for integrating biomedical with social factors to achieve optimal medical care (see a recent study by Ben-Sira, 1990). These authors illustrate some of the important implications of communication factors in the caregiver-patient relationship, which extend beyond the biomedical emphasis that has dominated much of recent medical education and practice.

The essay by Friedman reviews findings on nonverbal factors in the health care context. Friedman reviews findings that indicate that facial expressions, touch, gaze or olfaction provide important communication cues both for practitioners and patients. Friedman suggests that nonverbal communication takes on a special importance in medical settings and may have an important impact on the outcomes of medical interactions.

The third section presents reports of studies in which the caregiver-patient relationship has been empirically observed and analyzed. These studies represent only a sample of a growing number of investigations that systematically analyze caregiver-patient interaction (e.g. see Fisher & Todd, 1984; O'Hair, 1989; Stewart & Roter, 1989). Clearly, the findings of these studies indicate that communication between caregivers and their patients is important both to the process and outcome of health care delivery. Essays by Frankel and Beckman, Waitzkin, and Fisher focus primarily on verbal or sociolinguistic aspects of the interaction. These researchers' findings demonstrate how medical encounters are often characterized as asymmetrical in terms of power, influence, and information exchange. Typically health care encounters are dominated by the caregiver, and consequently critical medical decisions may be made with little regard to patients' priorities, concerns, or values. Moreover, the practitioners' assumptions regarding the patients or their attributions regarding patients' behavior influence clinical decisions. The latter is dramatically illustrated in Fisher and Millman's observations. Millman describes how practitioners' presentation of "what went wrong" with patients who were misdiagnosed, directly relates to communication factors: these particular patients' symptoms were ignored because the practitioners assessed them as communicatively incompetent, or as morally irresponsible.

Kaplan, Greenfield and Ware's research is provocative and intervention oriented. These researchers suggest that better health related outcomes can be achieved by improving physician-patient communication. Specifically, they designed controlled experimental interventions to increase the participation of the patients in their encounters with physicians by enhancing particular communication competence skills. Their findings indicate that patients in the experimental group were more effective in obtaining information which was also related to better health status measures. The problematic factors related to information exchange between providers and patients, and the importance of enhancing participative decision making in medical encounters (e.g. see Ballard-Reisch, 1990) are reviewed in the essay by Guttman.

The topic of the fourth section is patient compliance. Patient compliance refers to the extent to which patients follow the treatment regimen or the medical recommendations prescribed by caregivers. Mounting evidence persuasively indicates that patients often do not follow medical recommendations. As the readings suggest, issues related to noncompliance and strategies available to encourage patients to follow medical recommendations are numerous and complex, and are burdened with practical as well as ethical dimensions.

Byham and Vickery review numerous studies, often of contradictory conclusions regarding patient compliance with medical recommendations, and offer suggestions on how to improve outcomes. These authors propose that compliance should not be viewed as coercive obedience to practitioners' orders, but "as a negotiated agreement." This echos the participatory theme that emerges in the biopsychosocial perspectives. Trostle, however, challenges us to consider patient compliance as an ideology which promotes physician control over medical care. He concludes with suggestions that we should examine the assumptions underlying the notion of medical compliance, and that our conceptualization of what it means to "comply" should be made more explicit.

Quality of care and patient satisfaction with health care delivery has become a growing concern in health care delivery. The essays in the fourth section suggest that communication factors are at the heart of patient satisfaction, which in turn can be related to the outcome of care—whether these outcomes relate to memorable experiences as discussed by Ruben, or to malpractice prevention, as discussed in the essay by the Midwest Medial Insurance Company Risk Management Committee.

The analyses of the research findings on the caregiver-patient relationship indicate that communication in the medical context is important but often unsatisfactory. The fifth section presents essays on the topic of enhancing the communication competencies of the parties involved. Greenfield, Kaplan and Ware's research has focused on enhancing some of the communication competencies of patients. However the traditional and most common approach has been to focus on enhancing the communication skills of providers. Cline presents an overview of this topic, discusses the importance of adopting a communication perspective, and offers suggestions on how medical practitioners can enhance their relationship with their clients. Rowland-Morin and Reuben turn to the patients and offer them suggestions on what they can do to make the most from their medical encounter. Essays by Hunt and Schuman and Wiles suggest that the issue of patients' rights treads a delicate balance between patients' right to know, and their right not to know, as well.

The final section shifts the discussion on the nature of the caregiver-patient relationship to the more general context of health care. Although Engel in his biopsychosocial model urges the consideration of the social context of caregiving, he does not address the cultural implications of medical caregiving in a highly technocratic and technological environment. Social critics such as Ivan Illich, argue that modern medicine as it is practiced today is big business, and that it has changed the way human beings relate to living and dying, to pain or pleasure, and to various social institutions. The question that we are asked to consider is whether society has become over-medicalized, which in turn might create unrealistic expectations on the part of patients relative to their medical practitioners (Gibbs, 1989). The essays by Fox and Illich provoke us to consider whether the medical caregiver is expected to provide us with unlimited biomedical solutions to a wide gamut of emotional, social and even moral issues that are an inevitable part of the fabric of human existence. Illich, in the book *Medical Nemesis*, suggests that medicine as it is practiced today may do us more harm than good; it is accompanied by an essay by Renée Fox that provides an analysis and critique of this perspective.

Although the essays by Illich and Fox do not focus on the communication between caregivers and patients, the implication of their analyses clearly suggests that practitioner-patient communication is influenced by the cultural context of medical practice. These authors do not elaborate on how relationships between medical practitioners and laypersons are related to changing norms and cultural expectations. However, the progression of practitioner-patient communication models as reviewed by Perry in this volume suggest that in order to better understand the challenges that face health care encounters we must contextualize them in an institutional and cultural milieu. As a journalist (Gibbs, 1989, p. 49) recently observed:

> the physicians, victims of their own success, are finding that however swift the advance of medical knowledge, it is still outpaced by public expectations. 'The public thinks that all diseases should be treatable, all disabilities repairable' observes John Stoeckle, chief of the medical clinics at Massachusetts General Hospital. 'And there should be no pain and suffering.'

Clearly, this observation confirms Illich's prediction that modern medicine will contribute to what he labels cultural iatrogenesis, or escalating expectations of medical technology and practitioners to "fix" and eliminate a wide gamut of human problems. Unfortunately, these are expectations which modern medicine cannot fully meet, leading to frustration and dissatisfaction among the various parties involved.

The final essay takes us a step into the future, and presents a scenario of how patients could be medically diagnosed at their homes, via computer technology, without the necessity of a visit to a health practitioner. In fact, current technology can offer us similar services today, as those described by Watson. Readers may want to consider the implications of the use of this type of technology for medical practice and patient communication. Might we be better off interacting with a "smart" system, and eliminating the difficulties associated with face-to-face medical encounters?

Since the use of computer technology raises the potential for "self-care" and enhanced access to expert opinion, one might ask about possible benefits and implications. However, with increased use of this type of technology for health care delivery, issues such as privacy, liability and increased inequity of access to health care among different members of society will need to be addressed as well.

The purpose of this book is to introduce the reader to some of the major issues in caregiver-provider communication, and to offer conceptual frameworks and empirical findings to help guide and challenge our own observations and reservations.

The essays in the volume are presented from different perspectives and by authors who come from different backgrounds. These include physicians, patients (e.g. Norman Cousins who after an illness, became very interested in studying the relationship of emotions to clinical aspects of care), communication scholars, sociolinguists, sociologists, anthropologists, management specialists and social critics.

Few topics are as complex and touch the lives of as many of us as health communication. And few topics, therefore, are more deserving of our thoughtful attention as professionals, students, and laypersons. Our hope is that this volume will contribute meaningfully to dialogue on this important topic.

References

Ballard-Reisch, S.S. (1990). A model of participative decision making for physician-patient interaction. *Health Communication*, 2(2), 91-104.

Ben-Sira, Z. (1990). Primary care practitioners' likelihood to engage in a bio-psychosocial approach: An additional perspective on the doctor-patient relationship. *Social Science and Medicine*, 31(5), 565-576.

Calnan, M. (1987). *Health and illness: The lay perspective*. London: Tavistock Publications.

Brickman, P., Rabinowitz, V.C., Karuza, J., Coates, D., Cohn, E., & Kidder, L. (1982). Models of helping and coping. *American Psychologist*, 37(4), 368-384.

Engel, G.L. (1978). The Biopsychosocial model and the education of health professionals. *Annals of the New York Academy of Sciences*, 310, 169-181.

Fisher, S. & Todd, A.D. (Eds.). (1983). *The Social Organization of Doctor-Patient Communication*. Washington, DC: Center for Applied Linguistics.

Gibbs, N. (1989). Sick and Tired. *Time*, July 31, 48-53.

Kaplan, S. H. (1987). Patient reports of health status as predictors of psychologic health measures in chronic disease. *Journal of Chronic Disease*, 40(Suppl. 1), 27S-35S.

Lau, R.R., Bernard, T.M., & Hartman, K.A. (1989). Further explorations of common-sense representations of common illnesses. *Health Psychology*, 8(2), 195-219.

Northouse, P.G. & Northouse, L.L. (1985). *Health Communication: A Handbook for health professionals*. Englewoods Cliffs, NJ:Prentice Hall.

O'Hair, D. (1989). Dimensions of relational communication and control during physician-patient interaction. *Health Communication*, 1(2), 97-115.

Ruben, B. D. (1990). The health caregiver-patient relationship: pathology, etiology, treatment. In E.B. Ray & L. Donohew (Eds.), *Communication in Health Care Contexts: A Systems Perspective*. Hillsdale, NJ: Lawrence Erlbaum Associates.

Ruben, B. D. (1992). "What Patients Remember: A Content Analysis of Critical Incidents in Health Care." *Health Communication* 5(2), 1992 in press.

Stewart M. & Roter D.(Eds.). *Communicating with Medical Patients*. Newbury Park, CA: Sage.

Models of Caregiver-Patient Relationship

The Basic Models of the Doctor-Patient Relationship

Thomas S. Szasz and Marc H. Hollender

When a person leaves the culture in which he was born and raised and migrates to another, he usually experiences his new social setting as something strange—and in some ways threatening—and he is stimulated to master it by conscious efforts at understanding. To some extent every immigrant to the United States reacts in this manner to the American scene. Similarly, the American tourist in Europe or South America "scrutinizes" the social setting which is taken for granted by the natives. To scrutinize—and criticize—the pattern of other peoples' lives is obviously both common and easy. It also happens, however, that people exposed to cross cultural experiences turn their attention to the very customs which formed the social matrix of their lives in the pant. Lastly, to study the "customs" which shape and govern one's day-to-day life is most difficult of all. (Ref 1).

In many ways the psychoanalyst is like a person who has integrated from one culture to another. To him the relationship between physician and patient—which is like a custom that is taken for granted in medical practice and which he himself so treated in his early history—has become an object of study. While the precise nature and extent of the influence which psychoanalysis and so-called dynamic psychiatry have had on modern medicine are debatable, it seems to us that the most decisive effect has been that of making physicians explicitly aware of the possible significance of their relationship to patients.

The question naturally arises as to "What is a doctor-patient relationship?" It is our aim to discuss this question and to show that certain philosophical preconceptions associated with the notions of "disease," "treatment," and "cure" have a profound bearing on both the theory and the practice of medicine.[1]

What Is a Human Relationship?

The concept of a relationship is a novel one in medicine. Traditionally, physicians have been concerned with "things," for example, anatomical structures, lesions, bacteria, and the like. In modern times the scope has been broadened to include the concept of "function." The phenomenon of a human relationship is often viewed as though it were a "thing" or a "function." It is, in fact, neither. Rather it is an abstraction, appropriate for the description and handling of certain observational facts. Moreover, it is an abstraction which presupposes concepts of both structure and function.

The foregoing comments may be clarified by concrete illustrations. Psychiatrists often suggest to their medical colleagues that the physician's relationship with his patient per se helps the latter.

Szasz, T. S. and Hollender, M.C. The basic models of the doctor-patient relationship. Archives in Internal Medicine, 97, p. 585-592.

1 In our approach to this subject we have been influenced by psychologic (psychoanalytic), sociologic, and philosophic considerations. See in this connection References 2-4 and Szasz, T.S.: On the Theory of Psychoanalytic Treatment, read before the Annual Meeting of the American Psychoanalytic Association, Atlantic City, N.J., May 7, 1955; *Internat. J. Psychoanal.*, to be published.

This creates the impression (whether so intended or not) that the relationship is a thing, which works not unlike the way that vitamins do in a case of vitamin deficiency. Another idea is that the doctor-patient relationship depends mainly on what the physician does (or thinks or feels). Then it is viewed not unlike a function.

When we consider a relationship in which there is joint participation of the two persons involved, "relationship" refers to neither a structure nor a function (such as the "personality" of the physician or patient). It is, rather, an abstraction embodying the activities of two interacting systems (persons). (Ref. 5).

Three Basic Models of the Doctor-Patient Relationship

The three basic models of the doctor-patient relationship (see Table 1), which we will describe, embrace modes of interaction ubiquitous in human relationships and in no way specific for the contact between physician and patient. The specificity of the medical situation probably derives from a combination of these modes of interaction with certain technical procedures and social settings.

1. The model of activity-passivity

Historically, this is the oldest conceptual model. Psychologically, it is not an interaction, because it is based on the effect of one person on another in such a way and under such circumstances that the person acted upon is unable to contribute actively, or is considered to be inanimate. This frame of reference (in which the physician does something to the patient) underlies the application of some of the outstanding advances of modern medicine (e.g., anesthesia and surgery, antibiotics, etc.). The physician is active; the patient, passive. This orientation has originated in—and is entirely appropriate for the treatment of emergencies (e.g., for the patient who is severely injured, bleeding, delirious, or in coma). "Treatment" takes place irrespective of the patient's contribution and regardless of the outcome. There is a similarity here between the patient and a helpless infant, on the one hand, and between the physician and a parent, on the other. It may be recalled that psychoanalysis, too, evolved from a procedure (hypnosis) which was based on this model. Various physical measures to which psychotics are subjected today are another example of the activity-passivity frame of reference.

Table 1 Three basic models of the physician-patient relationship

	Model	Physician's Role	Patient's Role	Clinical Application of Model	Prototype of Model
1.	Activity-passivity	Does something to patient	Recipient (unable to respond or inert	Anesthesia, acute trauma, coma, delirium, etc	Parent-infant
2.	Guidance-cooperation	Tells patient what to do	Cooperator (obeys)	Acute infectious processes, etc.	Parent-child (adolescent
3.	Mutual participation	Helps patient to help himself	Participant in "partnership" (uses expert help)	Most chronic illnesses, psychoanalysis, etc.	Adult-adult

2. The model of guidance-cooperation

This model underlies much of medical practice. It is employed in situations which are less desperate than those previously mentioned (e.g., acute infections). Although the patient is ill, he is conscious and has feelings and aspirations of his own. Since he suffers from pain, anxiety, and other distressing symptoms, he seeks help and is ready and willing to "cooperate." When he turns to a physician, he places the latter (even if only in some limited ways) a position of power. This is due not only to a "transference reaction" (i.e., his regarding the physician as he did his father when he was a child) but also to the fact that the physician possesses knowledge of his bodily processes which he does not have. In some ways it may seem that this, like the first model, is an active-passive phenomenon. Actually, this is more apparent than real. Both persons are "active" in that they contribute to the relationship and what ensues from it. The main difference between the two participants pertains to power, and to its actual or potential use. The more powerful of the two (parent, physician, employer, etc.) will speak of guidance or leadership and will expect cooperation of the other member of the pair (child, patient, employee, etc.). The patient is expected to "look up to" and to "obey" his doctor. Moreover, he is neither to question nor to argue or disagree with the orders he receives. This model has its prototype in the relationship of the parent and his (adolescent) child. Often, threats and other undisguised weapons of force are employed, even though presumably these are for the patient's "own good." It should be added that the possibility of the exploitations of the situation—as in any relationship between persons of unequal power—for the sole benefit of the physician, albeit under the guise of altruism, is ever present.

3. The model of mutual participation

Philosophically, this model is predicated on the postulate that equality among human beings is desirable. It is fundamental to the social structure of democracy and has played a crucial role in occidental civilization for more than two hundred years. Psychologically, mutuality rests on complex processes of identification—which facilitate conceiving of others in terms of oneself—together with maintaining and tolerating the discrete individuality of the observer and the observed. It is crucial to this type of interaction that the participants (1) have approximately equal power, (2) be mutually interdependent (i.e., need each other), and (3) engage in activity that will be in some ways satisfying to both.

This model is favored by patients who, for various reasons, want to take care of themselves (at least in part). This may be an overcompensatory attempt at mastering anxieties associated with helplessness and passivity. It may also be "realistic" and necessary, as, for example, in the management of most chronic illnesses (e.g., diabetes mellitus, chronic heart disease, etc.). Here the patient's own experiences provide reliable and important clues for therapy. Moreover, the treatment program itself is principally carried out by the patient to help himself.

In an evolutionary sense, the pattern of mutual participation is more highly developed than the other two models of the doctor-patient relationship. It requires a more complex psychological and social organization on the part of both participants. Accordingly, it is rarely appropriate for children or for those persons who are mentally deficient, very poorly educated, or profoundly immature. On the other hand, the greater the intellectual, educational, and general experiential similarity between physician and patient, the more appropriate and necessary this model of therapy becomes.

The Basic Models and the Psychology of the Physician

Consideration of why physicians seek one or another type of relationship with patients (or seek patients who fit into a particular relationship) would carry us beyond the scope of this essay.

Yet, it must be emphasized that as long as this subject is approached with the sentimental viewpoint that a physician is simply motivated by a wish to help others (not that we deny this wish), no scientific study of the subject can be undertaken. Scientific investigation is possible only if value judgement is subrogated, at least temporarily, to a candid scrutiny of the physician's actual behavior with his patients.

The activity-passivity model places the physician in absolute control of the situation. In this way it gratifies needs for mastery and contributes to feelings of superiority, (Ref. 6 and 7.) At the same time it requires that the physician disidentify with the patient as a person.

Somewhat similar is the guidance-cooperation model. The disidentification with the patient, however, is less complete. The physician, like the parent of a growing child, could be said to see in the patient a human being potentially (but not yet) like himself (or like he wishes to be). In addition to the gratifications already mentioned, this relationship provides an opportunity to recreate and to gratify the "Pygmalion Complex." Thus, the physician can mold others into his own image, as God is said to have created man (or he may mold them into his own image of what they should be like, as in Shaw's "Pygmalion"). This type of relationship is of importance in education, as the transmission of more or less stable cultural values (and of language itself shows. It requires that the physician be convinced he is "right" in his notion of what is "best" for the patient. He will then try to induce the patient to accept his aims as the patient's own.

The model of mutual participation, as suggested earlier, is essentially foreign to medicine. This relationship, characterized by a high degree of empathy, has elements often associated with the notions of friendship and partnership and the imparting of expert advice. The physician may be said to help the patient to help himself. The physician's gratification cannot stem from power or from the control over someone else. His satisfactions are derived from more abstract kinds of mastery, which are as yet poorly understood.

It is evident that in each of the categories mentioned the satisfactions of physician and patient complement each other. This makes for stability in a paired system. Such stability, however, must be temporary, since the physician strives to alter the patient's state. The comatose patient, for example, either will recover to a more healthy, conscious condition or he will die. If he improves, the doctor-patient relationship must change. It is at this point that the physician's inner (usually unacknowledged) needs are most likely to interfere with what is "best" for the patient. At this juncture, the physician either changes his "attitude" (not a consciously or deliberately assumed role) to complement the patient's emergent needs or he foists upon the patient the same role of helpless passivity from which he (allegedly) tried to rescue him in the first place. Here we touch on a subject rich in psychological and sociological complexities. The process of change the physician must undergo to have a mutually constructive experience with the patient is similar to a very familiar process: namely, the need for the parent to behave ever differently toward his growing child.

What Is "Good Medicine"?

Let us now consider the problem of "good medicine" from the viewpoint of human relationships. The function of sciences is not to tell us what is good or bad but rather to help us understand how things work. "Good " and "bad" are personal judgments, usually decided on the basis of whether or not the object under consideration satisfies us. In viewing the doctor-patient relationship we cannot conclude, however, that anything which satisfies—irrespective of other considerations—is "good." Further complications arise when the method is questioned by which we ascertain whether or not a particular need has been satisfied. Do we take the patient's word for it? Or do we place ourselves into the traditional parental role of "knowing what is best" for our patients (children)?

The shortcomings and dangers inherent in these and in other attempts to clarify some of the most basic aspects of our daily life are too well known to require documentation. It is this very complexity of the situation which has led, as is the rule in scientific work, to an essentially arbitrary simplification of the structure of our field of observation. (We omit any discussion of the physician's technical skill, training, equipment, etc. These factors, of course, are of importance, and we do not minimize them. The problem of what is "good medicine" can be considered from a number of viewpoints (e.g., technical skill, economic considerations, social roles, human relationships, etc.). Our scope in this essay is limited to but one—sometimes quite unimportant—aspect of the contact between physician and patient.)

Let us present an example. A patient consults a physician because of pain and other symptoms resulting from a duodenal ulcer. Both physician and patient assume that the latter would be better off without these discomforts. The situation now may be structured as follows: healing of the ulcer is "good," whereas its persistence is "bad." What we wish to emphasize is the fact that physician and patient agree (explicitly or otherwise) as to what is good and bad. Without such agreement it is meaningless to speak of a therapeutic relationship.

In other words, the notions of "normal." abnormal." "symptom," "disease," and the like are social conventions. These definitions often are set by the medical world and are usually tacitly accepted by others. The fact that there is agreement renders it difficult to perceive their changing (and relativistic) character. A brief example will clarify this statement. Some years ago—and among the uneducated even today—fever was regarded as something "bad" ("abnormal," a symptom"), to be combated. The current scientific opinion is that it is the organism's response to certain types of influences (e.g., infection) and that within limits the manifestation itself should not be "treated."

The issue of agreement is of interest because it has direct bearing on the models of the doctor-patient relationship. In the first two models "agreement" between physician and patient is taken for granted. The comatose patient obviously can not disagree. According to the second model the patient does not possess the knowledge to dispute the physician's word. The third category differs in that the physician does not profess to know exactly what is best for the patient. The search for this becomes the essence of the therapeutic interaction. The patient's own experiences furnish indispensable information for eventual agreement, under otherwise favorable circumstances, as to what "health" might be for him.

The characteristics of the different types of doctor-patient relationships are summarized in Table 2. In this connection, some comments will be made on a subject which essentially is philosophical but which continues to plague many medical discussions; namely, the problem of comparing the efficacy of different therapeutic measures. Such comparisons are implicitly based on the following conceptual scheme: We postulate disease "A." from which many patients suffer. Therapies "B," "C," and "D" are given to groups of patients suffering with disease "A," and the results are compared. It is usually overlooked that, for the results to be meaningful, significant conceptual similarities must exist between the operations which are compared. The three categories of the doctor-patient relationship are concretely useful in delineating areas within which meaningful comparisons can be made. Comparisons between therapies belonging to different categories are philosophically (and logically) meaningless and lead to fruitless controversy.

To illustrate this thesis let us consider some examples. A typical comparison with which we can begin, is that of the various agents used in the treatment of lobar pneumonia: type specific antisera, sulfonamides, and penicillin. Each superseded the other, as the increased efficacy of the

Table 2 Analysis of the concepts of "disease," "treatment," and "therapeutic result"

Doctor-Patient Relationship	The Meaning of "Treatment"	The "Therapeutic Result"
1. Activity-passivity	Whatever the physician does; the actual operations (procedures) which he employs	Alteration in the structure and/or function of the patient's body (or behavior, as determined by the physician's judgment); the patient's judgment does not enter into the evaluation of results; e.g., T & A is "successful" irrespective of how patient feels afterward
2. Guidance-cooperation	Whatever the physician does; similar to the above	Similar to the above, albeit patient's judgment is no longer completely irrelevant; success of therapy is still the physician's private decision; if patient agrees, he is a good patient, but if he disagrees he is bad or "uncooperative"
3. Mutual participation	An abstraction of one aspect of the relationship, embodying the activities of both participants; "treatment" cannot be said to take place unless both participants orient themselves to the task ahead	Much more poorly defined than in the previous models; evaluation of the result will depend on both the physician's and the patient's judgments and is further complicated by the fact that these may change in the very process of treatment

preparations was demonstrated. This sort of comparison is meaningful because there is agreement to what is being treated and as to what constitutes a "successful" result. There should be no need to belabor this point. What is important is that this conceptual model of therapeutic comparisons constantly used in situations in which it does not apply; that is, in situations in which there is clearcut disagreement as to what constitutes "cure." In this connection, the problem of peptic ulcer will exemplify a group of illnesses in which several therapeutic approaches are possible.

This question is often posed, Is surgical, medical or psychiatric treatment the "best" for peptic ulcer? Such a question is roughly comparable to asking, "Is an automobile or an airplane better?"—without specifying for what. See Reference 8. Unless we specify conditions, goals, and the "price" we are willing to pay (in the largest sense of the word), the question is meaningless. In the case of peptic ulcer, it is immediately apparent that each therapeutic approach implies a different conception of "disease" and correspondingly divergent notions of "cure." At the risk of slight overstatement, it can be said that according to the surgical viewpoint the disease is the "lesion," treatment aims at its eradication (by surgical means), and cure consists of its persistent absence (nonrecurrence). If a patient undergoes vagotomy and an evidence of the legion disappears, he is considered cured even if he develops another (apparently unrelated) illness six months

The Notions of Disease and Health	In Medicine (Illustrative Examples)	In Psychiatry (Illustrative Examples)
The presence or absence of some unwanted structure or function. The actual state of affairs. The same state without the disability	1. Treatment of the unconcious patient; for example, the patient in diabetic coma; cerebral hemorrhage; shock due to acute injury; etc. 2. Major surgical operation under general anesthesia	1. Hypnosis 2. Convulsive treatments (electroshock, insulin, etc.) 3. Surgical treatments (lobotomy, etc.)
The presence or absence of "signs" and "symptoms"; the physician's particular concept of "Disease" (e.g., infection), "Health" (usually no disease; e.g., no infection)	Most of general medicine and the postoperative care of surgical patients (e.g., prescription of drugs, "advice" to smoke less, etc.)	1. "Suggestion," counseling, therapy based on "advice," etc. 2. Some modifications of psychoanalytic therapy 3. So-called psychotherapy "combined" with physical therapies (e.g., electric shock)
The notions of disease and health lose most of their relevance in this context; the notions of more-or-less successful (for certain purposes) modes of behavior, adaptation, or integration take the place of the earlier, more categorical concepts	The treatment of patients with certain chronic diseases or structural defects; for example, the management of diabetes mellitus or of myasthenia gravis; "rehabilitation" of patients with orthopedic defects, such as learning the use of prostheses, etc.	1. Psychoanalysis 2. Some modification of psychoanalytic therapy

later. It should be emphasized that no criticism of this frame of reference is intended. The foregoing (surgical) approach is entirely appropriate, and accusations of "narrowness" are no more (nor less) justified than they would be against any other specialized branch of knowledge.

To continue our analysis of therapeutic comparisons, let us consider the same patient (with peptic ulcer) in the hands of an internist. This specialist might have a somewhat different idea of what is wrong with him than did the surgeon. He might regard peptic ulcer as an essentially chronic disease (perhaps due to heredity and other "predispositions"), with which the patient probably will have to live as comfortably as possible for years. This point is emphasized to demonstrate that the surgeon and the internist do not treat the "same disease." How then can the two methods of treatment and their results be compared? The most that can be hoped for is to be able to determine to what extent each method is appropriate and successful within its own frame of reference.

If we take our hypothetical patient to a psychoanalyst, the situation is even more radically different. This specialist will state that he is not treating the "ulcer" and might even go so far as to say that he is not treating the patient for his ulcer. The psychoanalyst (or psychiatrist) has his own ideas about what constitutes "disease," "treatment," and "cure." (Ref. 9 and 10.)

Conclusions

Comments have been made on some factors which provide satisfactions to both patient and physician in various therapeutic relationships. In conclusion, we call attention to two important considerations regarding the complementary situations described.

First, it might be thought that one of the three basic models of the doctor-patient relationship is in some fundamental (perhaps ethical) way "better" than another. In particular, it might be considered that it is better to identify with the patient than to treat him like a helplessly sick person. We have tried to avoid such an inference. In our opinion, each of the three types of therapeutic relationship is entirely appropriate under certain circumstances and each is inappropriate under others.

Secondly, we will comment on the therapeutic relationship as a situation (more or less fixed in time) and as a process (leading to change in one or both participants). Most of our previous comments have dealt with the relationship as a situation. It is, however, also a process in that the patient may change not only in terms of his symptoms but also in the way he wishes to relate to his doctor. A typical example is the patient with diabetes mellitus who, when first seen, is in a coma. At this time, the relationship must be based on the activity-passivity model. Later, he has to be educated (guided) at the level of cooperation. Finally, ideally, he is treated as a full-fledged partner in the management of his own health (mutual participation). Confronted by a problem of this type, the physician is called upon to change through a corresponding spectrum of attitudes. If he cannot make these changes, he may interfere with the patient's progress and may promote an arrest at some intermediate stage in the evolution toward relative self-management. The other possibility in this situation is that both physician and patient will become dissatisfied with each other. This outcome, however unfortunate, is probably the commonest one. Most of us can probably verify it firsthand in the roles of both physician and patient (Ref. 11).

At such juncture, the physician usually feels that the patient is "uncooperative" and "difficult," whereas the patient regards the physician as "unsympathetic" and lacking in understanding of his personally unique needs. Both are correct. Both are confronted by the wish to induce changes in the other. As we well know, this is no easy task. The dilemma is usually resolved when the patient seeks another physician, one who is more attuned to his (new) needs. Conversely, the physician will "seek" a new patient, usually one who will benefit from the physician's (old) needs and corresponding attitudes. And so life goes on.

The pattern described accounts for the familiar fact that patients often choose physicians not solely, or even primarily, on the basis of technical skill. Considerable weight is given to the type of human relationship which they foster. Some patients prefer to be "unconscious" (figuratively speaking), irrespective of what ails them. Others go to the other extreme. The majority probably fans somewhere between these two polar opposites. Physicians, motivated by similar personal "conflict" form a complementary series. Thus, there is an interlocking integration of the sick and his healer.

Summary

The introduction of the construct of "human relationship" represents an addition to the repertoire of fundamental medical concepts.

Three basic models of the doctor-patient relationship are described with examples. The models are (a) Activity-passivity. The comatose patient is completely helpless. The physician must take over and do something to him. (b) Guidance-cooperation. The patient with an acute infectious process seeks help and is ready and willing to cooperate. He turns to the physician for guidance. (c) Mutual participation. The patient with a chronic disease is aided to help himself.

The physician's own inner needs (and satisfactions) form a complementary series with those of the patient.

The general problem usually referred to with the question "what is good medicine?" is briefly considered. Different types of doctor-patient relationships imply different concepts of "disease," "treatment," and "cure." This is of importance in comparing diverse therapeutic methods. Meaningful comparisons can be made only if interventions are based on the same frame of reference.

It has been emphasized that different types of doctor-patient relationships are necessary and appropriate for various circumstances. Problems in human contact between physician and patient often arise if in the course of treatment changes require an alteration in the pattern of the doctor-patient relationship. This may lead to a dissolution of the relationship.

References

1. Ruesch, J., and Bateson, G.: *Communication: The Social Matrix of Psychiatry*, New York, W. W. Norton & Company, Inc., 1951.
2. Dewey, J., and Bentley, A.F.: *Knowing and the Known*, Boston, Beacon Press, 1949.
3. Russell, B.: *Power: A New Social Analysis*. New York, W.W. Norton & Company, Inc., 1938
4. Szasz, T. S.: Entropy, Organization, and the Problem of the Economy of Human Relationships, *Internat. J. Psychoanal.* 36:289, 1955.
5. Dubos, R. J.: Second Thoughts on the Germ Theory, *Scient. Am.* 192:31, 1955
6. Jones, E.: The God Complex, in Jones E.: *Essays in Applied Psychoanalysis*, London, Hogarth Press, 1951, Vol. 2, p. 244.
7. Marmor, J.: The Feeling of Superiority: An Occupational Hazard in the Practice of Psychotherapy, *Am. J. Psychist.* 110:370, 1953.
8. Rapoport, A.: *Operational Philosophy*, New York, Harper & Brothers, 1954.
9. Zilboorg, G.: *A History of Medical Psychology*, New York, W. W. Norton & Company, Inc., 1941.
10. Bowman, K. M., and Rose, M.: Do Our Medical Colleagues Know What to Expect from Psychotherapy? *Am.J.Psychiat.* 111:401, 1954.
11. Pinner, M., and Miller, B. F., Editors: *When Doctors Are Patients*, New York, W. W. Norton & Company, Inc., 1952.

The Biopsychosocial Model and the Education of Health Professionals

George L. Engel

Over the past 50 years, medical education has grown increasingly proficient in conveying to physicians sophisticated scientific knowledge and technical skills about the body and its aberrations. Yet at the same time it has failed to give corresponding attention to the scientific understanding of human behavior and the psychological and social aspects of illness and patient care (1-4). The average physician today completes his formal education with impressive capabilities to deal with the more technical aspects of bodily disease, yet when it comes to dealing with the human side of illness and patient care, he displays little more than the native ability and personal qualities with which he entered medical school. The considerable body of knowledge about human behavior which has accumulated since the turn of the century and how this may be applied to achieve more effective patient care and health maintenance remain largely unknown to him. Neglect of this important dimension of the physician's education lies at the root of frequently voiced complaints by patients that physicians are insensitive, callous, neglectful, arrogant, and mechanical in their approaches.

There undoubtedly are many reasons for this situation, but the most important is the pervasive influence of the biomedical model of disease. Rasmussen traces the philosophic origins of this model back three or four centuries when established Christian orthodoxy lifted the prohibition against physicians dissecting the human body as long as they did not presume to deal with man's soul, morals, mind, and behavior (5). This compact helped determine that Western Medicine be based upon dualism and reductionism. Dualism predicates separation of mind from body, of the psychological from the somatic, and provides no conceptual framework, other than reductionism, whereby the two can be related. Reductionism assumes that the understanding of a more complex entity can be best achieved by its analysis into its component parts and therefore that the complexities of life and biological phenomena, including behavior and mental processes, are to be studied and explained by the methods and in the language of physics and chemistry. Reductionism fosters a view of nature as involving interactions of discrete entities in a linear causal fashion, simple cause-and-effect relationships. This influence is expressed in the habit of speaking of diseases not as dynamic processes but as discrete entities, the elimination of which awaits only discovery of their causes. The pledge of the ultimate conquest of disease, upon which biomedicine solicits support from the public, merely panders to a deep-seated human desire for paradise on earth. We are already paving the price for promises that have not and cannot be fulfilled.

Engel, G. L. (1978) THE BIOPHYCHOSOCIAL MODEL AND THE EDUCATION OF HEALTH PROFESSIONALS. Annals of the New York Academy of Sciences, 310, 169-181.

Biomedical Model

Yet it is not to be gainsaid that as a scientific framework within which to elaborate the disordered bodily mechanisms involved in disease, the biomedical model has been extraordinarily fruitful. But this very success has served not only to entrench dualism and reductionism but also to encourage its more enthusiastic advocates to promote the biomedical model as ultimately capable of explaining all aspects of health and disease. The dogmatism inherent in such blind faith in and exaggerated claims for the model has been a powerful factor in deflecting scientific interest and attention from problems that do not readily yield to the biomedical approach. Outstanding among these have been the more personal, human, psychological, and social aspects of health and disease, the caring rather than curing function of the physician. These aspects biomedicine considers neither accessible to rigorous scientific evaluation nor essential for the education of the physician. Small wonder that what patients have to report and what physicians can observe with their own senses are given less credence than are data measured in the laboratory or established through sophisticated instrumentation; that many medical students are being awarded their medical degrees without ever having been supervised in the complete interview and physical examination of even a single patient; that there is excessive and inappropriate "shotgun" use of laboratory and diagnostic procedures with their corresponding discomfort and cost to patients and increased risk of mishap and malpractice actions; that patients feel used, abused, and dehumanized and become resentful of physicians and the system which subjects them to such experiences; and that physicians feel bewildered, inept, frustrated, and angry when sophisticated instrumentation fails to yield answers and patients persist in feeling ill and making demands in the face of the laboratory demonstration of "no disease." These are all penalties we are paying for tolerating the degradation of a productive scientific model into a dogma.

Public Dissatisfaction

As public dissatisfaction with the quality of medical care once again becomes more vocal and articulate, thoughtful physicians are beginning to question wherein our present medical educational system is failing to fulfill its responsibility to prepare physicians satisfactorily to care for the sick. For it is clear that even patients with ready access to health facilities have complaints about the quality of care they receive from physicians and medical institutions (6). But so far, the main response from the leaders of American medical education has been a curiously regressive romanticism. Writer after writer pays homage to the triumphs of biomedical science and urges no compromise in the scientific preparation of the future doctor, but few seem aware that a major part of the medical student's scientific education, namely, that concerned with the human dimensions of illness, has been largely, if not totally, neglected (1). Instead, the typical response of medical educators to the complaints of patients and the increasing questions of students and young physicians is to recommend a sentimental return to the past. For them, what is required to enable the physician of tomorrow to escape the alleged dehumanizing influence of "science" and acquire the human skills and sensitivities said to characterize the humble practitioner of old is to expose students earlier to practitioners caring for patients. Ignored is the necessity to develop scientific principles and to apply the scientific method to the human dimensions of medicine. The picture naively conjured up is that the scientific competence of today's physician can be blended with the legendary warmth, compassion, and common sense of the kindly family doctor of yesteryear.

Unfortunately, this notion is both false and devoid of logic. There is in fact no historical support for the claim that physicians of past generations were any more endowed with compassion and concern than are physicians of today (2). In each era, whether the 1970s, the 1920s, the

1880s, or the 1850s, one finds physicians of the preceding generation praised for their humanity while physicians of the day are accused of insensitivity and ineptness in personal dealings with patients and of excessive zeal in their application of the therapeutic measures in vogue at the time. The cry always is that the "modern" physician has lost the human touch and become too mechanical or too scientific in his approach.

Furthermore, even less evidence exists to support the claims of those who believe that mere exposure to or exhortation from an idealized older physician will somehow or other inculcate better attitudes and result in more effective practices. For no matter how inspiring a personal example a physician may set for students, without a scientific understanding of the psychosocial aspects of illness and patient care, the doctor's ability to communicate principles upon which others can build will be limited.

Herein lies the dilemma. For while medicine recognizes the need to be more responsible to growing public dissatisfaction with how individual care is being provided, the model upon which medical education and research is based does not include the patient. The biomedical model is disease oriented, not patient oriented. To be patient oriented the model must include psychosocial dimensions. But even the term "psychosocial" has a strange and esoteric ring for biomedically trained physicians. For most, "psychosocial" means problems primarily of concern to the psychiatrist or the social worker. Whatever else has to do with the patient and his care is classified as the "art of medicine" and is based on intuition, professional rules, aphorisms, and maxims from the accumulated wisdom of experienced clinicians. A recent survey of family practice concluded that emphasis on psychosocial studies in the education of the family physician is unwarranted, since among 23,000 cases only 1300 (5.7%) could be classified as psychosocial problems" (7). But in that study psychosocial problems were defined as problems with psychologic and social origins and psychologic or social manifestations," and turned out to include only depression, marital problems, and anxiety neurosis, hardly even representative of psychiatric morbidity. A much better perspective is to what psychosocial encompasses can be derived from the complaints of the public about doctors and medical care, for it is patients and families who are most painfully aware of what is missing. They are the ones who complain that doctors don't communicate well, that they don't really listen, that they seem insensitive to personal needs and individual differences, that they neglect the person in the zeal to pursue diagnostic and treatment procedures. They stress the unavailability of the physician and health services, often as much indicative of psychological remoteness as of economic barriers or geographical distances.

Different Health Criteria

All of such complaints-and many more-bespeak the public's awareness of grave deficiencies in the medical establishment's knowledge and ability to handle rationally all that is encompassed in the human experience of being ill. Central to this gap between medicine and the public it is meant to serve is that the criteria for health and well-being applied by the patient are fundamentally different from those applied by the physician, even though culturally and intellectually both patient and physician adhere to the biomedical model of disease. For the patient, the ultimate criteria are psychosocial, even when the complaint is physical. Patients' criteria have to do with how one feels, how one functions, how one relates; with the ability to love, to work, to struggle, to seek options, and to make choices. The physician, in contrast, while ostensibly attentive to such concerns, nonetheless is wont to consider such criteria as merely subjective. For the physician, the real criteria for status and outcome are physical measures, for which increasingly elegant and sensitive instruments are available. No comparable conceptual tools or intellectual skills are available for the physician to resolve the discrepancies between what the patient has to say and what the laboratory has to report. Even the organization of health care delivery is predicated on the assumption that the doctor, that is, the laboratory, is right and the patient is wrong.

For hundreds of years, Western Medicine has brushed aside the complaints of patients, yet herein lies the key to what is missing, the-understanding of what comprises the psychosocial dimensions of illness and health care. But as long as the biomedical model prevails, unscientific and simplistic solutions to resolve the complaints of patients will be promoted. Currently, the most seductive holds that since nothing more than compassion, a humane attitude, and good common sense are required to meet the more personal needs of patients and their families, these functions can be delegated to other health professionals, leaving diagnosis and treatment of disease to the biomedically qualified physician.

Role of Nurse

For physicians to solicit the assistance of others is hardly novel; medicine has a long tradition of developing aides with various specialized technical skills and knowledge to assist physicians in patient care. But there is a subtle difference in how ancillary health professionals evolved in the past and what is happening today. For the most part, these aides, beginning with the trained nurse in the last century, evolved from the needs of physicians to perform their functions more efficiently. Moreover, nurses remained dependent on the doctor for basic medical knowledge and skills as well as, to a large extent, for the definition of professional tasks and roles. For example, early nineteenth century nursing care commonly was provided by women from religious orders in institutions or by female relatives or servants in the home, often with little or no medical supervision.

As medicine became more scientific and technical, the value of a specially trained cadre of women to provide nursing services in hospital and at home became obvious. In this way, nursing came under the aegis of medicine rather than religion, and the "trained nurse" emerged not only to assist the doctor with procedures but also to implement his orders and to attend to the bodily and personal needs of the sick. As nursing education became more formalized and nursing achieved status as a profession, educational and preceptorial roles became increasingly the responsibility of nurses themselves. And as nurses progressively evolved new roles and activities which were natural outgrowths of what nurses, rather than doctors, do for and with patients, nursing achieved a professional identity of its own. And while physicians could only welcome this extension of the range of nurses' competencies and nurses' capacities for independent action and-judgment, there rarely was any question that ultimately, the nurse's responsibility was to the physician whose patient he was caring for. For the physician had not only the more extensive educational background and scientific qualifications but also the most thorough scientific understanding of the *disease* for which the patient came for treatment.

But note carefully my language: the physician *had the most thorough and scientific understanding of the disease for which the patient came for treatment, not the most thorough and scientific understanding of the patient who came for help.* Here is the crux of the matter: It is now becoming clear that in this one area, the understanding of human needs and human behavior, physicians are by no means any more qualified or competent than are those whose aid they solicit as health care extenders. In fact, in this understanding, neither the physician nor the health care extender, whether nurse or other, is necessarily much more qualified than any other reasonably educated, sensitive layperson. Those professionals more knowledgeable than laypeople in psychosocial matters, namely, the psychiatrist, the psychiatric nurse, the psychiatric social worker, the clinical psychologist, and the mental health aide, are the exceptions that prove the rule, because their professional responsibility generally includes the care of the mentally ill and the seriously deviant not the everyday aspects of patient care.

At the heart of this situation are two factors. The first factor is the apparent intransigence of the "biomedical establishment" in its refusal or inability to consider human behavior as a subject accessible to scientific study and understanding other than in reductionistic terms. This serves to entrench the view, not only among health professionals but among the general public as well, that no special training or expertise is required to deal with the "human side" of patient care. "Anyone can do it" and "We have always done it" are typical but unwarranted claims.

The second factor is the widespread dissatisfaction of many patients and their families with the quality of personal attention and understanding they receive from physicians and medical institutions. This has obliged the medical establishment to consider, even to acknowledge, that a problem exists, that the contributions of biomedicine, indispensable and remarkable as they are, do not suffice, that something is missing. To the extent that this constitutes a challenge to examine critically cherished beliefs, policies, and practices and is an inducement to seek new approaches and solutions, it can only be welcomed. But to the extent that it generates defensiveness and provokes an adversary atmosphere, alarm must be expressed.

Adversary Atmosphere

Unfortunately, it is the latter, an adversary atmosphere, which is prevailing within medicine as well as between medicine and other health-related disciplines. The notion that the diagnosis and treatment of disease should be the responsibility of physicians while the care of the patient and maintenance of health may be delegated to other health providers is fostering a dichotomy, well illustrated in a diagram from a current nursing text (8). Even with medicine, such a division of tasks is being promoted. Thus, the various primary-care disciplines, e.g., family medicine, general internal medicine, and general pediatrics, now fervently proclaim their commitment to the patient, almost as though-they "had rediscovered compassion and the art of medicine and had some monopoly on altruistic, principles" (9). In taking such a position, they unjustifiably equate their wish and motivation to understand and meet the more personal needs of patients with their actual ability and knowledge to do so.

Some nurses, too, are militantly laying claim to a superior knowledge and feeling for the patient, some even arrogating to themselves the responsibility to protect the patient from the "cold, insensitive" physician. Unfortunately, this concern often evolves from the false premise that science and humanism are somehow in opposition. Such a posture promotes rivalry, if not antagonism, between and among health professionals. But the care of the sick calls for collaboration and smooth interaction between professionals, with complementary roles to fulfill and tasks to perform. This is impossible as long as the dominant model is one which philosophically denies the application of science to the care of the patient, places science and humanism in opposition, and divides health professionals into a "superior" group who treat disease and a "lesser" breed who care for the sick.

No resolution of the above divisive situation will be forthcoming until a model is developed that can be shared by all who are involved in the care of the sick, one which encompasses all the elements involved in health and disease, from the molecular to the psychosocial. Without such a common conceptual framework, only more conflict and chaos will ensue, with the patient the ultimate loser. For the key to optimal patient care is *collaboration, communication,* and *complementarity* among all branches of 'he health profession. Given the varieties of tasks to accomplish and the differing skills, techniques, and approaches required to accomplish them, collaboration, communication, and complementarity are only possible when the various disciplines share in common a basic set of assumptions and principles. Otherwise, each of the different health professions is tempted to evolve its own more limited model, suitable for its own purposes, but in practice likely to inhibit collaboration, confuse communication, and substitute competition for complementarity.

Biopsychosocial Model

To meet the existing need, I have proposed guidelines for a more inclusive model, a biopsychosocial model, based on general systems theory (3, 10-14). As the name suggests, its intent is to provide a framework within which can be conceptualized and related as natural systems all the levels of organization pertinent to health and disease, from subatomic particles through molecules, cells, tissues, organs, organ systems, the person, the family, the community, the culture, and ultimately the biosphere.

In nature, such organized systems are hierarchically arranged in order of complexity, the simplest and developmentally the oldest being subordinate to the more complex. Thus, processes at the cellular level are subordinate to those at the tissue or organ level, which in turn are subordinate to those at the person or community level. Yet, while each system in the hierarchy is functionally integrated and relatively autonomous, it is also interconnected with every other system by information flow through feedback arrangements. Hence, disturbances at any system level may be communicated to and affect any other system level, with those in the closest functional relationship likely to be the first affected.

Predicated on the systems approach, the biopsychosocial model dispenses with the scientifically archaic principles of dualism and reductionism and replaces the simple cause-and-effect explanations of linear causality with reciprocal causal models. Health, disease, and disability thus are conceptualized in terms of the relative intactness and functioning of each component system on each hierarchical level. Overall health reflects a high level of intra- and intersystemic harmony. Such harmony may be disrupted at any level, at the cellular, at the organ system, at the whole person, or at the community levels. Whether the resulting disturbance is contained at the level at which it is initiated or whether other levels become implicated is a function of the capacity of that system to adjust to change. For example, a modification in an individual's social environment, impacting first on the psychological functions of perception and appraisal, may be successfully accommodated at the psychological level and hence give rise to no perceptible reverberations elsewhere. Similarly, a molecular substance introduced into the body might be broken down, excreted, neutralized, or inactivated without implicating any but the particular molecular, cellular, tissue, or organ system required for its disposal. In both instances, the systems involved have the capacity to handle the imposed change without disruption.

Yet, under different circumstances or with another individual with a different past history, the very same social change or the very same molecules may induce profound disruptions involving many systems in the hierarchy. Such contrasts between smooth functioning and disruption provide the basis upon which health, disease, illness, and disability may be differentiated (10, 11). Central to this perspective are not only the dynamic interrelations that determine relative degrees of intra- and intersystemic harmony or disruption but also the fact that every change becomes part of the history of each system, rendering it different at every successive point in time. In the biopsychosocial model there can be no return to status quo ante. Health restored is not the former state of health but represents a different intersystemic harmony than existed before the illness, with characteristics based on all the system changes incurred during the illness. By virtue of the illness not only is the individual changed as a person, but so too may be changed others in relationship to him, in the family as well as the community (14).

The advantages of such a systems-oriented biopsychosocial model over the traditional biomedical model may be illustrated by contrasting the clinical approaches of adherents of each model. When a patient presents a problem, how the physician goes about its solution is determined not just by past experience and knowledge but even more by the working conceptual models in relationship to which the physician organizes such experience and knowledge. The following is an actual clinical event that examines how the conceptualizations of a biomedical dualist-reductionist and a biopsychosocial systematist, respectively, might influence the approach of each to the same clinical situation:

A 55-year-old real estate salesman was admitted to the Strong Memorial Hospital Emergency Room with symptoms and findings consistent with the diagnosis of acute myocardial infarction. While the intern was attempting an arterial puncture, ventricular fibrillation abruptly developed. The patient was promptly and successfully resuscitated.

To begin with, the language each uses to characterize and think about the problem would differ, in itself indicating how differently issues are conceptualized by each. The biomedical model focuses on the disease as an entity which can be understood and treated independently of the person afflicted. Hence, the familiar impersonal language tit the reductionist physician would characterize the problem as "a case of acute myocardial infarction with ventricular fibrillation." In contrast, for the systematist physician, the person must be the primary frame of reference, leading to a more wordy but also more human and personal reference, e.g., "A middle-aged real estate salesman with an acute myocardial infarction developed ventricular fibrillation while the intern was attempting an arterial puncture." However, note a salient difference. The reductionist sees the problem as a discrete entity while the systematist deals with it as part of a series of ongoing dynamic events. Hence, for the systematist, even the identifying characterization must include some - sense of sequences and circumstances, that is, the dimensions of time and space.

Of course, when it comes to the acute emergency and how the cardiac arrest is to be handled, differences between the -reductionist and systematist temporarily vanish. Both institute identical resuscitation procedures, which, if successful, would be followed by efforts to establish the reason for the cardiac arrest. Both, too, would in subsequent care of the patient attend not only to remote biochemical or physiological events that might unfavorably affect the function and electrical stability of the heart but also to remote consequences for other organs of the cardiac malfunction. But again, differences emerge in how each conceptualizes the place of the patient in these processes.

This is dramatically demonstrated by how the biomedically oriented staff responded to the arrest and subsequent successful resuscitation; they congratulated each other and the patient on the good fortune that he happened to be in the ER at the time of the arrest. The possibility that the two circumstances may not have been entirely fortuitous was not even considered.

The systematist physician, in contrast, ever aware of the potential for disruption at any system level, would always have in mind the possibility that psychological disruption might be precipitated by the setting of the care, including his own behavior with the patient.

Interview of this particular patient documented this indeed to have been the case. The dogged persistence of the intern in persevering in his efforts to perform the arterial puncture, without either explanation to the patient or attention to his distress and pain, induced intense patient anger and frustration, an abrupt loss of confidence in those providing care, followed by a growing sense of impotence to do anything about the situation in which he found himself (4).

The occurrence of ventricular fibrillation at that point is in keeping with well-established knowledge documenting the ability of increased autonomic activity and catecholamine secretion to lower threshold for ventricular fibrillation in the presence of an existing substratum of myocardial electrical instability, in this instance based on myocardial infarction (15).

The systematist does not stop with consideration of how perturbations at other levels might have contributed to cardiac arrest. Of equal concern is how the cardiac arrest may be impacting or might in the future impact on the stability or instability of other systems. Thus, while the reductionist thinks in terms of cause and effect, of final consequences and discrete entities, the systematist is thinking in terms of ongoing, progressive sequences of intra- and intersystemic interactions, with the stability of each system being ultimately determined through multilevel feedback arrangements. And while the reductionist would tend to view restoration of sinus rhythm as an end in itself, the systematist sees it as a possible source of new perturbations as well as a step toward establishment of new levels of intersystemic harmony.

The experience for the patient of having suffered an arrest is seen by the biomedical physician as separate from the disease process. Not so for the biopsychosocial physician, who not only recognizes that events in the patient's life might set in motion disturbances at the psychological level ultimately capable of affecting the electrical stability of the heart, but also considers how the personality structure of the patient might determine such an outcome and how such knowledge may be helpful in the patient's care (4).

Whether the patient lives or dies, the biopsychosocial model further provides the physician with the conceptual tools with which to include in thinking and planning the implications of the cardiac arrest not only for the patient but also for the family, the community, and even for the health care providers as well. Within the framework of the biopsychosocial model, all of these are legitimate as well as assimilable concerns for those who man the health care system. A biopsychosocial physician even finds it logical to ask to what extent the death or permanent impairment of the victim of cardiac arrest might affect the health and well-being of those who survive, whether they be the family left bereft, the employer deprived of a valuable worker, or the health care provider who was involved in the unsuccessful attempt at resuscitation.

It is hoped the example, with all its oversimplifications, will indicate how adoption of a biopsychosocial model can contribute to the unity of the health professions and render collaboration, communication, and complementarity a reality rather than mere sloganeering. Through sharing basic knowledge and a common way of looking at Man, from the organization of his body to the determinants of his behavior to the social structures of which he is an integral part, health professionals would have in common the languages essential for communication and cooperation and for the complementarity inherent in the need for the special knowledge and skills required for the many varied activities involved in providing high-level health care.

Competence

To buttress collaboration, communication, and complementarity, the fourth indispensable attribute of health care professionals must be competence. How stubborn and pernicious the influence of biomedical dogma can be is betrayed by those who say, "I fully agree with your position *but*, when I get sick, I would rather have for my physician one who is conversant with the most up-to-date biomedical knowledge and techniques than one who understands my psyche." Again, dualism intrudes, as though competence in one sphere precludes competence in the other. The proper distinction is between a general level of competence and specialized competencies. Criteria for specialized competencies already exist for most categories and subcategories of the health profession. What is generally lacking now is the requirement that general competency include the psychosocial sphere. Current biomedical dogma designates psychosocial knowledge and skills a special competency, training for which is expected only of psychiatrists and other mental health professionals.

With the biopsychosocial model as its foundation, general competency for all health professionals would derive from their shared understanding that all three levels, biological, psychological, and social, must be taken into account in every health care task. Accordingly, for any particular task, the hierarchical arrangement of responsibilities among the different health professionals should be determined by the levels of general competency and the types of special competency possessed by each of the various professionals available in the setting and at the time.

Thus, for some tasks, any health professional, regardless of discipline, might be competent, while for other more specialized or complex tasks, only a professional with the knowledge and skills needed for that particular task would be qualified, be it a speech therapist, a surgeon, a nutritionist, a nurse, or a psychiatric social worker.

Similarly, for tasks that require the collaboration of several professional disciplines, hierarchical relationships at any point should depend upon which individual, regardless of discipline, has the superior or unique competency required for that particular task at that particular time. . . .

Conclusion

Educators for the health professions are confronted with choices that could have momentous significance for the future of health care. Educators can continue to try to force medicine into the Procrustean Bed of the biomedical model, with all the divisiveness and fragmentation encouraged by its inherent reductionism and dualism, or they can consider a more comprehensive model that emphasizes psychosocial skills based on a systems approach, with its potential to enhance collaboration, communication, and complementarity among the various health professions and enhance the general level of competence of each. That choice and opportunity are especially crucial for those just beginning their education, because how the health sciences and health care evolve in the future is to a large degree determined by the approach health profession educators take in training fledgling providers-to-be.

References

1. Engel GL: The best and the brightest: The missing dimension in medical education. *The Pharos* 36:129-133, 1976
2. Engel GL: Too little science: The paradox of modem medicine's crisis. *The Pharos* 39:127-131, 1976
3. Engel GL: The need for a new medical model: A challenge for biomedicine. *Science* 196:129-136, 1977
4. Engel GL: The care of the patient: Art or science? *Johns Hopkins Med J* 140:222-232, 1977
5. Rasmussen H: Medical education: Revolution or reaction. *The Pharos* 38:53-59, 1975
6. Duff RS, Hollingshead AB: *Sickness and Society*. New York, Harper and Row, 1968
7. Warrington AM, Ponesse DJ, Hunter ME, Grant DA, Grasset AV, Gray DW, Hayward CD, Long BF, Morrison GEC, Sutherland D, What do family physicians see in practice? *Can Med Assoc J* 117:354-356, 1977
8. Mitchell PH: Nursing in the context of health care. *In* Mitchell PH (ed). *Concepts Basic to Nursing*, 2nd Ed. New York, McGraw-Hill, 1977, pp. 22-36
9. Sundwall DN: Family practice, here today, gone (again) tomorrow. *JAMA* 238:217, 1977
10. Engel GL: A unified concept of health and disease. *Perspect Biol Med* 3:459-485, 1960

11. Engel GL: *Psychological Development in Health and Disease*. Philadelphia, W. B. Saunders Co., 1962
12. Von Bertalanffy L: *General System Theory*. New York, George Braziller, 1968
13. Laszlo E: *The Systems View of the World*. New York, George Braziller, 1972
14. Brody H: The systems view of man: Implications for medicine, science, and ethics. *Perspect Biol Med* 17:71-92, 1973
15. Lown B, Verrier RL, Rabinowitz SH: Neural and psychologic mechanisms and the problem of sudden cardiac death. *Am J Cardiol* 39:890-902, 1977

Models of Physician-patient Interaction: Paternalism to Mutual Participation

Claudia A. Perry

Given the interdisciplinary nature and theoretical plurality of research in health communication, the availability of a common framework may provide some guidance for health communication scholars. One integral aspect of health communication which has been a focus of attention from various fronts is the nature of practitioner-patient interaction. Not only is the practitioner-patient relationship central to the health communication process, it also has received renewed interest in recent years. Growing dissatisfaction with the traditional paternalistic model of physician-patient interaction has led to what D. H. Smith has described as "a paradigmatic shift . . . toward patient participation in health care" (1989, p. 20). Existence of an alternative paradigm does not, however, guarantee its acceptance among either health care practitioners or their patients. In order to understand the evolution of the patient participation model, this paper reviews a number of models of physician-patient interaction: asymmetric models with the physician dominant, (e.g. Parsons); asymmetric models with the patient dominant, such as the consumer model; and models of relatively mutual participation (e.g. Szasz & Hollender, Siegler). The paper also examines the implications of the shift toward greater mutuality in the health care interaction in terms of possible topics for investigation by researchers in health communication.

In the inaugural issue of the journal *Health Communication*, Nussbaum (1989) and D. H. Smith (1989) noted the interdisciplinary nature and theoretical plurality of research in health communication. Relevant research spans such fields as psychology, sociology, anthropology, and marketing, not to mention nursing, medicine, speech and communication. With roots in so many disparate fields, and so many topics of potential interest to pursue, there is a need for a common base of understanding, a unified framework from which health communication scholars may proceed. Only by knowing the history of our field can innovations or resistance to alternative conceptualizations be fully appreciated.

One integral aspect of health communication which has been a focus of attention from various fronts is the nature of practitioner-patient interaction. Not only is the practitioner-patient relationship central to the health communication process, it also has received renewed interest in recent years (e.g. Brickman, et al., 1982; H. Brody, 1987; Childress & Siegler, 1981; Lazare et al., 1976; McCullough, 1988; Quill, 1983; Reeder,

Reprinted by permission of Claudia Perry

1972; Siegler, 1981; Smith & Pettegrew, 1986; Squier, 1990). Noting dissatisfaction with the traditional paternalistic model of physician-patient interaction, D. H. Smith described "a paradigmatic shift . . . toward patient participation in health care," at least among those who study health communication. But he also commented that "not all will find it easy to accept and work with the patient participation idea" (1989, p. 20). Similarly, Stoeckle and Billings characterized the "modern ideology for the doctor-patient relationship" as including patient choice in decision-making, negotiation between patient and physician, promotion of health education and the communication of information, and concern with patient and physician values (1987, p. 125). These concepts may be conveyed implicitly to students in the language of medical textbooks and in the behaviors of clinical instructors, and explicitly recommended by such groups as the President's Commission for the Study of Ethical Problems in Medicine and Biomedical and Behavioral Research (1983). Nonetheless, this ideology represents a normative ideal rather than an accurate reflection of practice.

"While such guidelines suggest how modern doctors and patients should behave, both may diverge from these prescriptive ideals" commented Stoeckle and Billings (1987, p. 125). The patient participation model may entail a perceived loss of power for physicians, and greater responsibility for patients, which many may actively resist. Further, successful adoption of this perspective is likely to depend on the development of appropriate skill levels, relevant training, and support mechanisms which must be developed over time. Despite the call by theorists for a new model of physician-patient interaction, research in health communication must take account of the lingering influence of more traditional interaction models. Therefore, it may be useful to review the various conceptualizations of the physician-patient relationship, and the implications these models may have for needed communication and information skills in both patients and their doctors.

Traditional Model

Parsons and the Sick Role

Traditional models of the provider-patient relationship emphasize the essential asymmetry of the interaction. Parsons introduced the influential "sick role" model in 1951, which despite substantial criticism (see Bloom & Summey, 1978; Segall, 1976) has had a lasting impact on the way in which the provider-patient relationship has been conceptualized. The sick role, in Parsons' view, consisted of a set of institutionalized expectations concerning the responsibilities of the patient and his or her relationship to the medical establishment and society (1951, reprinted in 1984). The sick person has the right to be excused from normal societal demands and obligations (e.g. should stay home in bed) and should not be considered responsible for the development of illness. At the same time the sick person is obligated to want to "get well" and to seek technically competent help and cooperate in the process of recovery. The sick role is thus assumed to be a temporary state, with the patient occupying a passive role vis-a-vis the medical establishment.

In a later paper Parsons attempted to counter criticisms concerning the limits of his approach (1976). He commented that the degree of patient participation is very much dependent on the patient's state of illness: "the less acute the mediate situation, the more likely it is that participation will be substantial" (p. 270). Parsons acknowledged that chronically ill patients are far more likely to assume responsibility for an active role in their treatment than those suffering acute illness, and that friends and family members might also play a fairly major role in health maintenance, as for example assisting in home dialysis of the patient suffering kidney failure. Even so, because of differences in formal technical training and experience, he maintained that "the relation of sick person and health care agency is inherently asymmetrical on the hierarchical axis" (p. 276), much like the relationship of teacher and student. Parsons did not allow for change in relationships over time, nor the possibility that the relationship of patient and doctor might assume a very different configuration in a preventive or health maintenance context.

Balint and the Long-term Relationship

By comparison, Balint (1957) examined the physician-patient interaction in the context of the continuing, long-term relationship, as for example between a general practitioner and his or her patients. In such a relationship, the physician is likely to get to know patients as individuals in health as well as in illness, with a detailed knowledge of family, work habits, and community. A major theme in his work is the essential role played not so much by whatever therapy is prescribed, but by "the doctor himself" and the way in which doctor and patient relate to each other.

Like Parsons, Balint noted that "there are many factors in every doctor-patient relationship which will push the patient into a dependent-childish relationship to his doctor" (1957, p. 248). The degree of dependence will vary according to "the nature of the illness, the patient's personality, and—we propose to add—the doctor's individual apostolic beliefs" (1957, p. 248). Balint conceived of the physician's "apostolic" beliefs as a set of vague but firm ideas concerning how patients ought to behave when sick. As a corollary, he proposed that doctors act as though it was part of their responsibility to convert patients to share these views. At the same time, he recognized the "mutual influencing" of patient and doctor, "the persistent hard work on both sides to gain the other's confidence and convert him to one's beliefs", especially in the long term relationship (p. 249-250).

Balint noted the essential differences between the patient-specialist interaction in a short-term consultation, and the "mutual investment" relationship between patient and general practitioner, developed over many years. There would tend to be far less "mutual influence" in the short-term consultation, an observation of particular interest given the increasing rarity of the long-term physician-patient relationship. However, while referring to the inevitability of the dependent-childish relationship in certain circumstances, Balint, unlike Parsons, left open the possibility that there was potential for alternative, more symmetrical approaches to develop between patients and their doctors. He also clearly recognized that there is more to the practice of medicine than simply the diagnosis and treatment of physical signs and symptoms.

The Biopsychosocial Model

In a like manner, Engel acknowledged that there is a great deal more to the experience of illness than is explained by the manifestations of disease. Despite impressive advances in science and technology, Engel recognized that medicine has had limited success in dealing with illness and patient care. He blamed many of the problems in medicine on "the pervasive influence of the biomedical model of disease" (1978, p. 169). Engel claimed that the model upon which research and education in medicine is based is disease-centered and does not include the patient. He argued that until psychosocial concerns are included in the conceptualization of disease, problems in medicine will persist.

A central point in Engel's argument is that patients and physicians hold fundamentally different criteria for health and well-being. "Patients' criteria have to do with how one feels, how one functions, how one relates; with the ability . . . to seek options and make choices. . . . For the physician the real criteria for status and outcome are physical measures" (Engel, 1978, p. 172). In response to these perceived gaps between the patient's and the physician's views, Engel proposed the biopsychosocial model, based on general systems theory. In this model, the patient is considered as part of an ordered framework incorporating levels of organization ranging from subatomic particles to cells, through organ systems, family, culture and biosphere. Disruptions to any part of this system, whether social or molecular, have the potential to result in disease, although this is not inevitable. Different individuals may react to similar stresses in very different ways, a situation of which physicians must be cognizant in order to be effective.

"For the systematist physician the person must be the primary frame of reference", and he or she must be aware of the potential for disruption at any level, even including the impact of his or her own behavior on the patient (Engel, 1978, p. 178). His argument favors a more holistic approach to the practice of medicine, much like Balint. However, despite his call for a patient-centered conception of disease, Engel's work does not necessarily imply a more symmetrical physician-patient model. Engel advocated a more collaborative, complementary role for all health professionals on the health care team, and stressed the importance of communication, ("among all branches of the health professions", p. 175) but he did not explicitly address the role of the patient in the interaction, nor how a physician's knowledge of the patient's personality and disturbances in a patient's personal life is to be gained. The model, while far more reflective of reality than the biomedical model, still implies an essentially paternalistic and asymmetric view of the provider-patient relationship, although it does not necessarily preclude the more active participation of the patient. It should also be acknowledged that the model is proposed as a way of viewing disease, not specifically as a model of interaction.

The Health Belief Model

The biopsychosocial model incorporates the subjective as well as the objective aspects of illness, with an emphasis on the physician's perceptions of the patient. A complementary approach, which concerns patients' perceptions of disease and recommended health-enhancing responses, is the Health Belief Model (HBM). King characterized this approach as "the most extensively validated model of patients' health behavior" (1983, p. 114), which has been widely used to explain and predict patients' adherence or nonadherence to medical advice. It continues to evolve based on feedback obtained from relevant research in preventive as well as in specific illness-related contexts.

The HBM incorporates a number of factors pertaining to the patient's subjective evaluation of the health condition and the advocated health behavior, cues to action or motivation, and various modifying and enabling factors (Becker, 1976; Becker et al., 1979). Components include measures of the patient's perceptions of his or her susceptibility to the disease and its severity, patient's views of the costs and benefits of the health advice, and such factors as the physician-practitioner relationship, continuity of care, demographic/social variables, attitudes, prior experiences, social pressures, advice from others, and the patient's concern about health matters in general. In discussing limitations of the model, King noted that related research has focused little attention on the stability or acquisition of beliefs, and that for the model to be useful, all its components need to be considered (1983, p. 120). The value of the model for the present discussion lies not so much in its prediction of adherence, but rather for its depiction of the role of the patient as more than simply a passive recipient of medical help.

The HBM views patients as essentially responsible for their own health, based on actions they themselves have decided upon, which may or may not include consulting with physicians or following their advice. Hence, as David H. Smith commented,

> the patient becomes an active, interpreting, choosing creature rather than a passive one dependent on health care professionals. People are viewed as doing things about their health, and one of these might be to consult the formal system and professional care givers. Noncompliance can then be redefined as a reasonable

expression of the patient's own health beliefs and values (1989, p. 19).

The HBM thus extends the focus of attention in the health care interaction to the patient even more than was the case in the biopsychosocial model. While the components of the HBM might also be used by physicians as part of a persuasive arsenal designed to convince patients to "follow orders", an integral assumption of the model is that individual differences have a major impact on what patients choose to do or not do. The HBM asserts that patients, at least in a fair number of circumstances, have a far greater potential for exercising power than has traditionally been assumed.

A Range of Models

A classic paper by Szasz and Hollender (1956, reprinted in 1987) was one of the first to outline a range of possible models of the physician-patient relationship. These incorporated a variety of conceivable roles for physician and patient: 1) activity-passivity, 2) guidance-cooperation, and 3) mutual participation. Aspects of these models incorporate many of the above-mentioned conceptualizations. The "activity-passivity" model is historically, "the oldest conceptual model" (Szasz and Hollender, p. 167), and is based on the parent-infant prototype. The physician takes action to treat the patient, who is completely helpless and passive, as for example, when one is delirious or severely injured. Such a model would be particularly suitable in cases of acute trauma, coma, or surgery under anesthesia, when a more active patient role would be impossible, at least in the short term.

Szasz and Hollender considered the model of guidance-cooperation to be the dominant one in medical practice. In this model, both participants are active, but the physician is still in a position of greater power, akin to the parent of an adolescent child. The physician is expected to act as leader, while the patient's role is to cooperate and obey, as in Parsons' description of the sick role. "Moreover, [the patient] is neither to question nor to argue or disagree with the orders he receives" (Szasz and Hollender, 1987, p. 168). While the physician is expected to have the patient's best interests at heart, the guidance-cooperation model presents the opportunity for the physician to try to convert the patient to his own goals and beliefs, (the "apostolic" role, in Balint's view) rather than be influenced by the beliefs that may be held by the patient.

Unlike most of the preceding perspectives, the "mutual participation, model is one of fundamental equality between physician and patient, where the physician is viewed as helping the patient to help himself. Szasz and Hollender considered this model to be especially appropriate in the case of chronic illness and for those well-able to take an active role in managing their own care. The authors acknowledged, however, that this model was "essentially foreign to medicine" (p. 169), a situation that has been slow to change.

In the mutual participation model, both physician and patient are assumed to have something important to contribute. "The physician does not profess to know exactly what is best for the patient. The search for this becomes the essence of the therapeutic interaction. The patient's own experiences furnish indispensable information for eventual agreement, under otherwise favorable circumstances, as to what 'health' might be for him" (Szasz & Hollender, 1987, p. 171), an approach consistent with the assumptions of the HBM. Further, the relationship is viewed as a process, "leading to change in one or both participants" (p. 175), and one in which different types of doctor-patient relationship are appropriate in various circumstances. Inevitably, this implies that both patient and physician may be required to adapt their attitudes and behaviors to accommodate changes in health status or changes in the other party, a potentially threatening prospect.

The models proposed by Szasz and Hollender, as well as a number of other models discussed here, are most appropriately viewed as points on a continuum, rather than as specific alternatives existing only in pure form. For example, one can easily envision a range of behaviors extending between the guidance-cooperation and mutual participation models. Like Szasz and Hollender, several authors have emphasized the need for a plurality of models appropriate for different circumstances and individuals (Siegler, 1981; Smith & Newton, 1984). It is therefore not surprising that others have continued to propose alternative formulations, which might more closely approximate the range of human behavior in the health care interaction.

Models of Helping and Coping

Brickman, Rabinowitz, Karuza, Coates, Cohn and Kidder reviewed four models of helping and coping, each potentially applicable to the health care setting (1982). In each example, the attributions of responsibility for the problem and/or the solution are variously assigned to either the self or to others. The authors note that the assumptions implicit in these models can have a major impact on the subsequent behaviors and attitudes of the individuals, those trying to help them, and society at large.

The Medical Model

In the medical model, the traditional, paternalistic approach described by Parsons, the individual is assumed not to be responsible for either causing the illness, or curing it, as already discussed. While such assumptions may facilitate some aspects of the healing process (e.g. adhering to advice, relieving guilt), they can interfere with others, such as the ability of patients to assert their own point of view or take an active role in their own recovery.

The Enlightenment Model

In the enlightenment model, exemplified by Alcoholics Anonymous, individuals are similarly viewed as being unable to solve their own problems, but at the same time they are held responsible for causing those problems. "These attributions require people to accept a strikingly negative image of themselves and, in order to improve, to accept a strong degree of submission to agents of social control" (Brickman et al., 1982, p. 373). In either model, the patient is viewed as passive, with little capacity to assist himself except by submitting to a higher authority. Both models maximize the control of the health professional and provide the potential for the abuse of this power.

The Moral Model

The moral model, in contrast, holds the individual responsible for both creating and solving his or her problems, an approach basic to erhard seminars training (est) and other self-help groups. While the high expectations held of individuals are likely to increase their competency and sense of control over their lives, the model can also result in a "blame the victim" mentality, the sort of thinking behind Bernie Siegel's question to cancer patients: "Why did you need this illness?" (quoted in Konner, 1988, p. 49). While the moral model can be effective in efforts to lose weight or stop smoking, a failure to improve implies a lack of effort or ability, an approach which seems particularly unsuitable in the face of serious illness.

The Compensatory Model

The final model in this series is the compensatory model, in which individuals are held responsible for solutions, but not for problems. Jesse Jackson's exhortations to disadvantaged audiences that "You are not responsible for being down, but you are responsible for getting up" (quoted in Brickman, 1982, p. 372) epitomize this perspective. An advantage, according to Brickman and colleagues, is that this approach justifies individuals being provided with the help they need to solve their problems without blame, while at the same time encouraging in them an active sense of control.

However, the authors also noted that individual preferences for a particular model might not always lead to the best outcome. One study referenced reported that "the elderly preferred to apply the medical model, perhaps as the one justifying the most substantial form of help, yet were better off (in terms of positive affect and self-perceived coping) when other models were applied" (Brickman et al., 1982, p. 376). Like many of the authors discussed above, Brickman and colleagues considered whether different models may be appropriate for different individuals or for the same individuals in different circumstances, although they stated their own preference for the compensatory model. They also noted that "many of the problems characterizing relationships between help givers and help recipients (may) arise from the fact that the two parties are applying models that are out of phase with one another" (p. 375). They clearly stated the need for research to provide insight into issues such as these.

The Patient Sovereignty/Consumer Model

While a number of the above perspectives provide a somewhat more symmetrical way of perceiving the provider-patient relationship, the consumer model shifts the power balance in the opposite direction. The model, also referred to as "patient sovereignty", is in some ways the mirror image of the paternalistic medical model (Childress & Siegler, 1984; Haug & Lavin, 1979; President's Commission, 1983; Siegler, 1981). In the most extreme conceptualization of this perspective, the physician is viewed as no more than a technician or engineer, called in to fix the broken human machine at the behest of the customer. The concept apparently has its roots in the consumer movement of the sixties, during a time when many in society were challenging traditional authority figures. However, Reeder (1972) suggested that consumerism in health care arose also in response to changes in the health care system itself.

Reeder noted that structural changes in the health care system have led to a shift from curative care to preventive services, resulting in a buyer's market for health care. "When prevention of illness is emphasized, the client has to be persuaded that he has a need for medical services such as periodic checkups" (1972, p. 407), a point supported by the aggressive marketing efforts of health maintenance organizations and hospitals. At the same time, even with excellent preventive care, the need for curative and emergency services is hardly eliminated. At most, the consumer perspective will only be appropriate in selected instances.

Childress and Siegler (1984) commented that while a problem with the paternalistic model is the patient's "moral abdication", the reverse is true of the consumer model, which "offers autonomy to the patient, whose values dominate (at least in some settings) at the expense of the professional's moral agency and integrity" (p. 21). In either asymmetrical model, the gains to one partner are offset by losses experienced by the other, a process in which the ultimate goal—improved health status—is likely to suffer. Similarly, the President's Commission for the Study of Ethical Problems in Medicine and Biomedical and Behavioral Research, in reviewing both the concept of medical paternalism and that of patient autonomy, noted that "neither extreme adequately reflects the current nature and needs of health care" (1983, p. 36). Rather, they recommend a shift to "a relationship between patients and professionals characterized by mutual participation and respect and by shared decision-making" (p. 36). This recommendation is consistent with much of the related literature on the subject, although formulations of a mutual participation model day differ in degree.

Although in its pure form, as an "ideal-type", the consumer model exhibits major flaws, some aspects of the approach certainly warrant consideration in an amended model. Lazare, Eisenthal and Wasserman (1975) proposed that a "customer approach to patienthood", in which the physician explicitly asks the prospective patient what he or she wants, can provide valuable diagnostic information as well as ensuring that patient expectations are dealt with. Hornstra and colleagues (1972) similarly suggest the possible utility of market analysis and the importance of adjusting treatment options to patients' needs and expectations. Implicit in both these papers is the point that there often may be more than one viable perspective in medical treatment and care, and that the patient's preferences and participation are essential components of the process. Perhaps the chief value of the patient autonomy/consumer model is as a reminder that asymmetry in either direction in the health care interaction is potentially problematic, but that the patient's perspective must in some way be incorporated.

Mutual Participation/Negotiation Models

At the root of many of the models which will be classed here as examples of "mutual participation" is the understanding that perhaps inevitably, as a result of differences in training, status, knowledge, socialization, and access to information patients and health professionals are likely to have different goals and different expectations, and that an imbalance of power continues to exist (e.g. D. S. Brody, 1980; Lazare et al., 1976; Stone, 1979). In most cases, drawing on the theoretical perspectives which have already been discussed, these models assume that differences exist much if not all of the time, and that both parties have something to contribute to the therapeutic encounter. Further, they assume that constraints, such as time and resources, have an impact on the decision-making that must go on in the health care setting. As a result, in order for the perspectives of both parties to be considered, some sort of negotiation or accommodation process is often necessary.

Szasz and Hollender acknowledged that the mutual participation model is likely to work best "the greater the intellectual, educational, and general experiential similarity between physician and patient" (1987, p. 169). Yet as already indicated, such similarity may exist in a minority of situations. Lacking such social and intellectual equality, implementation of a mutual participation model becomes a greater challenge. As a result, models consistent with mutual participation which can incorporate dissimilarity of goals and characteristics are needed.

The Patient's Role in Clinical Decision-making

David Brody (1980), drawing on the work of Lazare and colleagues (1975, 1976) and the mutual participation model of Szasz and Hollender, discussed the patient's role in clinical decision-making, and the steps the physician can take to encourage this process. He noted the importance of providing a conducive atmosphere, eliciting patient goals and expectations, educating the patient concerning the illness and the costs and benefits of treatment, and finally, "eliciting the patient's informed suggestions and preferences and negotiating any disagreement" between the two parties (Brody, 1980, p. 720). Lazare and colleagues, similarly, noted the inherent role of conflict in the clinician-patient relationship, and the critical role of conflict resolution in the development of successful helping relationships (Lazare, Eisenthal, Frank & Stoeckle, 1976, p. 127). Although many patients and physicians may lack the skills or inclination for involving the patient in the decision-making process, Lazare, Eisenthal, Frank and Stoeckle (1976) frankly stated that they believed "that the use of the negotiation concept . . . is part of the physician's job" (p. 133). A similar point of view was expressed by Stone (1979).

The Health Transactions Model

Stone described a "Health Transactions Model", which extends the Health Belief Model and its conception of compliance to include not only patient beliefs but also the role and beliefs of the expert (1979). The expert-client interaction is viewed as a "problematic social situation" which can be dealt with in progressive stages: problem definition and reformulation, generation and selection of alternatives, implementation and evaluation. Stone stressed that this is a cycle involving both patient and physician, so that responsibility and input are shared, though perhaps not equally at every stage. This shared participation ensures that the burden of adherence to the therapeutic regimen is not given over to the patient unfairly, to be blamed for failing to comply. Rather, if for some reason the patient fails to follow advice it is viewed as a mutual failure of both parties, to be addressed by both. Further, the paper points specifically "to an expansion of the knowledge and skills needed by the provider", in terms of his or her communication and education roles, as being an integral part of the responsibilities of the physician.

Physician-patient Accommodation

Siegler (1981), like Stone (1979), asserted the importance of balancing the respective rights and responsibilities of both parties in the physician-patient relationship. He contended that "the physician-patient accommodation. . . . is both a process and an outcome" (Siegler, 1981, p. 61), and that it includes both communication and negotiation. In common with Engel, he viewed the entire interaction from a holistic perspective. The accommodation process depends on all aspects of the encounter, including the nature, characteristics, and beliefs of both the patient and the physician, the nature of the medical problem, and the clinical setting. The approach attempts to be sufficiently flexible to be able to adjust to the different needs, styles and expectations of a wide variety of participants.

Further, the accommodation model is dynamic, and constantly changing, with no requirement that the agreement at one point in time necessarily holds for alternative circumstances. Siegler suggested that the traditional view of the static, enduring physician-patient relationship—such as that described by Balint—was perhaps really a series of repeatedly negotiated interactions built up over time. Such a relationship might better be viewed as a specific and increasingly rare variation of the accommodation model, whose decline parallels the increase in medical specialization, technology, and fragmentation of care.

Mutual Participation and Shared Decision-making

The recommendations of the President's Commission for the Study of Ethical Problems in Medicine and Biomedical and Behavioral Research (1983) for a model of mutual participation and shared decision-making relied heavily on Siegler's description of the accommodation model, which they characterized as essentially contractual. Yet the Commission noted that the unequal status of patients and professionals raise serious questions about the ability of many patients to have an effective role in shaping the relationship" (p. 37). This necessitates a certain degree of regulation by society—such as the requirement for informed consent—in the interests of patients. The Commission acknowledged the importance of flexibility in the relationship and further indicated that health professionals are not obligated to accede to the demands of patients that violate the standards of acceptable medical practice or their own deeply held moral beliefs.

However, given the disparities between the participants, in the Commission's view, the responsibility for ensuring full patient understanding and involvement lies more with the physician than with the patient.

> The interaction should, at a minimum, provide the patient with a basis for effective participation in sound decisionmaking regardless of the particular form of accommodation. . . . Simply put, this means that the physician or other health professional invites the patient to participate in a dialogue in which the professional seeks to help the patient understand the medical situation and available courses of action, and the patient conveys his or her concerns and wishes (1983, p. 38).

Like Stone (1979), the President's Commission viewed the physician's leadership role in facilitating patient understanding as one of his or her primary responsibilities.

The Mutual Persuasion Model

In advocating a "Mutual Persuasion Model" of doctor-patient communication, Smith and Pettegrew (1986), like many of the other authors discussed above, agreed with the concept of mutuality inherent in the report of the President's Commission. Smith and Pettegrew's approach, "a rhetorical view of doctor-patient communication" emphasizes free choice based on reason, brought about by discourse which considers the beliefs and values of both parties. Aspects of their model are strikingly similar to many of the central points of models proposed or described by Siegler (1981), Stone (1979), D. Brody (1980) and Lazare and colleagues (1975, 1976), as well as the President's Commission (1983).

Nevertheless, Smith and Pettegrew strongly criticized what they saw as undue concern with the potential for physicians to manipulate their patients in the Commission's report. They commented that "the Commission's admonition [regarding manipulation] would seem to require a neutral, expressionless monotone by the physician delivered in a wooden, motionless way" (p. 135), and discussed at length the impossibility of emotional neutrality in communication, especially if shared decision-making is an important goal.

This point is emphasized disproportionately in their paper. Less than two pages of the Commission's 180 page report dealt with the potential for manipulation, a concern that seems totally reasonable in view of the power asymmetry which has so long characterized the physician-patient relationship. In discussing influence and manipulation the Commission made the simultaneous point that "health care professionals should . . . present information in a form that fosters understanding" (Commission, 1983, p. 67), a process unlikely to be achieved if information is delivered in an expressionless monotone. Furthermore, subsequent sections of the Commission's report stressed the importance of discussion and dialogue concerning medical status and treatment alternatives, along with the physician's statement of his or her professional opinion as to the best course of action. Such recommendations hardly seem consistent with a call for emotional neutrality.

Although Smith and Pettegrew present a convincing case for a mutual participation model with roots in the rhetorical tradition, it is not at all clear why this argument was framed in distinct contrast to certain aspects of the shared decision-making perspective of the President's Commission. As the present paper has attempted to demonstrate, the concepts of "mutual influence" and "mutual participation" in doctor-patient interaction have existed at least since Balint and Szasz and Hollender wrote on the topic in the 1950s. In advocating "mutual persuasion", Smith and Pettegrew noted many of the problems others have found with the medical model and the consumer model. In my view they have articulated an approach which is consistent with, rather than distinctly different from, the ideal of mutuality expressed by the President's Commission. This same ideal appears to be achieving increasingly wide consensus among those concerned with the therapeutic relationship.

Model of Empathic Understanding

Previous models in the patient participation tradition have stressed the importance of dialogue and an awareness of the beliefs and values of both parties. A recognition of the concurrent importance of affective-motivational and cognitive-informative aspects of practitioner-patient relationships led Squier (1990) to propose a model of empathic understanding and adherence to treatment regimens. Although Engel (1978) is not cited in Squier's paper, his model has a holistic emphasis that is entirely consistent with Engel's biopsychosocial model. Both cognitive and affective components are viewed as inherently interactive. For example, "whilst the informational exchange and feedback process is leading to increasing cognitive understanding of the illness in both practitioner and patient, the affective climate is reducing the anxiety connected with the symptoms and decreasing any stress contributing either primarily or secondarily to the illness" (Squier, 1990, p. 334). Squier's approach extends the biopsychosocial model to provide a means of conceptualizing the interaction itself, and not just a way of thinking about the disease process.

As might be assumed from the label "empathic understanding", a major emphasis is on the responsibility of the health practitioner to see things from the patient's perspective, and on the verbal and non-verbal behaviors which might enable practitioners to convey that understanding to others. Somewhat less attention is devoted to informational aspects of the model, perhaps because of the relatively greater emphasis on this component of adherence in the literature. Squier's review of the role of empathy provides yet another dimension to consider in conceptualizing the physician-patient relationship, but the model still appears to perpetuate a relatively passive role for the patient.

A Focus on the Patient Role in Participation

While it is not surprising that much of the literature addresses the role of the physician in the participation model, a few authors also have addressed aspects of the patient's responsibilities in this regard. Quill (1983) enumerated several responsibilities associated with patients, following Lazare and colleagues (1975); these include defining the nature of the problem and interventions sought, considering seriously (although not necessarily adhering to) the recommendations of the physician, and paying for the physician's time and expertise. Quill noted that "the ideal medical partnership encourages the patient to be independent and responsible for as much of his own care as possible" (1983, P. 231), but like many other theorists he agreed that this level of control is likely to vary depending on the patient's degree of sickness or health. Both participants must therefore be willing to be flexible.

Similarly, McCullough (1988) commented that "models of shared responsibility imply accountability on the patient's part, not just the physician's" (p. 462), but acknowledged that further research is needed to identify these responsibilities. Does the public availability of health information imply that it is duty of patients to read and understand information about their health situations? The report of the President's Commission mentioned the growing demand for such information, but also the fact that access varied tremendously in different settings (1983, pp. 123-6). McCullough noted the difficulty presented by the fact that not all patients are equally capable of evaluating such information, particularly that dealing with medical uncertainty. "It would be a dubious form of progress if we doubled the burden of patients, adding to illness a failure to genuinely empower their autonomy" (1988, p. 462). McCullough, like many others describing variations on the participation model, thus stressed the importance of the teaching, counseling, communication and negotiating roles of the physician.

Just as patients vary in their cognitive abilities to understand and evaluate medical information, they are likely to vary in their negotiation and communication skills, particularly when not feeling well. A fully participative model implies some responsibility on the part of society to "develop patients with increased abilities and expectations for a partnership in health care" (McCullough, p. 464). Although Roter noted that "self-care and patient activation programs are gaining popularity throughout the country, (1977; p. 304), it is likely that most of the training which will take place will continue to occur between participants in the physician-patient interaction for some time to come. Society's responsibility may therefore lie in ensuring that medical education provides suitable training for the physicians expected to fill these new roles, while at the same time enhancing access to health information for the layperson, and expanding more innovative efforts to develop patient competencies.

Conclusion

A gradual change has been under way in the conceptualization of the physician-patient relationship, from a model of paternalism to one in which, ideally, both participants in the interaction negotiate a mutually acceptable agreement as to how they will cooperate in the health care process. But rather than supporting one, relatively monolithic perspective, the proponents of the evolving consensus share a number of similar values, assumptions and expectations, but allow their models to differ in various details, often reflective of particular concerns and backgrounds, or in awareness of the changing nature of the health care interaction.

With the possible exception of Smith and Pettegrew, who take issue with one aspect of the report of the President's Commission, most theorists stress their similarities with other participation perspectives, acknowledging that different approaches—even including the paternalistic model—are likely to be useful in some conceivable situation. The one requirement of overriding importance is the potential for discussion, negotiation, and informed decision-making on the part of the patient, even if that choice is for an authoritarian relationship; along with the possibility for change, as the situation warrants it.

As D. G. Smith and L. Newton (1984) commented,

> There are no fixed models. The Siegler model of 'accommodation' requires continued negotiation between patient and physician to establish their relationship at each state of their encounter. In this 'model', a plurality of models exists in the relating, and whatever the parties are comfortable with at any given time simply is the model, for them, then. In its recognition of the integrity of human mutuality, this model may be the most useful one for the future of this discussion (p. 58).

Similarly, Howard Brody noted that while the proponents of different models and their critics may differ in important ways, "an emerging point of agreement is the importance of 'dialogue', or what Katz (1984) has referred to as 'conversation', (H. Brody, 1987, p. 218). So long as patients and physicians have a respectful opportunity to talk over their expectations, requirements, constraints, and needs, it is proposed that some degree of mutually acceptable accommodation, and an outcome acceptable to both parties, will be at least theoretically possible. It remains to be seen if empirical research will support these expectations.

The accompanying table summarizes the various aspects of the models discussed in the body of this paper. Substantial differences are found even among those models grouped within the same section, as well as many similarities. However, one of the most striking patterns lies in the notion of effective communication within each category, as suggested above. In nearly every case within the asymmetrical models discussed, communication is viewed in a linear, directive or one-way manner, with information envisioned as a bullet to be delivered to the recipient. The assumption is that the patient need merely absorb the information transmitted by the physician, or convey required information concerning symptoms to the physician, for an effective outcome. The fact that these assumptions have only rarely worked as expected is perhaps besides the point.

Conversely, in each of the symmetrical models, communication is viewed as a process between relative equals, affected by each party's beliefs, values and expectations. The interaction is voluntary, ongoing, and subject to negotiation. Information may be tailored to the needs of the recipient or not provided at all, depending on individual preferences. Although the dates of the different models vary, generally the older models reflect a more asymmetrical, focus, linear focus, while more symmetrical models were proposed in more recent papers.

The table provides a relatively straightforward illustration of the "paradigm shift" toward patient participation described by D. H. Smith (1989, p. 20). Although even in the 50s there was recognition that for some patients and some physicians in certain circumstances, a model of mutual influence (Balint, 1957) or mutual participation (Szasz and Hollander, 1956, reprinted in 1987) might be appropriate, the trend toward a greater acceptance of the participative model, at least among scholars, appears clear.

It remains for researchers in health communication to explore whether this shift in perspective is actually reflected in the expectations and behavior of practicing physicians and their patients. Are medical students receiving the sort of training that will prepare them for an expanded role in teaching, counseling, and negotiating with patients? What proportion of clinical instructors are providing role models for a patient participation approach to the medical encounter? Do opportunities exist for more experienced physicians to acquire these sorts of skills? How might patients be prepared for a more active role in their own health care? Are demands for improved access to consumer health information being met? As Brickman and colleagues propose, do problems in physician-patient relationships stem from a mismatch in role expectations, or are some patients better served by model which they might not prefer? What will be the role of society in regulating the physician-patient interaction, through requirements such as informed consent? How will this be monitored? Finally, given an increasingly rapid pace of change in the health care system, what will be the impact on the practitioner-patient relationship? There appears to be an important role for health communication researchers to fill in exploring the extent to which the ideal of mutual participation between physician and patient is found in practice, and the implications for society.

Models of provider-patient interaction

Model Name	Citation(s)	Patient role	Physician Role	Prototype	Identifiers/ application	Notion of effective communication	Major focus	Other comments
Asymmetrical models with Provider dominant:								
Medical; Biomedical	Brickman et. al (1982) Smith & Pettegrew (1986)	Passive; cooperative	Active; directive	Parent-child	Scientific, rational	directive, "bullet" approach, information = communication	physician role	Traditional, dominant model; little consideration of patient values; patient responsible for neither problem or solution
Sick role	Parsons (1975)	Cooperative	Active	Fiduciary relationship	acute as well as chronic illness	directive	patient role	Level of patient activity depends on severity of illness, but built-in, institutionalized superiority of physicians exists
Biophsychosocial	Engel (1978)	Passive; cooperative	Directive	Parent-adolescent	General Systems Theory	information exchange	physician role	like medical but considers patient's psychosocial attributes; more holistic, more patient-centered than the medical model
Activity-Passivity	Szasz & Hollender (1956)	Passive	Active	Parent-infant	acute trauma, coma	no interaction	physician role	Essentially synonymous with the Biomedical model.
Guidance-Cooperation	Szasz & Hollender (1956)	Cooperative	Directive	Parent-adolescent	acute infectious disease	directive, "bullet" approach	physician role	More Active model than above, but unequal power relationship
Enlightenment	Brickman et al. (1982)	Submissive	Directive	Parent-child	AA, evangelicals	directive; controlling	patient role	Patient responsible for problem but not solution
Asymmetrical models with Patient dominant:								
Patient sovereignty	Pres. Commission (1982) (Vol.1)	Decision-maker	Informer	Attorney-client	patient autonomy	doctor as "informer" only; "value-free" information	patient role	Artificial & difficult to implement; ignores importance of provider-patient relationship.
Consumer	Siegler (1981)	Decision-maker	Technician	Agent-client	patient "rights"	doctor as "informer" only	patient role	Response to traditional paternalistic model

Model Name	Citation(s)	Patient role	Physician Role	Prototype	Identifiers/ application	Notion of effective communication	Major focus	Other comments
Models of relatively mutual participation:								
Mutual Participation	Szasz & Hollender (1956) Brody (1980)	Participant	Helping	Adult-adult	chronic illness	symmetrical	mutuality	Assumes relatively equal competence and power.
Moral	Brickman et al. (1982)	Active	Encouraging	Adult-adult	est, self-help groups	encouragement	patient role	Patient responsible for problem and solution.
Compensatory	Brickman et al. (1982)	Active	Helping	Adult-adult	Jesse Jackson	problem-solving	patient role	Patient responsible for solution but not problem
Health Belief (HBM)	Becker; King; Smith	Active	Variable	Adult-adult	adherence/prevention	congruent with beliefs	patient role	Importance of patient beliefs and values
Mutual Persuasion	Smith & Pettegrew (1986)	Mutual influence	Mutual influence	Adult-adult	Rhetorical tradition	discourse; free choice	mutuality	Importance of both patient & provider beliefs & values; autonomy plus beneficence; patient more powerful
Health Transactions	Stone (1979)	Active; negotiable	Helping; negotiable	Adult-adult	focus on the transaction	process-oriented	physician role	Importance of both patient & provider beliefs & values; extends HBM but emphasizes physician role
Physician-patient Accommodation	Siegler (1981)	Active; negotiable	Helping; negotiable	Adult-adult	negotiation & joint decision-making	process-oriented	mutuality	Emphasis on voluntariness, respect for autonomy
Ethical	McCullough (1988)	Collaborative	Collaborative	Adult-adult	Normal pregnancy	process-oriented	physician role	What ought to be
Empathic Understanding	Squier (1990)	Cooperative participant	Helping	Adult-adult	role-taking/sensitivity	understanding patient frame of reference	physician role	Needs further development of cognitive component

References

Balint, M. (1957). *The doctor, his patient and the illness*. London: Pitman Medical Co.

Becker, M. H. (1976). Sociobehavioral determinants of compliance. In D. L. Sackett & R. B. Haynes (Eds.), *Compliance with therapeutic regimens* (pp. 40-50). Baltimore: Johns Hopkins University Press.

Becker, M. H., Maiman, L. A., Kirscht, J. P., Haefner, D. P., Drachman, R. H., and Taylor, D. W. (1979). Patient perceptions and compliance: Recent studies of the Health Belief Model. In R. B. Haynes, D. W. Taylor, & D. L. Sackett (Eds.), *Compliance in Health Care* (pp. 78-109). Baltimore: Johns Hopkins University Press.

Bloom, S. W. & Summey, P. (1976). Models of the doctor-patient relationship: A history of the social system concept. In E. B. Gallagher (Ed.), *The doctor-patient relationship in the changing health scene* (DHEW Publication No. (NIH) 78-183), (pp. 17-41). Washington, D. C.: U.S. Government Printing Office.

Brickman, P., Rabinowitz, V.C., Karuza, J., Jr., Coates, D., Cohn, E., & Kidder, L. (1982). Models of helping and coping. *American Psychologist, 37*(4), 368-384.

Brody, D. S. (1980). The patient's role in clinical decision-making. *Annals of Internal Medicine, 93*(5), 718-722.

Brody, H. (1987). The physician-patient relationship: models and criticisms. *Theoretical Medicine, 8*, 205-220.

Childress, J. F. & Siegler, M. (1984). Metaphors and models of doctor-patient relationships: Their implications for autonomy. *Theoretical Medicine 5,* 17-30.

Engel, G. L. (1978). The Biophychosocial model and the education of health professionals. *Annals of the New York Academy of Sciences, 310*, 169-181.

Hague, M. R. & Lavin, B. (1979). Public challenge of physician authority. *Medical Care 17*(8), 844-858.

Hornstra, R. K., Lubin, B., Lewis, R. V., & Willis, B. S.

(1972). Worlds apart: Patients and professionals. *Archives of General Psychiatry 27,* 553-557

Katz, J. (1984). The silent world of doctor and patient. New York: Free Press.

King, J. (1983). Health beliefs in the consultation. In D. Pendleton & J. Hasler (Eds.), *Doctor-patient communication* (pp. 109-125). New York: Academic Press.

Konner, M. (1988, March 13) Laughter and hope. *New York Times Magazine*, p. 49-50.

Lazare, A., Eisenthal, S., Frank, A., & Stoeckle, J.D. (1976). Studies on a negotiated approach to patienthood. In E. B. Gallagher (Ed.), *The doctor-patient relationship in the changing health scene* (DHEW Publication No. (NIH) 78-183), (pp. 119-139). Washington, D. C.: U.S. Government Printing Office.

Lazare, A., Eisenthal, S., Wasserman, L. (1975). *Archives of General Psychiatry 32,* 553-558

McCullough, L. B. (1988). An ethical model for improving the patient-physician relationship. *Inquiry, 25* 454-468.

Nussbaum, J. F. (1989). Directions for research within health communication. *Health Communication, 1*(1), 35-40.

Parsons, T. (1984). The functional setting of medical practice and cultural tradition. In N. Abrams & M. D. Buckner (Eds.), *Medical Ethics* (pp. 99-106). Cambridge, MA: MIT Press. (Reprinted from The Social System, New York, The Free Press, 1951).

Parsons, T. (1975). The sick role and the role of the physician reconsidered. *Milbank Memorial Fund Quarterly, 53*(3), 257-278.

President's Commission for the Study of Ethical Problems in Medicine and Biomedical and Behavioral Research. (1983). *Making health care decisions: The ethical and legal implications of informed consent in the patient-practitioner relationship* (Vol. 1). Washington, D. C.: U.S. Government Printing Office.

Reeder, L. G. (1972). The patient-client as consumer: Some observations on the changing professional-client relationship. *Journal of Health and Social Behavior, 13*, 406-412.

Segall, A. (1976). The sick role concept: Understanding illness behavior. *Journal of Health and Social Behavior, 17*, 162-169.

Siegler, M. (1981). Searching for moral certainty in medicine: A proposal for a new model of the doctor-patient encounter. *Bulletin of the New York Academy of Medicine, 57*(1), 56-69.

Smith, D. G. & Newton, L. (1984). Physician and patient: respect for mutuality. *Theoretical Medicine, 5*(1), 43-60.

Smith, D. H. (1989). Studying health communication: An agenda for the future. *Health Communication*, 1(1), 17-27.

Smith, D. H. & Pettegrew, L. S. (1986). Mutual persuasion as a model for doctor-patient communication. *Theoretical Medicine, 7*, 127-146.

Squier, R. W. (1990). A model of empathic understanding and adherence to treatment regimens in practitioner-patient relationships. *Social Science and Medicine, 30*(3), 325-339.

Stoeckle, J. D., & Billings, J. A. (1987). A history of history- taking: The medical interview. *Journal of General Internal Medicine, 2*(2), 119-127.

Stone, G. C. (1979). Patient compliance and the role of the expert. *Journal of Social Issues, 35*(1), 34-59.

Szasz, T. S.& Hollender, M. H. (1987). A contribution to the philosophy of medicine: The basic models of the doctor-patient relationship. In J. D. Stoeckle (Ed.), *Encounters between patients and doctors: An Anthology* (pp. 165-177). Cambridge, MA: MIT Press. (Reprinted from 1956 *AMA Archives of Internal Medicine, 97*, 585-592.)

Dimensions of Caregiving

The Mystification of Meaning: Doctor-Patient Encounters

Dean C. Barnlund

The words "mystique" and "mystify" have a curious affinity in language and life. "Mystique" refers to the magical aura that surrounds objects or persons which endows them with talismanic and magical influence. To "mystify" is to confuse, perplex, or make obscure or difficult to understand. They go together. Mystification is simply the means by which persons are endowed with mystique. While professional mystique seems to be an elusive idea, the process of communication that creates it is capable of systematic analysis.

Examining communicative relationships within the medical profession requires some broad appreciation of the communicative process itself. A good starting point might be this: every person from birth until death is engaged endlessly in a search for meaning. To survive physically and psychically, people must inhabit a world that is fairly stable, relatively free of ambiguity, and reasonably predictable. Though people tolerate occasional doubts, few can accept continuing meaninglessness.

To aid in coping with a chaos of fleeting sensations—what William James called this "blooming, buzzing confusion"—we seek to give events some structure that will render them intelligible. Repeated success in interpreting events contributes to an accumulating set of assumptions on which all future acts depend. These assumptions, as George Kelly once noted, provide templates or guides which every person fits over the realities of life.[1] Gradually people within a culture and within a profession acquire specialized frames of reference which, though they speed the process of judgment, often induce a certain blindness. What is "information" to the specialist may be only "noise" to the lay-person; what the physician regards as "noise," his patient often treats as "information." To the patient excessive thirst may be only an inconvenience, but to the doctor it is a symptom of diabetes; to the examining physician the color of the patient's chart may seem irrelevant, but to the patient it is an ominous sign.

All knowledge of the world is inescapably subjective. In effect, each person stands at the center of his or her own universe of meaning, transforming the flow of sensations into organized and intelligible events. Each of us views the world selectively and fits it to our own past experience and changing purposes. Each notes some details and overlooks others; each finds plausible some relationships and rejects others. Since every interpretation of events rests on fallible senses and personal motives, what is known is always incomplete and always subject to error.

Barnlund, D.C. The mystification of meaning: Doctor-patient encounters. *Journal of Medical Education* (retitled *Academic Medicine* in 1989) 51 (1976): 716-725.

1 Kelly, G. *The Psychology of Personal Constructs*. New York: Norton, 1955.

It is tempting in the daily clash of words to forget that it is the perceived world—not the real world—that we talk about, argue about, laugh about, cry about. It is not scalpels and crosses and bedpans that regulate human affairs, but how people construe them that determines what they will think, how they will feel, and what they will do about them. Meanings do not come from the world but are assigned to it by every interpreter, and it is he who is the final arbiter of events.

Symbols and Meanings

Language plays a critical role in the construction of the frames of reference through which we view events. It is the most elaborate and most flexible system humans have devised for transforming shapes and sounds into meaningful events. There is wide recognition that the single species-distinguishing attribute of humanity is the capacity to transform experience into symbols. As Langer[2] has emphasized, the brain works as naturally as the kidneys, carrying on a constant process of ideation, even when we are asleep. It follows its own internal law of translating sensory data into symbols to feed our insatiable appetite for meaning.

Life is so permeated with symbolism that it is difficult to imagine any human experience that is not mediated by language. Language tells us what to look for and what to disregard. It suggests causality here and denies it there. It can paralyze us or rouse us to act. It triggers fear and moments later transforms that fear into hope. It is the slender thread by which we overcome our isolation from each other. Yet if words sometimes clarify, they may also distort. If they induce trust, they may also arouse suspicion. If they contribute to insight, they can also lead into error.

Symbolic Dimensions

Symbolic mediation, the intervention of words between people and their experiences, would seem to be an especially sensitive problem in the treatment of human beings. A physical mechanism, a clock or computer, may break down; but any damage to the mechanism is easily identified and repaired without complications. To an animal, injury or disease is simply another physical state. Any suffering is tied directly to disturbances of normal function. Diagnosis has no influence upon the course of the disease, nor does the prognosis complicate recovery.

This is not the case with human beings. Human illness is not only a physical condition but a symbolic one as well. No animal talks itself into becoming sick, suppresses its symptoms because it fears a diagnosis, prolongs recovery because of the symbolic payoff it receives, or spontaneously recovers because it has redefined its situation.

Yet humans do all of these things. They avoid critical examinations that might save their lives. They seek unnecessary treatments and disregard essential ones. They often suffer more from the name of their illness than the physical pain it produces. They suppress some symptoms and invent others. They convert discomfort into excruciating pain and transform extreme suffering into tolerable discomfort. They can go into shock without physical justification and accept a painful death with serenity.

In short, every medical problem is in part a symbolic one. One cannot damage the physical self without injuring the symbolic self, nor can one inflict insult repeatedly on the symbolic self without damaging the physical self. Research on "experimenter influence" and the "placebo effect" convincingly demonstrates that neither physicians nor patients are free of the influence of the way they define their situation. Diagnosis and treatment are in large part symbolic problems,

2 Langer, S. *Philosophy in a New Key*. Cambridge, Mass.: Harvard University Press, 1957.

and to ignore this fact may distort or defeat their aims. There is little doubt that how people think about themselves can alter their blood pressure, oxygen needs, and blood chemistry.

The notion that there are a limited number of "psychosomatic" illnesses has gradually given way to the idea that every illness has some psychosomatic reverberations. The broken leg of a young skier may mean a minor inconvenience amply compensated for by increased attention, a flood of sympathetic concern from acquaintances, and special privileges at home and at school. To an older person the same fracture may signal a loss of physical coordination, a sign of aging, or an omen of approaching dependence.

It was once thought that pain was directly proportional to the amount of physical tissue damaged. According to Melzack,[3] this can no longer be assumed, for pain itself depends on the meaning attributed to physical incapacity. This meaning in turn reflects the past experiences and future expectations of the patient. Higher brain functions are capable of modifying or even suppressing signals that accompany physical distress. If every experience of the organism is invested with symbolic significance, it is naive to assume that the most dramatic of life experiences—those involving physical survival itself—are immune to such effects.

To put this another way, for the patient there is no distinction between perceived pain and real pain and between perceived health and real health. This is a dichotomy implied by language but one without counterpart in human experience. It is perceived malfunctions that bring patients to seek care. It is the persistence of such perceptions that keep them in treatment. It is a change in these perceptions that causes them to terminate treatment.

Similarly for the medical profession, it is a perceived disturbance of normal function that mobilizes the physician. He, in turn, acts upon this perception. Through elaborate procedures there is a search to confirm this perception. Investigation may modify or strengthen an initial interpretation. Ultimately it may be shared in part or in full with the patient. Eventually both share a perception of recovery. But all who are involved in the treatment process will base every question, every inference, every recommendation upon meanings assigned to their impressions through the symbols they impose on them. As Friedson has remarked,[4] "illness is a meaning assigned to behavior" and "illness behavior is ordered by that meaning."

One is forced to conclude that there is no patient who does not present the medical profession with, at least in part, a symbolic problem. No illness lacks its semantic dimension. The professional who feels involved exclusively in the maintenance of a physical mechanism and who dismisses the communicative aspect of this work operates on a simplistic and even dangerous premise. Human beings are not merely symbol users; every moment of life is permeated with symbolism.

Obstacles to Communication

The study of communication is concerned with the process by which people attribute meaning to their experience and with their efforts to share such meanings. It focuses upon factors that undermine or facilitate the achievement of common meanings through an exchange of messages. The complexity of medical communication may be intimated by examining some of the more common and more serious barriers to interpersonal understanding in medical settings.

Ego involvement. Less complete communication is likely whenever the topic of conversation is highly ego-involving, such as when one or

---

3 Melzack, R. The Perception of Pain. *Scientific American* 264 (February 1961): 41-49.
4 Friedson, E. *The Profession of Medicine*. New York: Dodd, Mead, 1972, p. 224.

both parties are fearful of the matter under discussion. Few subjects would appear to arouse as intense feelings as adequacy of the physical or symbolic self. Recent crosscultural research suggests that the least talked about of all topics are those relating to physical inadequacy, illness, and disease.[5] The anxiety associated with such matters triggers a number of defensive maneuvers, most of which interfere with a clear exchange of meaning. Some people flee and others attack, some refuse to listen and others refuse to talk, some exaggerate and others minimize. But rarely do people comprehend clearly when they are emotionally upset.

Differences in knowledge. Another factor complicating communication resides in the respective power of the communicants. We are beginning to appreciate that information is power. Where knowledge is unequal, where some people have access to the facts and others do not, equality of human relationships is impossible. It is not surprising, therefore, that incomplete and distorted communication surrounds so many encounters between specialists and lay people. To be uninformed is to be communicatively impotent, and this dependent state is not one mature people tolerate gracefully. Rarely is this condition absent between doctors and patients.

Social status. Difficulties are likely, also, when the social distance separating two communicants is great. The greater the disparity in education, income, and social standing, the less people are capable of hearing or of hearing what was said as it was intended. The presence of higher status figures—parents, teachers, supervisors, police—provokes fear quite apart from whatever they may happen to say. White,[6] found his cardiac patients manifesting significantly different levels of tension when he discussed their cases with them in status-aggravating or status-minimizing settings. When status distinctions are emphasized, people avoid contact with each other, withhold information, and distort the meanings intended by the words of others.

Communicative purposes. Status differences are complicated further by differences in point of view arising in part from differences in position and authority. Rarely do communicative purposes overlap completely. Because of distinctive motives, student and teacher do not argue about the "same" grade; nor do husband and wife discuss the "same" child; nor for that matter do physician and patient talk about the "same" X-rays, the "same" disease, the "same" operation, or the "same" fee. Messages acquire much of their meaning from the perspective from which they are uttered. Unless people are sensitive to such differences in purpose or unless these are explicitly discussed, meanings will not coincide since they are anchored in discrepant motives.

Emotional distance. Through conversation people seek some similarity of thought, some congruence of feeling. Words like "rapport," "intimacy," empathy," and "closeness" are used to describe satisfying encounters with others. But any such meeting of minds is difficult unless both communicants are willing to be "present," not merely available intellectually but totally present as persons. In the interaction of roles, in the encounter of facades, there is no commitment to communication. To give patients the feeling that they are a problem, a disease, or an intriguing curiosity rather than a human being is to undermine the process of sharing meanings. No one has put this point as cogently as Martin Buber.[7] The "I-It" relation, he argues, is demeaning and frustrating for it rests on perceptions of the other as no more than an object. It is only when people confront each other in an "I-Thou" relation that they meet as human beings with respect and

5 Barnlund, D. *Public and Private Self in Japan and U.S.* Tokyo: Simul Press, 1975.

6 White, A. The Patient Sits Down. *Psycoso. Med.* 15 (1953): 256-57.

7 Buber, M. *I and Thou.* New York: Scribners Sons, 1958.

mutual concern. When people cultivate emotional distance, they not only prevent any deep sharing of meaning but also arouse animosity and even hatred.

One-way communication. Once communication was regarded as a linear process. Someone, a sender or speaker, transmitted messages to a receiver or listener. Meanings obtained by the receiver were due to the skill of the sender. The sender did the work and the receiver merely paid attention. Any idea could be deposited in the nervous system of another person if one only chose the right words. Now we know better. No one deposits any meaning in the mind of others. Receivers do not passively absorb the intentions of others but creatively interpret what they hear in the light of their own perspectives, their own needs, their own expectations. Reaching any degree of interpersonal understanding requires a process of mutual accommodation. Each person must provide the other with clues to his or her meanings via words and actions. Each must attend to the clues of the other. And each must be prepared to clarify and elaborate his meaning from the viewpoint of the other. This process succeeds to the extent that both parties assume equal responsibility for achieving common meanings.

Yet the prevailing style of interaction from the clinic to the classroom is one-way rather than two-way. And, unfortunately, such channel restrictions impoverish the process and leave receivers confused and impotent. Laboratory studies supply dramatic evidence of the seriousness of this phenomenon; where communication flows in only one direction. The simplest instructions are misinterpreted, errors are compounded rather than corrected and morale and human relationships deteriorate. It is easy to appreciate the source of such distortion and friction. Nothing is more demoralizing than to be placed in critical situations and then be prevented from clarifying obscure and confusing messages.

Verbal manipulation. Many efforts to communicate are prompted not by the desire to share or create new meanings but to maneuver the other person into a predetermined decision. Whatever the form of such efforts, from verbal seduction to verbal coercion, they derive from an assumption of moral superiority on the part of one communicant. They also involve disrespect for the integrity of other persons and appropriation of their right to determine their own destiny. Enlarging the communicative responsibility of one person requires some surrender of responsibility by the other. And while such dependency is tolerated by children, adults often find it demeaning and insulting. In a highly manipulative society it is not surprising that most people become adept at recognizing their manipulators. They become suspicious and verbally devious themselves. Thus, communication is often subverted and people antagonized when the authority of their own experience is denied equal weight in the process of making decisions affecting their own survival.

Ambiguity of language. Language itself may introduce barriers to mutual understanding. Through a system of symbols with culturally sanctioned definitions, people seek to share their experience and establish grounds for cooperative action. Yet every communicative code forces the infinity of events into a limited set of categories and fixes appropriate labels to them. "Illness" has perhaps a hundred meanings. "Surgery" may have several dozen. "Fracture" is imprecise. "Cancer" is inexact. If so many words are vague in their reference, messages composed of such ambiguous elements will be even less precise. Nearly every statement can support many legitimate and even contradictory interpretations. In some respects the vocabulary of illness constitutes a special case. Anyone who has attempted to describe a sickness knows the frustration of searching for words to convey the subtle inner disturbances called symptoms. As the great English novelist, Virginia Woolf, once said, "let a sufferer try to describe a pain in his head to a doctor and language at once runs dry." Most people have experienced the communicative paralysis induced by a poverty of words for inner states combined with innocent insistence upon clarity from the doctor.

Language by itself solves nothing. Words can confuse as easily as they clarify. As we have seen, communication is not accomplished by mere listening; it requires a persistent and sensitive effort to solve a mystery whose major clues are provided by words. Common meaning is achieved only through repeated and mutual checking of interpretations. Where people have little appreciation of the ambiguity of words, they remain unaware of the extent to which their remarks can be misunderstood. And they are unlikely to adapt their communicative style to this fact of life.

Role of jargon. Language isolates in another way. Not only do Chinese and Russians speak different languages but also so do males and females, young and old, soldiers and civilians. Every subculture, every trade, and every profession cultivates a dialect of its own. Lawyers, engineers, scientists, accountants and physicians foster their private jargons. These are neither ornament not luxury; they serve genuine needs; they increase the efficiency of communication within the group; they cultivate rapport among members; they provide a sense of common identity. While contributing to communication within a group, these same dialects when turned outward confuse, frighten, stupefy, alienate. And the more sensitive the topic of conversation, the more such private languages undermine the function for which language was designed. If medical personnel are occasionally puzzled or irritated by the words of economists, lawyers, insurance agents, or musicologists, they might consider the extent to which these same people may be mystified by the diagnostic remarks of physicians.

Pressures of time. Compounding these difficulties is the factor of time. In some ways our humanity seems threatened more by the pace of our lives than by any other single factor. There is no human relationship, no communicative act, that is enriched or improved by speeding it up. It takes time to explain, time to listen, time to dissipate fears, time to assimilate frightening facts, time to prepare for crises, time to enter the experiential world of another person. The urge to hurry must be overcome if people are really serious about preserving the human community.

Significance for Treatment

The factors that complicate the process of sharing meanings are nearly all present in doctor-patient encounters. And most are found here in their most extreme and destructive form. It is here that emotionally disturbing matters, sometimes of life and death, are discussed. It is here that the immense authority and power of one communicant faces the ignorance and impotence of the other. It is here that the need for rapport is largest, yet the emotional distance is likely to be greatest. It is here, too, that critical choice must be made with information which is clothed in an esoteric jargon that obscures and mystifies. And it is here that words are uttered rapidly, even unintelligibly, with little time to clarify or assimilate their meaning. Some of these obstacles to understanding are inherent in illness itself; some derive from the historical roles of physician and patient; others result from the personal communicative style of the physician or are a matter of cultivation by the medical profession.

Yet if people are really serious about improving medical communication, they must resist the appeal of conspiratorial approaches. It is always easier to take sides than to understand—to align ourselves simplistically with child against parent, worker against management, student against teacher, patient against physician. The temptation to search for demons is an addiction the human race has not overcome even in this sophisticated age. The number of villains in the world is probably overestimated, and they are by no means the exclusive property of the medical profession.

Human acts nearly always make sense. They arise from some compromise between private impulse and social expectation. If human behavior is to change, it may be less because we substitute virtue for vice than because we deepen the awareness of people to the total context from which they derive their meanings and motives. The communicative manner of medical specialists may spring less from any malevolent effort to claim omniscience and prestige than from an accident of the role in which medical professionals have cast themselves and been cast by society and from the process by which people are selected and prepared to assume medical responsibilities.

The doctor, as well as the patient, must cope with anxieties surrounding treatment. The doctor may be aware of the seriousness of the case and may know the real limitations of medical knowledge and skill. He may be sensitive to past errors and the possibility of committing further mistakes. There is the danger of making the wrong choice among alternative treatments. There is risk of patient criticism and peer disapproval. If medical personnel sometimes emphasize their authority and status, assert opinions as if they were unassailable, manipulate patients, maintain emotional distance, and discourage patient collaboration, are these not some of the same tactics most people use when threatened and unaware of viable alternatives? Mystification may seem the only constructive way of protecting the patient from undue anxiety in view of the limited assistance that medicine and surgery can provide. It may be used in the hope that mystique can accomplish what science cannot. Mystification permits physicians as well as patients some escape from anxiety, embarrassment, and frustration. This does not justify it, but it may identify its source in the human psyche.

Medical Education

Consider acculturation into the medical profession. How much of this process is designed to promote respect for or insight into human personality? There appears to be minimal effort to assess candidates on their capacity to sustain extensive or intensive human relationships. Yet no profession has daily contact with so wide a spectrum of subcultures, and none exerts influence over such sensitive matters. How many courses are concerned with exploring the ways illness threatens the symbolic as well as physical self? How many class periods focus upon the communicative strategies patients use to cope with imminent threats to their survival? How much time is spent exploring the physician's own communicative style, the assumptions on which it rests, the impulses it reflects, the consequences for those he or she treats?

Throughout training the future physician is preoccupied with the physical properties of the body. Medical training is concerned with anatomy, chemical processes, manifestations of dysfunction, and the consequences of medical and surgical techniques. A vast array of instruments and technologies must be mastered. Is it surprising if later when faced with patients the physician should prefer to deal with physical their rather than psychic symptoms? Will medical specialists not be likely to feel more comfortable and competent handling X-rays, blood samples, printouts, and pathology reports than coping with frightened and distraught personalities? In some offices one gets the impression the physician would prefer never to meet or know the person being treated. If only somehow one could avoid dealing with the human being at all. It is understandable that few patients can effect so neat a surgery between illness and self.

A person's communicative manner derives from his view of human beings. Values are not elusive abstractions; they are manifest in every word. It is difficult to respect the integrity of others and the validity of their experience and at the same time manipulate them—as difficult as it is to see others as mindless children and still collaborate with them as equals. But commitment to humane values is rarely enough, any more than the simple desire to relieve suffering automatically confers diagnostic or surgical talent. Skill must be acquired to translate respect for patients as persons into capacity to engage them communicatively as equals. Communicative skills must be cultivated that respect patients' intelligence, acknowledge their needs, accept their feelings, value their opinions, and promote collaboration in decision-making. To achieve this sort of mature relationship demands some recognition of what often occurs under the guise of medical communication and of alternatives for building more effective encounters between physicians and patients.

Research

When one turns to ask what is currently known about communication between medical personnel and patients, the answer is itself mystifying. A phrase will suffice—very little. Here is a profession founded on science, dedicated to truth, committed to inquiry, concerned with the relief of suffering, yet either oblivious to or unwilling to examine its own communicative behavior. Is this simply a mote in an otherwise scientific eve? Or is it a defensive assertion of the medical mystique and the preference to do as one pleases?

If the suffering caused by communicative negligence were a result of some physical disorder, the response would be predictable: organize medical research, underwrite exploratory studies, encourage testing of alternative treatments, and counter the disorder. But when the suffering is a consequence of symbolic disorder—when it arises from the failure to listen, the failure to comprehend, the failure to respect and collaborate—even when such failures result, as they sometimes do, in suffering or death, should there not be an equally vigorous effort to remedy it? It is unfortunate that we have no clear idea of the precise extent of injury to the human personality—or for that matter to the body itself—by the unsought diagnosis, the unasked question, the unreported symptom, the uncomprehended explanation, the disregarded treatment, the incorrectly followed medication. We have only the horror stories so many tell, offset by occasional reports of sensitive and empathic collaboration. While we have some conception of the suffering imposed by broken bones and diseased tissue, we have only the vaguest notion of the damage done through communicative negligence.

This is an area of medicine where the questions far outrun the answers. And the reason there are so few answers is that so few within the field of medicine have raised questions about medical communication. Nearly everyone inside and outside the medical profession affirms that communication with patients deserves study, but few institutions have offered to support such research. To know little about something as complex as interactions between physicians and patients is nothing to apologize for. But to know little and to choose to remain ignorant about it is tragic for the patient and demeaning for the profession.

What are some of the questions that press for answers? We need to know more of the various types of patients and the manner in which they present their condition. There is no reason to assume that high and low income groups, females and males, blacks and whites, educated and uneducated respond in the same way to illness. To claim to respect all patients is nonsense unless medical personnel are willing to meet them on their own communicative terms. There is little reason, also, to assume that all types of illness and injury provoke similar reactions and similar questions or demand similar kinds of involvement. What is a helpful remark in one context may be frightening in another. If patients' reactions bear little resemblance to what seems appropriate, physicians must remember that it is patient's perceptions, not their own, that are the focus of treatment.

We need to know what types of communicative defenses are triggered by illness. It has been suggested that patients tend to be "copers" or "deniers," with the former seeking information in order to assimilate it and the latter avoiding information to keep from being overwhelmed by it. There may be many more ways of handling threatening news than this simple dichotomy suggests. There are, finally, a lot of questions concerning the dominant style of the physician. Should it be primarily investigative, informative, supportive, persuasive, collaborative, or therapeutic? At what point and with which patients might each of these contribute to recovery and self-esteem?

Some indication of the kind of investigative work that is possible and its potential is found in a simple exploratory study undertaken in 1970 by Thomas Lonner for a master's thesis at San Francisco State University. It focused on the preoperative and postoperative contacts between one physician and several patients undergoing surgery. The findings are suggestive rather than definitive. But they illustrate the possibilities of such studies.

What the investigator found was this: the physician was genuinely interested in his patients, earnestly tried to provide the care they needed, and attempted to be as clear and informative as possible. His motives were impeccable and his approach was constructive. But it was also clear, in spite of this, that he had only one approach to all patients; that he failed to recognize differences in their reactions to stress; that he was unable to predict their postoperative responses; that he made little effort to confer with them; that he did not adapt verbally, often using words that had no meaning for them; and that when he failed, he sought no explanation for his failure nor did he consider varying his behavior to adapt to this failure. Yet to unsophisticated observers, including some of his patients, he appeared to be an adequate example of the doctor communicating with his patient.

Medical educators, it would appear, must recognize the symbolic and semantic aspects of illness and injury. They must recognize, as well, that all treatment involves a communicative relationship with patients. It is important not only that more intensive efforts be made to investigate this critical relationship between persons seeking treatment and those providing it but also that part of medical training should be developing sensitivity and flexibility in human interaction.

If, as was once written, it is more important to know what manner of man has the disease than to know what disease he has, one might add that to know the manner of man is impossible without appreciating the way he symbolizes his situation. This is a communicative problem of no small dimensions but one for which the medical profession cannot escape some responsibility. It is meanings, not merely physical symptoms, that prompt people to seek or avoid examination, that cause them to withhold or describe their condition, that intensify or minimize their physical discomfort, that prompt them to report or distort reactions to treatment, that lead them to obey or contradict medical advice, that determine ultimately whether they assist or sabotage efforts to cure them. The entire process, from the onset of illness to recovery or death, is invested with symbolism, with meanings that are unique, to every person and to every physical condition. And these meanings, in turn, complicate the conditions that are the focus of treatment. If medical personnel are concerned with the relief of suffering, they can no longer disregard their communicative style with patients. Suffering and the relief of suffering are influenced by symbolic as well as physical acts. Medical personnel are inescapably involved in influencing meanings in some of the most traumatic moments of human existence. Mystification would appear to be a questionable substitute for communicative sensitivity.

Intangibles in Medicine: An Attempt at a Balancing Perspective

Norman Cousins

Understandably, reaction has set in against efforts to emphasize the importance of psychological factors in the treatment of patients. Medical periodicals have carried articles and letters from physicians who feel they are being pushed by imponderables in the wrong direction. The following letter is a composite of reactions:

> *I am not interested in charming or entertaining my patients or running popularity contests. I want to give them the benefit of my special knowledge and ability. If I myself were seriously ill, I would have no difficulty in expressing my preference for a physician who is capable of making an absolutely correct diagnosis and who would know exactly what has to be done—rather than choose a physician who is adept at sweet talk, or in making friends and influencing people, or in gaining recognition as one hell of a fine fellow.*

This letter and dozens like it are the understandable response to the flurry of recent books, articles, and statements emphasizing the importance of psychological factors in the management of disease. Physicians are concerned, and rightly so, that some people may regard positive emotions as a substitute for essential medical attention.

It becomes necessary, therefore, to create a balanced perspective, one that recognizes that attitudes such as a strong will to live, high purpose, a capacity for festivity, and a reasonable degree of confidence are not an alternative to competent medical attention but a way of enhancing the environment of treatment. The wise physician favors a spirit of responsible participation by the patients in a total strategy of medical care. It is a truism that compliance is strengthened in an atmosphere of patient understanding and involvement.

Most of all, the wise physician understands that there is no contradiction between compassion and competence; between the arts of reassurance where reassurance is possible and cautionary notes where required; between personal observation and technological data; in short, between respect for the intangibles of medical care and respect for scientific quantification.

Results of Current Research

In this light, it may be useful to review recent research bearing on the connection between emotional and physiological factors. The University of California at Los Angeles School of Medicine recently sponsored a world conference at Lake Arrowhead, Calif., for the purpose of reviewing new research on the interactions of the brain, the endocrine system, and the immune system. Investigators in the field of psychosomatic medi-

---

Cousins, N. Intangibles in medicine: An attempt at a balancing perspective. *Journal of the American Medical Association* 260, (11), pp. 1610-1612.

cine have developed substantial evidence on the physiological effects of emotional factors but it is only in recent years that specific pathways and mechanisms have come into view.

Not that the probes in this field are entirely contemporary. More than half a century ago, Cannon[1] reported his observation that the emotions could stimulate the spleen, resulting in an increase of from 10% to 15% in the population of red blood cells. At that time, knowledge of the immune system was far less developed than it is today. The fact of splenic stimulation of the immune system carries Cannon's observations into the contemporary arena. At the Lake Arrowhead conference, several researchers detailed the role of the spleen in activating or potentiating immune function.

Ever since Galen made his observations about melancholy as a contributory cause of breast cancer, medical researchers over the years have called attention to such possibilities. Research in progress at the University of California at Los Angeles indicates that a decline in depression among cancer patients leads to increases in specific measures of immune function.

Any review of new advances in the understanding of the interactions of the nervous system, the endocrine system, an the immune system must also take into account the work of Ader et al.[2] in demonstrating that immune response can be central nervous system conditioned; or the work of Besedovsky et al.,[3] of Schweizerisches Forschungsinstitut in Davos-Platz, Switzerland, discovering complementary function of the endocrine and immune systems as demonstrated by disturbances in one arena producing changes in the other, or the work of Blalock,[4] of the University of Alabama, Birmingham, finding hormonal receptors on leukocytes and observing that immune cells are capable of producing hormonelike substances; or the work of Bulloch et al.[5] of the University of California, San Diego, and Felten et al.[6] of the University of Rochester (NY), documenting the innervation of immune organs by the nervous system; or the work of Kiecolt-Glaser and Glaser[7] of Ohio State University, Columbus, correlating varying types of stress with compromises in specific measures of immune function both within and across individuals; or the work of Pert et al.,[8] of the National Institute of Mental Health, Bethesda, Md, exploring the role and implications of neuropeptides and their receptors functioning as a communication link between the brain, glands, and immune system; or the work of Stein et al.,[9] of the Mount Sinai School of Medicine, New York, stepwise progression of studies that depression is associated with unfavorable changes in the immune system.

Out of current research, there is now emerging a picture of the way emotions, experiences, and

---

1 Cannon W: *Bodily Changes in Pain, Hunger, Fear and Rage.* New York, Harper & Row Publishers Inc., 1963.

2 Ader R, Grota LJ, Cohen N: Conditioning phenomena and immune function. *Ann NY Acad Sci* 1987;496:532-544.

3 Besedovsky HO, del Rey A, Sorkin E, et al: Immunoregulatory feedback between interleukin-1 and glucocorticoid hormones. *Science* 1986;233:652-644.

4 Blalock JE:A molecular basis for bidirectional communication between the immune and neuroendocrine systems. *Physiol Rev*, in press.

5 Bulloch K, Cullen MR, Schwarz RH, et al: Development of innervation within syngeneic thymus tissue transplanted under the kidney capsule of the nude mouse: A light and ultrastructural microscope study. *J Neurosci Res* 1987;18:16-27.

6 Felten DL, Felten SY, Bellinger DL, et al: Noradrenergic sympathetic neural interactions with the immune system: Structure and function. *Immunol Rev* 1987; 100:225-260.

7 Kiecolt-Glaser JK, Glaser R: Psychosocial moderators of immune function. *J Behav Med* 1987;9:16-20.

8 Pert CB, Ruff MR, Weber RJ, et al: Neuropeptides and their receptors: A psychosomatic network. *J Immunol* 1985;135:820-826.

9 Stein M, Keller SE, Schleifer SJ: Stress and immunomodulation: The role of depression and neuroendocrine function. *J Immunol* 1985;135:827-833.

attitudes can create physiological change. For example, the role of emotional tension in producing elevated cholesterol levels has come under scrutiny, embellished by well-known reports of accountants experiencing high cholesterol levels with approaching income tax deadlines or of medical students going into national examinations. More than a generation ago, however, Wolf et al.[10] documented the connection between emotional tensions and serum lipid levels. Similar observations were made by Thomas and Murphy[11] and by Grundy and Griffin.[12] In 1958, Friedman and colleagues[13] reported evidence that "lipid regulating mechanisms are responsive to situational stress."

Half a century ago, Cannon[14] demonstrated that sudden fright could produce a wide range of physiological effects, including constricted blood vessels, nervous vagal disturbances, catecholamine surges capable of rupturing muscle fibers in the heart, and blood pressure abnormalities. McClelland,[15] formerly of Harvard University, Cambridge, Mass, has been making correlations between human motivation and high blood pressure. He has also carried out interesting studies in immunoglobulin A secretions in saliva under varying emotional circumstances. Similar studies have been carried out at Western New England College, Springfield, Mass, by Dillon et al.[16] Levy,[17] at the University of Pittsburgh, has written about possible connections between lifestyle factors and cancer.

The fact that emotional distress could increase susceptibility to virus-related diseases, as well as facilitate tumor development and inhibit immune function, has been established by various studies.[18] Similarly, a series of other studies has shown that ability to control certain kinds of stress could confer physiological benefits. In a classic study, Sklar and Anisman[19] found that the ability to control shock could mitigate tumor growth, whereas uncontrollable shock did not. Visintainer et al.[20] confirmed this finding using a viral dosage half as likely to induce tumor growth. This phenomenon suggests that coping mechanisms play a vital role in buffering the adverse effects of stress. Laudenslager et al.[21] found that inescapable shock decreased immune response, an effect not produced by identical but escapable shock. The immune response was measured following five brief inescapable shocks administered 24 hours *after* the initial 80-shock session (one shock per minute). Because the repeated shock session only negatively affected the

---

10 Wolf S, McCabe WR, Yamamoto J, et al: Changes in serum lipids in relation to emotional stress during rigid control of diet and exercise. *Circulation* 1962;26:379-387.

11 Thomas CB, Murphy EA: Further studies on cholesterol levels in the Johns Hopkins medical students: Effect of stress at examinations. *J Chronic Dis* 1958:8:661.

12 Grundy SM, Griffin AC: Effect of periodic mental stress on serum cholesterol levels. *Circulation* 1958;17:862.

13 Friedman M, Rosenman RH, Carroll V: Changes in the serum cholesterol and blood clotting time in men subjected to cyclic variation of occupational stress. *Circulation* 1958;17:862.

14 Cannon W: *Bodily Changes in Pain, Hunger, Fear and Rage*. New York, Harper & Row Publishers Inc., 1963.

15 McClelland D: Inhibited power motivation and blood pressure in man. *J Abnorm Psychol* 1979;88:182-190.

16 Dillon K, Baker K, Minchoff 8: Positive emotional states and enhancement of the immune system. *Int J Psychiatry Med* 1985;15:13-18.

17 Levy S: Host differences in neoplastic risk: Behavioral and social contributors to disease. *Health Psych* 1983;2:21-44.

18 Riley V, Fitzmaurice MA, Spackman DH: Psychoneuroimmunologic factors in neoplasia: Studies in animals, in Ader R (ed): *Psychoneuroimmunology*. Orlando, Fla, Academic Press Inc, 1981, pp 31-102.

19 Sklar LS, Anisman H: Stress and coping factors influence tumor growth. *Science* 1979;205:513-515.

20 Visintainer MA, Volpicelli JR, Seligman MEP: Tumor rejection in rats after inescapable or escapable shock. *Science* 1982;216:437-439.

21 Laudenslager ML, Ryan SM, Drugan RC, et al: Coping and immunosuppression: Inescapable but not escapable shock suppresses lymphocyte proliferation. *Science* 1983;221:568-570.

inescapable shock group, the researchers concluded that the ability to view stress as a challenge prevented cellular immunosuppression and, conversely, that the immune system was compromised by "learned helplessness." These results were repeated in another study[22] that measured different immunological variables, thus strengthening the view that the immune system can be governed by complex psychological bars.

With respect to pathways and biochemistry involved in interactions between the nervous system and immune system, evidence is now at hand that nerve-cell endings, not associated with blood vessels and peptide neurotransmitters, are found in the thymus and spleen of animals.[23, 24] Other studies have suggested that peptide neurotransmitters are directly capable of modulating immune function. Likewise, any immunomodulatory peptides yield striking central nervous system effects.[25]

Drug and surgical procedures that affect the brain (central nervous system) have been shown to have direct immunological consequences.[26, 27, 28] The research of Pert et al.[29] shows that brain membranes and immune cells share similar receptorantigens. In pursuit of the application of these findings to the pathology of acquired immunodeficiency syndrome, they have identified an octapeptide that obstructs the human immunodeficiency virus from infecting T lymphocytes and attaching to brain membranes.

Ader and Cohen[30] found that the administration of saccharin alone (after it had been associated with cyclophosphamide, which decreases immune function) could elicit a conditioned reduction in immune response. They raise the following questions as a result of such findings: "What shaping influences do the early emotional experiences of an individual have on his or her immune system and how do they influence later susceptibility to disease? Are differences in how individuals respond to drugs a reflection of immune responses subtly conditioned over a lifetime?"[31]

Hormonal receptors have been found on immune cells. Also, immune cells have been shown to be capable of producing hormonelike substances.[32, 33] These findings plus the discoveries

---

22 Shavit Y, Ryan SM, Lewis JW, et al: Inescapable but not escapable stress alters immune function. *Physiologist* 1983;26:64.

23 Felten DL, Felten SY, Carlson S, et aL: Noradrenergic and peptidergic innervation of lymphoid tissue. *J Immunol* 1985;135:755-765.

24 Bulloch K, Moore RY: Innervation at the thymus gland by brainstem and spinal cord in mouse and rat. *Am J Anat* 1981; 162:157-166.

25 Morley J E, Kay NE, Solomon GF, et al: Neuropeptides: Conductors of the immune orchestra. *Life Sci* 1987;41:527-544.

26 Korneva EA, Khai LM: Effect of stimulating different mesencephalic structures on protective immune response patterns. *Fiziol Zh SSSR* 1967;53:42-47.

27 Jankovic BD, Isakovic K: Neuroendocrine correlates of immune responses: 1. Effects of brain lesions on antibody production, arthus reactivity and delayed hypersensitivity in the rat. *Int Arch Allergy Appl Immunol* 1973;45:372.

28 Keller SE, Stein M, Camerino MS, et aL: Suppression of lymph stimulation by anterior hypothalamic lesions in the guinea pig. *Cell Immunol* 1980;52:334-340.

29 Pert CB, Hill JM, Ruff MR, et al: Octapeptides deduced from the neuropeptide receptor-like pattern of antigen T-4 in brain potently inhibit human immunodeficiency virus receptor binding on T-cell infectivity. *Proc Natl Acad Sci USA* 1986;83.9254-9258

30 Ader R, Cohen N: Conditioned immunopharmacologic responses, In Ader R (ed): *Psychoneuroimmunology.* Orlando, Fla, Academic Press Inc 1981, pp 281-319.

31 Ader R, Cohen N: Conditioned immunopharmacologic responses in Ader R (ed): *Psychoneuroimmunology.* Orlando, Fla, Academic Press Inc, 1981. pp 281-319.

32 Hazum E, Chang KJ, Cuatrecasas P: Specific nonopiate receptors for betaendorphin. *Science* 1979;205:1033-1035.

33 Smith EM, Brosnan P, Meyer MJ, et al: An ACTH receptor on human mononuclear leukocytes. *N Engl J Med* 1987;317:1266-1269.

of complementary and even facilitory functions of the neuroendocrine and immune systems[34, 35] have led pioneer immunologist J. Edwin Blalock[36] to believe that the immune system, far from being autonomous, serves a sensory function and that the central nervous system and immune system convey similar information to each other through hormone signals. A wide array of neuroendocrines—growth hormones, thyroid hormones, sex hormones, insulin, histamine, and catecholamines, for example—are known to influence immune activity.[37]

In a series of short- and long-term studies on academic stress and immunity in medical students, immunologist Ronald Glaser and psychologist Janice Kiecolt-Glaser found emotional factors such as distress and loneliness to be related to reduced levels of gamma interferon, diminished numbers and responsiveness of NK cells and T lymphocytes, and increased antibody titers to latent viruses.[38, 39, 40, 41]

Patient-Physician Interaction

The implications of much of this work on medical practice are now coming into view and give emphasis to the ideas of medical thinkers and teachers such as O. W. Holmes, Sir William Osler, and Claude Bernard, who believed that the style of the physician can have a bearing on the outcome of a case. William Henry Welch was convinced that the moment his father, a country doctor, "entered a sick room, the patient felt better." Similarly, Rene Dubos believed that "there is a miraculous moment when the very presence of the doctor is the most effective part of the treatment." Such views have long since been accepted as conventional wisdom, but are now being confirmed by laboratory findings.

More specifically, perhaps, the physician's communication skills need no longer be regarded as theoretical assets. Being able to keep a patient free of panic after a serious diagnosis may enhance the environment of effective treatment and compliance. For the physician, such at least would appear to be one of the prime values of the new scientific data concerning the role of intangibles in affecting the management of human disease.

To be sure, not all the new research in mind-body connections is without flaws. Much additional research is needed. But there has been enough replication of research involving controlled studies to point to a presiding fact; namely, the physician has a prime resource at his disposal in the form of the patient's own apothecary, especially when combined with the prescription pad.

Obviously, intangibles and imponderables must not be allowed to distort the scientific treat-

---

34 Besedovsky HD, del Rey A. Neuroendocrine and metabolic responses induced by interleukin-1. *J Neurosci Res* 1987;18:172-178.

35 Smith EM, Meyer WJ, Blalock JE: Virus-induced corticosterone in hypophysectomized mice: A possible lymphoid adrenal axis. *Science* 1982;218:1311-1312.

36 Blalock JE: The immune system as a sensory organ. *J Immunol* 1983;132:1067-1070.

37 McLean D, Reichlin S: Neuroendocrinology and the immune process, in Ader R (ed): *Psychoneuroimmunology*. Orlando, Fla, Academic Press Inc, 1981, pp 475-520.

38 Kiecolt-Glaser JK, Garner W, Speicher C, et al: Psychosocial modifiers of immunocompetence medical students. *Psychosom Med* 1984;46:7-14.

39 Glaser R, Kiecolt-Glaser JK, Stout JC, et aL: Stress-related impairments in cellular immunity. *Psychiatry Res* 1985;16:233-239.

40 Glaser R, Kiecolt-Glaser JK. Speicher CE, et al: Stress, loneliness, and changes in herpes virus latency. *J Behav Med* 1985;8:249-260.

41 Glaser R, Rice J, Sheridan J, et al. Stress-related immune suppression: Health implications. *Brain Behav Immunity* 1987; 1:7-20.

ment of patients. It would be as much an error to suppose that intangibles dominate human health and disease as it is to suppose that they are altogether absent. The essential issue is whether it is possible to strike a sensible balance between psychological factors and biologic factors in the understanding and management of disease. How to keep the medical profession from being overwhelmed or undermined by mystical or metaphysical notions while at the same time maintaining a necessary respect for the impact of the emotions on illness and health? Nothing is more futile than to debate the relative importance of knowledge vs technique.

Recent studies provide important impetus for essential research even as they promote respect for the physician's awareness, to paraphrase Sir William Osler, that it may be at least as important to know what goes on in the mind of the patient as what is happening inside his body.

What Makes the Patient-Doctor Relationship Therapeutic? Exploring the Connexional Dimension of Medical Care

Anthony L. Suchman and Dale A. Matthews

Physicians do not receive from the medical model the same explicit guidance in relating to their patients as in making diagnoses and prescribing pharmacologic and other treatments. To meet this need, we offer a framework for expanding the model. Therapeutic contact takes place within a connexional, or transpersonal, dimension of human experience, within which basic human needs for connection and meaning are met. Although seldom explicitly recognized, connexional experience is basic to medical care. Awareness of this dimension of experience leads clinicians to appreciate that establishing a therapeutic relationship is one of the principal goals of medical practice. It also reframes the doctor's task to make clinical uncertainty more tolerable and situations in which there is no appropriate biomedical response (such as care of the terminally ill) less frustrating and more fulfilling.

Returning to my office from a meeting across town, I found my desk covered with messages: "Joyce wants to see you as soon as you get back"; "Call Joyce's husband ASAP—wants to know why she needs blood"; and, "Joyce called again—don't forget to see her." (The patient's name has been changed.)

Joyce is a 38-year-old woman, a midlevel executive in a local firm, and a mother of two. She was in the hospital convalescing from a second attack of binary colic and waiting to have both a cholecystectomy and a staging laparotomy the following morning. At the time of her first episode of biliary colic 2 months earlier, a large mediastinal mass was discovered on her chest film. An extensive biopsy through the supraclavicular fossa was non-diagnostic and quite painful. Two weeks later, she had a thoracotomy for excisional biopsy of the grapefruit-sized mass, which proved to be Hodgkin disease.

"Why do I need a transfusion?" she demanded when I entered her room. "With my luck, I'll get hepatitis."

I had checked Joyce's chart before seeing her to make sure nothing new had developed since morning rounds. I told her that the surgical team had ordered a type and cross-match, not a transfusion.

"Well, a person came around to draw more blood this afternoon. I asked why they needed more when they already took several tubes this morning. She told me that it was for a blood transfusion, and I started to get the feeling that nobody was telling me what's going on around here." Joyce pursed her lips; her arms were folded tightly across her chest.

Putting together the frantic phone messages, the worry about hepatitis, the frustration and anxiety of her protracted diagnostic evaluation

Suchman A.L., Matthews D.A.: What Makes the Patient-Doctor Relationship Therapeutic? Exploring the Connexional Dimension of Medical Care. Annals of Internal Medicine 1988, 108, pp. 125-130.

and her present body language, I realized how much more frightened she was than she wished to show, or know. "This has been a hard day for you, hasn't it?"

Her shoulders sagged. She lowered her head for a moment and then looked up at me, her eyes filling with tears. All at once, I could feel her fears of a painful postoperative recovery, of her children without a mother, and of losing her ability to work. But even more than that, I sensed her dismay. She had been trying so hard to remain in control and to hide these fears from herself and from her husband, who was on the threshold of panic. Now, suddenly realizing how desperate and exaggerated her response to this unexpected phlebotomy had been, she recognized the underlying panic of her own that it belied.

Then, in the next moment, I recognized that she knew I was feeling her worry and dismay and that it was reassuring to her, as if my feeling it meant that she wasn't crazy I felt my own eyes well up, and I had a slight chilly feeling with gooseflesh on my neck. It was a vivid, almost uncanny moment.

"There are no heroes here," I said, taking her hand, "just people."

Most clinicians, when invited to do so, have no trouble recalling special moments of closeness and intimacy with patients (1, 2). Although such moments may seem to be chance occurrences that are pleasant but sporadic by-products of clinical activity, they are perceived nevertheless as being both therapeutic and personally valuable. indeed, given their intensity and their widespread occurrence, they bear closer inspection.

Far from being happenstance, these moments may instruct us about a dimension of human experience that is basic to medical care yet seldom recognized or explicitly discussed: the connexional dimension (3-6). Possessed with rich, intuitive understanding of this dimension, a few gifted clinicians can make themselves therapeutic consistently. But most physicians, who are well intentioned but lack explicit guidance, move through this dimension all but blinded to its existence by a medical model that specifically directs their attention away from subjective experience. Therapeutic encounters thus seem to occur haphazardly. Many opportunities to heal are lost, and much unnecessary and unintended suffering is inflicted (3, 7).

The purpose of our article is to render connexional experience more visible to clinicians and to encourage the systematic exploration of its role in medical care. Such inquiry will result in a more complete medical model that will better guide our practice and teaching, helping us to relate to our patients more skillfully and effectively, even as we strive to provide ever-improving technical care.

Throughout this article, we will use the words "connexional," "transpersonal," and "spiritual" interchangeably. Embedded in the word "connexional" are the roots "co" (together) and "nexus" (a binding together of parts to form a whole) (8). We use this word to indicate a mutual experience of joining that results in a sensation of wholeness. "Transpersonal" suggests going beyond the boundaries of one's "self" to join with an "other," whereas "spiritual" pertains to the vital, animating, and universal source of one's being. Just as each of the fabled blind men captured the essence of one aspect of an elephant, so each word reflects an aspect of something that is, at least in our language, difficult to express. The more blind men, then, the better.

We will begin with a description of connexional experience and its historical relationship to medicine. We will then examine the experiences of both patients and doctors from a transpersonal perspective. Finally, we will consider the ways in which such a perspective might change the practice of medicine and offer solutions to situations that we currently find problematic.

Connexional Experiences Described

There exists within each of us a sense of isolation, which seems to be an unavoidable consequence of learning to distinguish "self" from "other" (9, 10). Out of this uncomfortable separateness arises a drive to reach beyond the boundaries of the self, to feel connected once again to other people and to the world. We refer to this sense of belonging in the world as "meaning." The need for connection and meaning often goes unrecognized within modern Western culture, yet it remains a need of every person nonetheless. It is through connexional experience that these needs are satisfied.

A group of clinicians recently attempted to characterize their connexional experiences with patients (See Acknowledgments). Such moments, as shown in the opening vignette, may be distinguished by a particularly intense awareness of another's feelings, of mutual closeness, which is accompanied often by a peculiar physical sensation, such as a chill, gooseflesh, or flushing (11). This moment may be followed by a lingering feeling of love, a sense of privilege at having been allowed into the patient's life so vividly, and a humble feeling that one is part of something bigger than oneself. Such experiences may feel somehow universal and enlarging. The patient, too, may be moved and awed by the feeling of being so profoundly understood, no longer all alone in his or her suffering. Both patient; and doctor feel a moment of peace and joy, while they also share the sadness of the suffering that brought them together in the first place.

Outside of medicine, transpersonal experiences again are characterized by a sensation of unusual connectedness to someone or something, of losing oneself in something else: another person, a group of people, a piece of music, an object, a phenomenon of nature, an activity. More than an ordinary feeling of liking or personal attachment, this feeling of connectedness is suffused with an awareness of deep harmony and resonance. It may be a feeling of deeply understanding or being understood by another person, as described previously. Or the sensation may occur during physical activity, as when one "feels" the path a basketball will take through the hoop even as the ball is being released, or in music, as when one "feels" a sonata flowing through one's fingers at the keyboard of a piano. For many people, the primary path to this type of experience is through religious ritual.

Common to all these experiences is a receding of our sense of distinct individuality and personal control as we find ourselves in continuity with an existence that is much larger than we are; foreground and background merge. We may feel our usual boundaries momentarily become porous, allowing us to include within our own awareness elements that ordinarily seem to be outside ourselves. Without explanatory models or rituals to call attention to connexional experiences and to help us integrate them with the rest of our lives, they may pass all but unnoticed, or worse, they may be experienced as distressing, embarrassing, or anomalous. However, when they are recognized and appreciated, these experiences are sources of inspiration, joy, and wonder.

In referring to such experiences as transpersonal, we distinguish them from both interpersonal and intrapersonal experiences. Events at the interpersonal level comprise interactions between two separate persons and depend on that separateness to occur. They are concerned with coexisting (either cooperatively or competitively), but not with joining or connecting. Intrapersonal events take place within private consciousness, the individual space of one person's mind. Although they may involve internalized symbolic representations of objects (human or otherwise), they do not involve direct connection with the object, opening of one's boundaries, or enlargement of one's awareness. Sensory experiences, memories, emotions, and personality are examples of intrapersonal phenomena.

Given a universal need for connection and meaning, we can identify a particular form of suffering that ensues when this need is not met: a sense of inner void, an absence of joy, or a vague feeling that something is missing in one's life. We can recognize this particular type of suffering at the heart of such current societal phenomena as alcoholism, drug dependence, religious cults, and even the aggressive, acquisitive materialism associated with "yuppies."

Having described connexional experience, we now see that it is a familiar part of our lives, if not previously recognized or labeled as such. Yet, it certainly is not identified as an essential part of ordinary medical practice. This was not always the case.

Connexional Experience and the History of Medicine

Medicine arose out of the magic and ritual of religious healing. The interpretation of illness and the response to suffering were originally religious matters. Throughout antiquity, cures were sought through direct appeal to a god (for example, Apollo) or through divinely inspired healers (for example, followers of Askelepios). At the advent of Christianity, with its emphasis on the healing miracles of Jesus Christ, healing of the body was one with healing of the mind and spirit. The first hospitals were established in the monasteries of the Middle Ages as havens for the physical as well as spiritual healing of supplicants. The missionary movement, when it began during the 15th and 16th centuries, and to this day, has included as one of its core tasks the care of the sick.

By the time of the Renaissance, however, with Descartes' assertion of the duality of mind and body, the separation of medicine from religion was well underway. From the initial anatomic studies of Vesalius, through the dawning of germ theory, and up to the present, the progress of empirical science has been spectacular, but not without a price. This science, which was concerned with the bodily half of Descartes' dualism, admitted only verifiable perceptions of the five senses as valid data, effectively barring transpersonal phenomena from the consideration of scientific clinicians. The spiritual dimension of illness could not be banished, however, from the experience of the sick. Exclusive attention to healing of the body could not meet the needs for healing of the mind or spirit. The conflict between scientific and holistic paradigms thus arose.

This conflict still continues. But neither a purely biological nor a purely spiritual approach can be complete in itself. Tillich expressed this in his description of particular healing, in which only one dimension of experience receives attention (as compared with complete healing, in which all the dimensions of experience are addressed) (12).

> Human finitude makes particular healing necessary ... but it has the tendency to provoke diseases in another realm ... successful surgery may produce a psychological trauma; effective drugs may calm down an uneasy conscience, and preserve a moral deficiency; the well trained athletic body may contain a neurotic personality; the healed patient of the analyst may be sick through a lack of ultimate meaning in his life; the conformist's average life may be sick through inhibited self-alteration, the converted Christian may suffer under repressions which produce fanaticism and may explode in lawless forms.

Yet, the spiritual dimension remains neglected by contemporary Western medicine because of its subjective nature. It is perceived as involving "magic, wishful thinking . . . and the abandonment of rational scientific practice" (13).

Wilber refutes this perception, pointing out that the disciplined acquisition of knowledge consists of the same processes—careful description (or replication) of methods, observation, and consensual validation—whether one is exploring spiritual phenomena or natural and physical science (14). The difference lies only in the tools. Biochemists follow meticulously described laboratory procedures, make observations using standardized instruments and compare their results with those of their peers through presentations in print and at scientific meetings. In a similar manner, students of Zen follow prescribed methods of meditation and compare their perceptions with those of others or with a master. In each instance, a common body of knowledge scientifically accretes from the experience of individuals through the process of careful consensual validation.

The notion that only those aspects of awareness arising from the five senses are fit for scientific inquiry is arbitrary and constraining. It forces us to maintain boundaries between body and mind, and it leaves us without a scientific understanding of large portions of our experience, with ill consequences, particularly for medicine (3, 14).

If incorporation of knowledge about connexional experience into the basic paradigm of medicine is to improve patient-doctor relationships, it should provide new insights and lead us to new attitudes and actions. To ascertain the changes that an enlarged medical model might bring, we will now examine the experiences of both patients and doctors.

Patients' Needs for Connection and Meaning

We know that when a patient seeks the care of a doctor, it is not only for the rectification of a disordered biological process (15). The biopsychosocial model reminds us to consider the illness within the context of the whole of the patient's life—family, work, community, and culture—and to respond to disruptions at each of these levels (16). In recognizing the transpersonal dimension of experience, we can now see that the "brokenness" of illness involves threats to connection and meaning, too (17).

Illness may threaten a patient's sense of connection to others and the world (18). It can interfere with his security, challenge his sense of control over his destiny, and produce feelings of alienation from himself, his family, his community, and his God (5, 19). Pain, loss of function, and other types of distress disrupt ordinary means of making contact, thus intensifying the isolation of everyday existence. Usual coping responses may be weakened or overwhelmed, and the patient may be left hopeless, powerless, and demoralized.

A feeling of connectedness with the doctor, of being deeply heard and understood, reduces this feeling of isolation and eases despair. This feeling is the very heart of healing. Wholly independent of whatever biotechnical treatment is offered, this deep, transpersonal connectedness between the patient and doctor ("emphatic witnessing," as Kleinman has called it [20]) is comforting and therapeutic. Patients know this. Heading the list of the physician attributes they value most are the demonstration of personal concern and willingness to listen (21). Caring acknowledgment of patients' suffering legitimizes their experiences and gives them a feeling of personal integrity, wholeness, and value.

Joyce's suffering was exacerbated by her isolation as she tried to keep her feelings from her family. A simple question from her physician conveyed to her his appreciation for her suffering, allowing them to connect through mutual recognition of her fears. Although the moment of connection was brief, its effect was enduring: it left her better able to cope and considerably uplifted. She went on to have surgery and made an uncharacteristically rapid recovery. The relationship she developed with her physician continued to be a therapeutic agent in itself, the dosage of which she regulated (in the form of telephone calls, as needed) to help her through the subsequent difficult months of her radiation therapy.

Illness also presents the patient with a problem of meaning. Patients need an explanation for their illness that connects their personal experience to their broader, culturally determined explanatory model. (For example, "It was God's will." Or, "My resistance was down because I was working so hard, so I caught a virus.") If a patient's worldview cannot accommodate the illness ("How could this happen to me? I've led a good life."), a patient may face a crisis of meaning, a bewildering realization that the world does not work in accordance with her long-held beliefs, thereby calling all knowledge into question. Or, she may be led to a dysfunctional meaning, one that causes more disability and suffering than the disease itself ("I must be very bad to deserve this.")

Sometimes the illness primarily is an expression of a lack of connectedness or meaning. Frankl has identified many patients suffering from a loss of interest and hope, an inner void or emptiness, an "existential vacuum" in which the "will-to-meaning" has been lost (22). Some cases involving somatization disorders or substance abuse begin to make sense when viewed in this way. When symptoms arise out of meaninglessness, alienation, and emptiness, a relationship that provides a deep feeling of connection is an important part of the cure. The therapeutic relationship may occur with a health professional or with peers (witness the effectiveness of Alcoholics Anonymous and other peer support groups).

Although illness may pose a threat to one's sources of connection, it can also offer an important opportunity to discover personal meaning, dignity, and value (23). Life needs tension and disequilibrium to produce growth (22, 24):

> Disease is a symptom of the universal ambiguity of life. Life must risk itself in order to win itself, but in the risking it may lose itself A life which does not risk disease, even in the highest forms of the life of the spirit, is a poor life ... (12)

If a perspective such as this can replace an impossibly inaccurate one that holds that illness, loss, and death are alien to normal life, then patients will have a much better opportunity to find wholeness, hope, and ultimate transcendence over their condition.

Doctors' Needs for Connection and Meaning

Doctors have the same fundamental needs as any other human beings. Like our patients, we seek connection. Medicine offers us the possibility of connection with a most extraordinary range of people. We are granted the privilege of access to all manner of human experiences, which, if we are open to them, cannot help but promote our own growth. Furthermore, even as we share our patients' journeys into illness, they sometimes share our difficult journey as heaters. What physician has not been comforted by a patient from time to time?

Like our patients, we also seek meaning and purpose in our lives. Our meaning as physicians is given to us by our patients-they empower us (13). When we see that our attention has instilled a sense of personal value in a patient who feels isolated and useless, we feel that our lives have value. Medicine offers us an opportunity to feel that we are making a contribution and devoting ourselves to a cause beyond ourselves.

Joyce's physician, after their moment of connection, felt uplifted and awed by the power of that moment. He felt happy to be a physician and to have the opportunity to see his skills and perceptions contribute so directly to the lessening of another person's suffering. He also felt privileged to have experienced so immediately another person's life. His own lifeworld seemed enlarged as a result.

Our needs must go beyond the ordinary search for connection and meaning. After all, we have been particularly attracted to an occupation that thrusts us more forcibly than most into confronting the most profound of human problems. Rosen suggests that it is because we ourselves are wounded (6). This notion suggests a bond between doctor and patient: each is suffering, in need of healing, and capable of transforming illness into an opportunity for growth. What are our wounds? We may harbor particularly intense fears of death, feelings of powerlessness, or anxieties about the basic uncertainty of life with an accompanying need for control. Perhaps we enter medicine to be needed, seeking the attention and authority that people grant us. Whatever the nature of our wounds, we heal to be healed.

When we feel connected to our patients and to our work, the long hours, the difficult decisions, and the many other demands are sources of fulfillment. Without this connectedness, however, we find the hours and the demands to be overwhelming and draining; we become burned out.

With greater frequency than most people, we seek refuge in dangerous places: drugs, alcohol, or even suicide (25).

A New Perspective on Medical Care

Awareness of a transpersonal aspect of the patient-doctor relationship brings with it a change in emphasis in medical care. We now can see that the relationship serves not only as a medium for collecting data and imparting instructions or advice, but also as an important therapeutic agent. Making the diagnosis and carrying out a plan of treatment, actions that will always be important in their own rights, are now seen to serve an additional purpose: they create a context for the formation of a therapeutic relationship to meet the needs for connection and meaning of patient and doctor alike. The establishment of a healing relationship (often signaled by a special moment of connection) is a fundamental clinical task, which is coequal with diagnosis and biotechnical treatment, whether the relationship is to last 5 minutes or 50 years. Our patients have wanted a healing relationship all along; this kind of relationship has been provided by successful healers in every culture.

This change in emphasis may lead, in turn, to a change in the way we feel about our work. To the extent that our sense of success currently depends on curing or at least controlling disease, fulfillment is beyond reach in many, if not most cases. Uncertainty and lack of control threaten our sense of mastery. Because we feel that we are "winging it" much of the time, clinical practice can become endlessly frustrating. Then, adding to the frustration, patients accuse us of being insensitive and of not caring, despite our conscientious efforts to do everything called for by the medical model. In contrast, when a model that incorporates the transpersonal aspects of "medical care is used and when one of the goals of medicine is to witness empathically the experiences of the patient and family, to maintain the therapeutic connection that dispels isolation and despair, success, if not always achieved, is nevertheless always within our grasp.

Our approach to terminally ill patients may also change. When confronted with disease that appears to be beyond treatment, we tend to feel helpless. We pull away from patients saying, "Nothing more can be done." If, instead, we can recognize the therapeutic value of simply being there, which is an important kind of "doing," we need not feel helpless. We will not feel tempted to withdraw, with all the iatrogenic suffering that withdrawal (dis-connection) creates. We can find meaning for ourselves in helping patients to maintain their connection as life ebbs.

Issues of connection and meaning do not emerge only in settings of life-threatening illness, nor do they find expression exclusively through intensely personal discussions of loneliness and longing. They are present to a degree in every medical encounter, whether explicitly addressed or not. The ever-present possibility of access to unifying experiences and moments of connection can impart a sense of discovery and excitement to even the most routine clinical situations.

A shift in the emphasis of the medical model would lead to changes in medical education. Relationship skills and connexional experience would receive the same attention during clinical teaching exercises as physical examination skills and diagnostic reasoning. Self-awareness and personal growth would be included among the explicitly stated goals of the educational process. Others have called for these changes already (26, 27). The necessary skills are already being defined (28), and the methods for teaching these skills are being developed and disseminated (29). The recognition of patients' connexional needs now strengthens the theoretical foundation of these activities and highlights their true importance.

Awareness of patients' connexional needs does not merely promote nice bedside manners; it represents the efforts of our profession to meet one of its most fundamental goals. Not only can students be taught to relate to their patients more therapeutically and effectively, but the educational process itself can become a source of connexional experience for both students and teachers.

With the foregoing advantages of a new model in mind, we should also consider several cautions. First, recognition and cultivation of spiritual experiences in medical care will not be a panacea for all the ills of medicine and physicians. Indeed, we may never all agree on a single, unified view of the proper place of these experiences in the care of patients any more than we now agree on the indications for blood transfusions or preoperative laboratory tests.

Second, increased awareness brings increased responsibility, which we may not want (30, 31). Barnard notes, "At the root of physicians' resistance to the priestly role is their profound unease at being at the receiving end of people's most intense existential fears and hopes" (13). Receiving our patients' most intense fears and hopes requires that we be willing to confront our own. We must have adequate personal strength and support to cope with the additional fears and losses we will encounter through our patients, and we must be willing to relinquish the illusions of personal power, mastery, and control that are afforded us by the narrower, traditional medical model. The less a physician is willing to meet these conditions, the less of the connexional dimension he or she will be able to experience, with an attendant diminution in his or her ability to be therapeutic.

Finally, we must be careful not to confuse connexional experience with personal, emotional attachment. Although the latter may include transpersonal elements, it also involves the satisfaction of personal needs for companionship, security, and physical contact (interpersonal and intrapersonal needs), which is not the proper domain of the patient-doctor relationship. That the distinction is not always clear speaks to the need for us to know how to monitor our own feelings as we work with patients and to feel comfortable seeking the observations, support, and advice of peers or supervisors when uncertainty arises.

Replacing Art with Science

With this bare foundation of a theory about what makes the patient-doctor relationship therapeutic, the task before us is to build it into a body of knowledge that is as detailed, as useful, and as rigorously derived as that of the rest of medicine. Assessment of and responses to the needs of patients for connection and meaning must be no less scientific than the diagnosis and treatment of Hodgkin disease and cholecystitis. To do this, we must be prepared to examine our patients' subjective experiences, as well as our own. We must learn how to observe, characterize, and verify these experiences, to shape them using various interviewing techniques, and to correlate them with clinical outcomes.

Awareness of connexional experience is prerequisite to beginning this task. From the very outset, it will help us to understand our patients and ourselves better and to find a welcome sense of wholeness in our work. With our

often maligned, but still respected place as conduits of the healing privilege in our era, we can be influential in furthering the reintegration of those aspects of experience—body and mind, science and spirituality—that were divided so long ago. Only when the medical model itself embodies the wholeness of a human being's experience can it guide clinicians and patients toward complete healing.

References

1. Radetsky M. Sudden intimacies. *JAMA.* 1985;254:1361.
2. Tierney WM. From a deeper well. *J Gen Intern Med.* 1986;1:350.
3. Cassell EJ. The nature of suffering and the goals of medicine. *N Engl J Med.* 1982;306:639-45.

4. Whitfield CL. *Alcoholism, Other Drug Problems, and Spirituality: A Transpersonal Approach.* Baltimore: The Resource Group; 1985:16-23.
5. Vastyan EA. Spiritual aspects of the care of cancer patients. *CA.* 1986;36:110-4.
6. Rosen DH. Modern medicine in search of its soul. *Med Heritage.* 1987. In press.
7. Engel GL. Physician-scientists and scientific physicians: resolving the humanism-science dichotomy. *Am J Med.* 1987;82:107-11.
8. Murray JAH, ed. *The Oxford English Dictionary.* Vol. 2. Oxford, England: The Oxford University Press; 1933:838-9.
9. Wilber K. *No Boundary.* Boulder: Shambhala Pubns., Inc.; 1979:75-6.
10. Buber M. *I and Thou.* 2nd ed. New York: Charles Scribner's and Sons; 1958:24-34.
11. Goldstein A. Thrills in response to music and other. *Stimuli Physiol Psych.* 1980;8:126-9.
12. Tillich P. The meaning of health. *Perspect Biol Med.* 1961;5:92-100.
13. Barnard D. The physician as priest revisited. *J Relig Health.* 1985;24:272-86.
14. Wilber K. *Eye to Eye.* Garden City, New Jersey: Anchor Press; 1983:39-61.
15. Barsky AJ. Hidden reasons some patients visit doctors. *Ann Intern Med.* 1981;94(4 pt 1):492-8.
16. Engel GL. The need for a new medical model: a challenge for biomedicine. *Science.* 1977;196:129-36.
17. Ashbrook J. The impact of the hospital situation in our understanding of God and man. *J Pastoral Care.* 1956; 10:1-15.
18. Rabin Dr. Occasional notes: compounding the ordeal of ALS: isolation from my fellow physicians. *N Engl J Med.* 1982;307:506-9.
19. Booth G. The voice of the body. In: Belgum D, ed. *Religion and Medicine: Essays on Meaning, Values and Health.* Ames, Iowa: Iowa State University Press; 1967:96-118.
20. Kleinman A. Interpreting illness meanings: the clinician's mini-ethnography. *Med Encounter.* 1986;3(3):5-7.
21. Matthews DA, Feinstein AR. A new instrument for patients' appraisals of physician performance [Abstract). *Clin Res.* 1985;33:758A.
22. Frankl VE. *The Doctor and the Soul: From Psychotherapy to Logotherapy.* New York: Alfred A. Knopf, Inc.; 1965.
23. Mack RM. Lessons from living with cancer. *N Engl J Med.* 1984;311:1640-4.
24. Peck MS. *The Road Less Traveled.* New York: Simon and Schuster; 1978:15-8.
25. McCue JD. The effects of stress on physicians and their medical practice. *N Engl J Med.* 1982;306:458-63.
26. Subcommittee on Evaluation of Humanistic Qualities in the Internist, American Board of Internal Medicine. Evaluation of humanistic qualities in the internist. *Ann Intern Med.* 1983;99:720-4.
27. Project Panel on the General Professional Education of the Physician and College Preparation for Medicine. Physicians for the twenty-first century. *J Med Educ.* 1984;59(11 pt 2):1-208.
28. Lipkin M Jr, Quill TE, Napodano RJ. The medical interview: a core curriculum for residencies in internal medicine. *Ann Intern Med.* 1984;100:277-84.
29. Duffy D, Barker LR, Levinson W, Rubenstein H. The faculty development course: a personal account. *Med Encounter.* 1986; 3(Winter): 1-4.
30. Peck MS. *The Road Less Traveled.* New York: Simon and Schuster; 1978:284-9.
31. Steiner R. *Knowledge of the Higher Worlds and its Attainment.* New York: Anthroposcopic Press: 1947:75-6.

Nonverbal Communication Between Patients and Medical Practitioners

Howard S. Friedman

Since ancient times, physicians and other healers have relied upon careful observation to diagnose illness, and have developed appropriate bedside manners to promote recovery. Medical education emphasizes the need for careful attention to the patient's subtle clues of pain, anxiety, emotion, and disease (O'Brien, 1974). Medical lore offers numerous suggestions for proper comforting of patients, for correct demeanor, and for appropriate reactions to patient behavior (DiMatteo, 1979). In practice, many experienced practitioners rely heavily on the subtleties of face-to-face interaction. However, although scientific procedures have replaced art in much of medical practice, the dynamics of interpersonal interaction remain mostly unattended by systematic research (Bennett, 1976). Even in the face of the past decade's advances in behavioral science and communication (e.g., Korsch, Gozzi, & Francis, 1968), intuition, faith, morale, empathy, sensitivity, caring, comfort, will to live, and similar pregnant but imprecise terms are still the by-words of nursing and direct patient care. Actually, there is a quantity of available scientific information on the use and meaning of *nonverbal communication* which can be applied to medical interactions.

Nonverbal communication involves those subtle cues which complement and illustrate aspects of the verbal interaction and often provide messages and express feelings that are not subject to direct conscious analysis by the interactants. A patient's grimace, smile, or expression of fear, as well as a nurse's comforting touch or facial expression of disgust, are communicative acts which may be even more important than the matter under verbal discussion.

For a number of reasons, nonverbal communication is especially crucial in medical settings. Medical care is increasingly complex. Doctors, nurses, patients, family members, and allied health personnel all affect each other, and systems approaches have become useful. Such approaches shift attention away from considering only what doctors prescribe for patients, and instead focus attention on the nature of the ongoing interaction, the responses of each interactant, and the *process* of health care-all areas where nonverbal communication becomes important (Daubenmire, 1976).

Health Care Transactions

Analysis of what actually occurs in health can be usefully divided into those cues which the patient receives and those which the patient expresses or sends.

Patient Sensitivity

A number of factors combine to make it likely that most patients will be especially observant of

Howard S. Friedman (1979), "Nonverbal Communication Between Patients and Medical Practitioners," Journal of Social Issues, Volume 35, No. 1, pp. 82-99.

and sensitive to the nonverbal communication of health practitioners. First of all, illness generally provokes fear, anxiety, and emotional uncertainty not only because of the possibility of disability or death, but also because of encounters with unfamiliar scientific terminology and medical jargon, reactions to drugs, the presence of imposing new machinery and novel environments, and separation from loved ones and familiar surroundings. Under these conditions, many patients will have a strong need for social comparison, and will look to those around them—health care personnel—for subtle clues as to how and what they are or ought to be feeling (cf. Schachter, 1959; Ellsworth, Friedman, Perlick, & Hoyt, 1978). Second, most patients are likely to be searching for factual information about the nature of their disease, its severity, its course, and their prognosis. Of course, some of this information is provided in the form of a verbal diagnosis, lab reports, and statements of current condition. However, this information may not be fully understood by patients. More importantly, it may not be fully believed. Furthermore, practitioners may withhold or distort the whole truth for a variety of legitimate and not-so-legitimate reasons and patients know that this may be true in their cases. Since people commonly believe that clues about possible deception are expressed and "leaked" through nonverbal channels (Knapp, Hart, and Dennis, 1974), such cues are likely to be afforded special consideration by patients. Furthermore, patients playing the role of the "good" patient (Taylor, 1979) may be hesitant to question a busy, high-status professional in detail and prefer to rely on messages left "unsaid" for clues about their medical condition. Third, patients are especially likely to attend to nonverbal cues because of their position of weakness. There is evidence that subordinates will closely monitor the nonverbal cues of their bosses, perhaps to assess the mood and ascertain which actions are having a positive and which a negative effect (Exline, 1972; Henley, 1977). Patients are often completely at the mercy of the practitioner and are probably especially motivated by such concerns. Finally, certain medical matters that interfere with normal verbal communication, such as speech or throat impairments, orders to hold still, attachment to a respirator, need for the practitioner to concentrate, and even a thermometer in the mouth, all limit the patient's ability to question the practitioner and increase the importance of nonverbal cues.

Patient Expressiveness

Some of these same factors and some additional ones make it likely that patients will be especially nonverbally expressive and that some important information will be emitted solely through nonverbal channels. First of all, patients are likely to experience a number of emotions, which are often more clearly revealed nonverbally than verbally, especially through facial expressions (Argyle, 1975; Ekman, Friesen, & Ellsworth, 1972). Furthermore, some of these emotional states, such as pain, fear, depression and various bodily disturbances, may be states that the patient rarely experiences otherwise and thus are not readily described in words. Second, patients are unlikely to have had much experience hiding or controlling these emotions, especially in medical settings. Thus, anger at an interpersonal slight in a supermarket may be controlled, but fear, surprise, or pain at a doctor's probing may be directly revealed. Third, patients may be hesitant to communicate their feelings about certain difficult matters—concerning death, embarrassing disabilities, desires for additional services, and so on—and thus communicate them only through channels that are not deliberate, that is, through nonverbal communication. Fourth, many illnesses affect a patient's movements, odors, facial expressions and other nonverbal signals in ways not fully recognized by the patient. Such cues cannot be described or controlled by the patient, but could be important clues to practitioners. Finally, various medical conditions resulting from disease, drugs, or other treatment may disrupt verbal communication and leave the patient communicating only by nonverbal means. For example, weakness of the seriously ill may make verbal conversation too difficult but leave nonverbal messages, such as a glance or gesture, still available (Blondis & Jackson, 1977).

Thus it is probable that patients will: 1) be especially observant of and sensitive to the nonverbal cues emitted by health practitioners; and 2) communicate a significant amount of important information through their own nonverbal cues. Since so much valuable information is revealed by the patient through nonverbal communication, the importance of practitioner sensitivity to these matters in diagnosis and monitoring of treatment is obvious. The relations of specific nonverbal cues to diagnosis and maintenance are presented throughout the remainder of this paper. The importance of practitioner nonverbal expressiveness—the other side of the coin of patient nonverbal sensitivity—is perhaps not so obvious: ignorance of this factor may be one of the most serious deficiencies of the practice of modern medicine.

Practitioner Communication and the Placebo Effect

In most medical research involving patients, the methodological safeguard known as the "double-blind" procedure is essential. In this procedure, neither the patient nor the physician (or clinician) knows whether the patient has received the experimental treatment or is in the control group. For example, in a pharmacological study of pain reduction, neither the patient nor the physician is told whether the patient is receiving a traditional analgesic such as aspirin or a new experimental narcotic. This procedure is necessary to protect the validity of the experimental design from the well-known but poorly understood placebo effect—the psychological or psychophysiological effect of a therapy that does not have specific activity for the condition being treated (Shapiro, 1971). Often, improvement results from the expectation of improvement. However, this research "problem" points up two processes essential to many aspects of healing: the patient's expectations and the practitioner's role in creating these expectations.

The placebo effect remains overlooked and underresearched, although it is central to the healing process. Much of the history of medicine before modern times was the history of the placebo effect, and it is understandable that medical practitioners would want to disavow any association between modern medicine and such therapies as bleeding, leeching, purging, shocking, and such drugs as crocodile dung, eunuch fat, and swine's teeth. Yet throughout history, physicians have retained relatively high status because such treatments often worked (Shapiro, 1960, 1971). They worked, in part, because of the importance of psychological and emotional factors to "physical" health. Yet such factors have been so belittled and have met such resistance in recent times that a 1975 article in the *Journal of the American Medical Association* urged physicians to reconsider this "neglected and berated aspect of patient care" (Benson & Epstein, 1975). Rather than a threat to the science of medicine, placebo effects are intimately related to the well-being of many patients. Placebos may produce definite, severe physiological effects (Shapiro, 1971) and placebo effects may disrupt the usual action of a treatment.

It is likely that one prime element of a placebo effect is expectation (Shapiro, 1971; Rosenthal, 1976; Jones, 1977; Frank, 1978). If the practitioner can transmit positive expectations to the patient, real benefits may ensue; negative expectations may produce negative effects. It is important to understand and keep in mind that placebo effects involve a therapy, with nonspecific activity for the condition being treated; drugs or pills may function as placebos but so may various other therapies, including psychotherapy (Shapiro, 1971). In fact, it seems likely that placebo effects more often result from procedures—exercise regimens, extensive testing, diets, and other medical rituals—than from pills. Certainly in such areas as pain reduction, which have relatively strong psychological components (Johnson, J. E., 1973), expectation can significantly influence outcome (cf. Jones, 1977). Yet, positive expectations do not arise miraculously. Patients' expectations arise from interactions with health practitioners. Expectations are social-psychological in nature. And, for the various reasons described above, patients are especially likely to obtain information on which these expectations are based through nonverbal cues. Patients will observe the nonverbal actions of the health providers and decide whether they are liked, respected, and expected to improve, or are repugnant, worthless, or untreatable.

Elements of Nonverbal Communication

A number of recent writers in medical psychology recognize the importance of the face-to-face practitioner-patient interaction itself, discussing such matters as tone, warmth, rapport, empathy, and support. They sometimes specifically refer to nonverbal communication (e.g. Adler, 1979; Blondis & Jackson, 1977; DiMatteo, 1979; Korsch et al., 1968; Stone, 1979; Wortman & Dunkel-Schetter, 1979). Unfortunately, relatively little use has been made of the advances of the last decade in the field of nonverbal communication. This field has identified specific nonverbal cues and has begun to examine how they combine with other cues and with the social situation to produce unique meanings. A number of ideas, hypotheses, and findings concerning facial expression, touch, smells, gestures, and related cues, are directly relevant to medical settings.

Touch

For hundreds of years during the Middle Ages, Europeans sought relief from the disease of scrofula (a tubercular lymphatic disease) through the "King's touch" or the "royal touch" (Bloch, 1973). The persistence of the belief in the curative powers of the royal touch, despite a very low "cure" rate, attests to the tremendous symbolic value of touch in healing as well as to the important role of expectation in health care. The healing power of the royal touch tended to wane with the disappearing divinity of kings, but it may in fact have been transferred to physicians. Patients may feel much better after a routine physical exam in which the doctor uses his or her special expertise to examine rather than merely question them. Certainly the desire to be touched by high-status political leaders, entertainers, sports figures, and the like, has not disappeared in this modern age; touch has retained its symbolic value as a kind of blessing involving the transfer of special powers.

Faith healers have long used the technique of the "laying on of hands" and this "therapy" is still popular in American society. Since its efficacy is supposedly derived from the transfer of a healing spirit, just as the King transferred the divine spirit, this technique is generally viewed as quackery by modern medicine. Some sophisticated proponents have explained it as involving the operation of electromagnetic fields, but it may be more fruitfully seen as a special sort of placebo effect (cf. Riscalla, 1975). The practitioner's touch may indeed promote healing if it is imbued with a special symbolic value. In the last two decades, the concept of touching as basic to the process of healing has been enthusiastically adopted by the so-called "human potential movement." In fact, even "the most timid and conservative T-groups are assailing cultural taboos against touching. It is rare to find a group whose members do not at some point take turns being lifted up in the air from below by the hands of others" (Howard, 1970, p. 146). At the very least, touching may have a significant psychological effect on many patients.

Not all benefits of touching are due to expectation. Since Harrow's classic studies of monkeys raised with wire and cloth surrogate mothers (Harlow & Zimmerman, 1959), the importance of touch to healthy social development has been widely accepted. The comfort of contact is physiologically based; indeed, lack of touch has been implicated in skin disease (Montague, 1978).

Certainly backscratching, patting, gentle massaging, and other touches can be tension-reducing. The successful use of waterbeds in hospitals, supposedly to reduce the incidence of bedsores ("Making Waves," 1975), may in fact partly result from an increased need for tactual stimulation in a tense atmosphere removed from usual family touching. In fact, nursing instructors will now acknowledge that "In nursing, touch may be the most important of all nonverbal behaviors" (Blondis & Jackson, 1977, p. 6). An ill, anxious patient, surrounded by cold equipment, may be especially reassured by a warm touch. A similar conclusion was reached by Ashley Montague (1978) who wrote that "in every branch of the practice of medicine touching should be considered an indispensable part of the doctor's art. . . . Touch always enhances the doctor's therapeutic abilities" (p. 223).

Although therapeutic touching has been left as a relatively unresearched "art," medical practitioners are well-trained to palpate, poke, feel, and otherwise touch their patients for purposes of diagnosis. Furthermore, diagnostic procedures such as temperature-taking, blood-testing, ear, nose and throat examinations, stethoscopic examination, blood pressure taking, and reflex testing all necessitate invading the patient's bodily integrity with a scientific instrument. Often, as in routine examination of the breasts, vagina, anus, prostate, and groin, the touch is in intimate areas not usually invaded by relative strangers. This touching will produce reactions on two levels: emotional and interpersonal.

There is little doubt that being touched is sometimes comforting and sometimes emotionally (or sexually) arousing. However, whether a certain type of touch at a certain part of the body can be shown to have a general, predictable effect is doubtful. First of all, there are tremendous individual differences in responses to different types of touches, ranging from the type of pat that is reassuring to the type of touch that is sexually arousing. Furthermore, many differences arise from interpersonal matters: the meaning of the touch for the specific matter at hand.

Two likely interpersonal meanings of touch involve intimacy and power. In usual interaction, the part of the body touched is generally clearly related to the intimacy of the relationship (Jourard, 1966); for example, the genitals are generally only touched by an opposite-sex close friend. Violation of such norms in the medical setting may produce confusion. Nurses often report incidents in which patients begin disclosing very personal information or become flirtatious during or after a backrub, a bath, or other usually "intimate" forms of touching, even though such behavior violates role constraints (Johnson, B. S., 1965). Touching also communicates power (Henley, 1977). Practitioners may touch patients routinely, but there is usually very little occasion for the patient to touch the practitioner. The practitioner is of higher status. Of course, most of this one-sided touching is for instrumental purposes in the technical side of medical care. But the implication of a power difference remains.

In sum, touch has various significant functions and meanings in medical settings. Touch may have symbolic value in healing, may create positive expectations, may have important physiological effects, and, even when used for strictly diagnostic purposes, may affect the interpersonal nature of the practitioner-patient interaction. Certainly this topic is deserving of much additional research which reflects the multidimensional meaning of touching.

Gaze

One of the most influential nonverbal cues is gaze. People generally know and respond when they are stared at (Ellsworth, 1975). Eye behavior is like touching in that its meaning depends upon other factors in the situation: a stare may be comforting if it intensifies a pleasant situation or opens communication in an uncertain situation, but a stare may be arousing or threatening if the context is negative (Ellsworth, 1975; Ellsworth et al., 1978). Glances from a sympathetic nurse or an unhurried doctor may encourage a patient who is having a difficult time or help a patient bring up a sensitive subject. Failure to look a patient in the eye, on the other hand, may be part of the process of dehumanization, common in medical settings, in which the patient is seen as (and comes to feel like) a body not a person.

Excessive staring at a patient, with no apparent cause, will likely have a negative effect, perhaps making the patient feel like a freak or like a bad person. Presumably, health providers will generally not stare at a patient's physical deformity, but constant eye contact to avoid so doing is also likely to be noticed and reacted to by a patient. Although studies have not found systematic effects of stigmata on eye contact behavior, interaction with a handicapped person (including eye contact) does tend to be less variable, that is, more rigid and unchanging (Kleck, 1968). Refusal to look at or constant staring at the chest of a mastectomy patient, or avoidance of or excessive eye contact with a dying patient, may have similar effects: a signal to the patient that something is awry in the interaction and an intensification of the emotions being communicated through other channels.

The Face and Facial Expression

The most specific and detailed information about states and emotions is communicated through facial expression (Izard, 1977). First of all, the face is a key area for diagnosis because it has many muscles, detailed ennervation, several sense organs, and high visibility. Long ago, Hippocrates urged the physician to study the patient's face first. A face with, "the nose sharp, the eyes sunken, the temples fallen in, the ears cold and drawn in and their lobes distorted, the skin of the face hard, stretched and dry, and the colour of the face pale or dusky," usually portends death (Hippocrates, 1950 ed., p. 113). In modern times, facial features have proved very useful in diagnosing genetic disorders (Goodman & Gorlin, 1970).

Facial expression is an important element in the communication of pain. While pain is not one of the basic facial expressions of emotion in current categorizations, it is closely related to them (Izard, 1977; Ekman & Friesen, 1975). There is little doubt that valuable information about the intensity and stage of pain and related negative feelings (fear, distress, sadness) is communicated to the health practitioner through the face, even when the patient is not fully conscious. For example, facial expression has been used to assess amount of distress of women in labor (Leventhal & Sharp, 1965). In fact, the concept of pain itself has a communicative component in that its expression generally brings help from others (Szasz, 1957); pain is, in part, a request for comfort. Facial expression of pain may thus be expected to vary in part as a function of the nature of interpersonal relationships. If the expression of pain brings rewards other than pain relief, the patient may show more and more pain. On the other hand, if the expression of pain is ignored or punished, it may decrease, though at the cost of the possibility of relief through treatment.

This communicative function of pain expression is especially important because recent theory and research suggest a role for facial expression in the perception and management of pain. At the very least, facial expression plays an important mediational role in the subjective experience of emotion (Izard, 1977). Controlling the facial expression of pain (hiding pain) may help to reduce the pain (Lanzetta, Cartwright-Smith, & Kleck, 1976). Thus it may be advantageous for health providers to reinforce patients' suppression of facial expressions of pain. However, since such suppression will, in turn, affect other responses of the health care providers, the issue is a complex one, and research efforts should continue in this field.

The practitioner's expectations are often clearly and forcefully communicated through facial expression. The human face is fantastically expressive and is most often the object of our attention (Vine, 1970). People can easily and quickly recognize distinct emotional states from facial expression (Ekman et al., 1972; Ekman & Friesen, 1975) and thus such expression can effectively communicate a nurse's disgust at a wound or deformity, a physician's anger at a patient's failure to follow treatment regimens, or a technician's fear of a patient's deterioration. On the other hand, facial expressions can be effectively controlled by most people (Ekman & Friesen, 1975). With proper training and motivation, practitioners' expressions might just as effectively communicate a nurse's sympathy and understanding or a physician's positive outlook and expectations. This psychological power of facial expression was not lost on tribal medicine men who wore elaborate masks during healing. In fact, in Ceylon, different masks were worn for each disease (Liggett, 1974). Patients, paying special attention to nonverbal cues and especially influenced by the affective nature of the interaction (Ben-Sira, 1976), will usually be heavily influenced by the provider's facial expression.

Voice

As with facial expressions, the specific emotional and motivational states of patients and practitioners may be revealed through their tone of voice (cf. Davitz, 1964). The tone of voice refers to those sounds, primarily pitch variations, which accompany the spoken word but are independent of the verbal content. Feelings like fear, anger, sadness, joy, and pain are readily transmitted through vocal cues. Furthermore, voice tone may be especially important where possible deception is involved (cf. DePaulo, Rosenthal, Eisenstat, Rogers, & Finklestein, 1978). However, the practitioner must be willing to spend some time talking to and listening to the patient in order to perceive and transmit many of these cues.

Although tone of voice is probably an important element of the overall "tone" the practitioner sets for an interaction, surprisingly little research has been conducted in this area. Voice has, however, been implicated in the transmission of experimenter expectancies (Duncan & Rosenthal, 1968) and thus is likely important in placebo effects. One study found a negative correlation between the amount of "anger" judged to be present in a doctor's voice and his success in dealing with alcoholic patients (Milmoe, Rosenthal, Blane, Chafetz, & Wolf, 1967). Another showed a relationship between a physician's ability to express emotions through voice tone or face and voice and the way the physician was evaluated by his or her patients (Friedman, DiMatteo & Taranta, in press). Thus, additional research should continue to address such questions as the effects of the voice tones of health care providers on the expectations and emotional reactions of various types of patients. Aspects of vocal communication that are unique to the health care setting should also be identified.

Olfaction

Although communication through odors is very important throughout much of the animal world, it appears relatively insignificant among humans, especially in American society (e.g., Knapp, 1978). However, the medical field may be an important exception. Some illnesses and treatments may act directly to produce unpleasant odors in the patient, while others affect patient odor through actions on the gastrointestinal tract. There is even some promise of a breathalyzer device for diagnosis ("Breath and body odors," 1978). On the other hand, practitioners too may be associated with particular odors. The use of disinfectants, chemical treatments, anesthesia, alcohol, and so on, as well as the lingering odors of other patients, may all transmit olfactory messages to the patient. And there is no doubt that many of these patient and practitioner odors arouse strong negative feelings.

In the area of person perception, negative personal attributes are often associated with malodor. A bad person may be labelled a "stinker" or "stinkpot." In fact, perceiving the outgroup as smelly is a prime characteristic of prejudice (Largey & Watson, 1972; Allport, 1954). Thus, the diseased person suffering from malodor may be reacted to with negative feelings. Some health care personnel may come to see foul-smelling patients as less good or moral, especially if the patient has at least some control over the odor. Such reactions of distaste are then likely to be transmitted to patients through facial expressions and the distances used in face-to-face interaction (cf. Hall, 1966).

The particular, uncommon smells of medical settings may also affect the health care process in another way. For unknown reasons, odors often have tremendous power to evoke memories of forgotten times and places (Meerloo, 1964; Allport, 1954). Hence, a doctor's office or a hospital or sickroom may evoke vivid memories of the previous negative experiences of an ill relative or a childhood trauma and thus may create significant negative expectations. The many implications of olfactory communication in medical settings remain to be systematically investigated. The first step probably should be the collection of impressions and observations regarding odor in medical settings to serve as a basis for more systematic research.

Other nonverbal cues

There are many other nonverbal cues which are important to face-to-face interaction and take on a special meaning in medical settings. Although relatively little is known about these cues (with a few exceptions), the terminology and approach of the field of nonverbal communication can do much to inform the untrained observer of medical interactions.

A major category of nonverbal communication involves body positions and gestures. Posture, hand movements, gait, lean, foot-tapping and so on are combined in this category because they generally receive little attention from the interactants and little is known about the meaning of individual actions. However, such behaviors do have important effects on the "immediacy" or mutual stimulation of an interaction (Mehrabian, 1972). One especially active area of research involves the nonverbal detection of deception. There is theoretical and empirical reason to suspect that cues of deception are often emitted through body behavior rather than through facial expression, presumably because the body is under less conscious control (Ekman & Friesen, 1969). Nurses learn to recognize a patient's squirming, gesturing, pacing, and similar body signs of general restlessness (Blondis & Jackson, 1977), but should also learn to watch these cues when questioning a patient. The issue of whether patients with their heightened vigilance can detect practitioner lying and thus develop negative expectations is unresearched but certainly deserving of immediate attention. Practitioners often speculate that certain patients who have been denied the whole truth really "know" it anyway, and if so, it is possible that deception actually hurts rather than helps treatment.

There are also a number of sounds which may affect the nature of face-to-face interaction and are more likely to appear among patients than in the general population. For example, stomach rumbles, belches, flatulence, sneeze, coughs, and so on may be especially common. Although these signs may be valuable for diagnostic purposes, they also may violate some subcultural norms of polite society. The effects of such disturbances on practitioner-patient interactions has not been investigated, but could be addressed using the paradigms established for studying other nonverbal cues.

Finally, many other factors in the health care environment, ranging from the clothing worn by practitioners and patients to the color and design of hospital rooms, will likely have a significant effect on the health care process. However, the present paper focuses mainly on the dynamic aspects of face-to-face practitioner-patient interaction, since these elements are likely to be psychologically most salient. Nevertheless, environmental factors are also deserving of increased research efforts.

Verbal and Nonverbal Communication

One of the most critical aspects of effective treatment involves neither just what is said nor just how it is said. Rather, what is often more important is the degree of consistency between verbal and nonverbal cues. Stigmatized people in general are quite vigilant in watching for clues as to how they will "really" be treated (cf. Goffman, 1963). As noted above, such vigilance probably even greater in the ill who are also seeking factual information about the nature and severity of their illness and social comparison information as to what they should be feeling in a time of emotional uncertainty. So even the slightest inconsistency is unlikely to go unnoticed.

A positive verbal communication such as "You're looking ;better today" accompanied by a negative nonverbal cue is likely to be perceived as insincere (Argyle, 1975; Friedman, in press). If there is some anger in the communicator's face, sarcasm and nastiness may be perceived. However, if the practitioner saying positive words shows a sad face, the overall message may be seen as one of indifference (cf. Friedman, in press). On the other hand, a relatively submissive, negative verbal message such as "I hope you won't mind if I tell you that you need some additional tests" will probably be perceived as sincere and sympathetic, despite the negative content, if accompanied by a sad face, but might be seen as patronizing if accompanied by a happy face. The degree and type of consistency between verbal and nonverbal cues create the "innuendo" that can be very distressing or comforting to an ill person. Additional research is needed before we can fully understand such subtleties of cue combinations but the illustrations given here show that we need not remain tied to vague notions of "empathy" and "sincerity" but can define specific behaviors and researchable questions.

It seems likely that nonverbal communication increases in efficiency and utility as a relationship between two people develops (Altman, 1974). Spouses are probably better than strangers at quickly communicating and detecting distress, encouragement, understanding. However, illness brings practitioners and patients into an intimate relationship (especially from the patient's perspective) involving verbal self-disclosure in which nonverbal communication channels have not been fully developed. The relationship is intimate but its development has been forced or abrupt. Confusions and omissions may result, as patients emit special cues that practitioner's miss or misunderstand. Unfortunately, an absence of research on such matters precludes any solution at present other than helping the parties involved recognize that mistakes in nonverbal communication are likely to occur.

Finally, it is important to note that in the name of increased efficiency, various modern forces tend to decrease the amount of face-to-face interaction between practitioners and patients. Such technological advances include the use of computer diagnosis (cf. Slack, 1971) and the use of telephone and even television in diagnosis and especially in treatment. Since patient-practitioner nonverbal communication may be disrupted or even eliminated by such techniques, the quality of health care may suffer.

Conclusion

For a number of reasons, nonverbal communication takes on a special importance in the medical setting. Although this importance is increasingly recognized, the topic is generally not approached with the scientific rigor applied to most other medical matters. Fortunately, it is no longer necessary for medical practitioners to rely solely on vague concepts like intuition, sincerity and empathy in dealing with the subtle interpersonal aspects of health care. Further, it is an oversimplification for behavioral scientists studying medical care to discuss the "tone," the "atmosphere," or the "rapport" of practitioner-patient' interactions. There is a growing scientific literature on the meaning and impact of touch, facial expressions, voice tone, and related elements of nonverbal communication. This literature provides the concepts, tools, and strategies necessary to learn more about the crucial face-to-face aspects of health care. Attention to nonverbal cues deserves a key place in diagnosis and monitoring, alongside the newest computerized, mechanized techniques. And appropriate expectancies and encouragement, communicated both verbally and nonverbally, must be an important part of medical regimens.

References

Adler, N. E. Abortion: a social-psychological perspectivc. *Journal of Social* Issues, 1979, 35,(1).

Allport, G. W. *The Nature of Prejudice.* Garden City: Addison-Wesley Publishing Company, Inc., 1954.

Altman, I. The communication of interpersonal attitudes: an ecological approach. In T. L. Huston (Ed.), *Foundations of Interpersonal Attraction.* New York: Academic Press, 1974.

Argyle, M. *Bodily Communication.* New York: International Universities Press, Inc., 1975.

Bennett, A. E. *Communication Between Doctors and Patients.* Oxford: Oxford University Press, 1976.

Ben-Sira, Z. The function of the professional's affective behavior in client satisfaction: a revised approach to social interaction theory. *Journal of Health and Social Behavior, 1976,* 17, 3-11.

Benson, H., & Epstein, M. The placebo effect: A neglected asset in the care of patients. *Journal of the American Medical Association,* 1975, 232(12), 1225-1226.

Bloch, M. *The Royal Touch* (F. E. Anderson trans.). Montreal: McGill-Queen's University Press, 1973. (Originally published, 1961.)

Blondis, M. N., & Jackson, B. E. *Nonverbal Communication with Patients.* New York: John Wiley & Sons, Inc., 1977.

Breath and body odors may be diagnostic tools. UPI (Chicago), December 3, 1978.

Daubenmire, M. J. Nurse-patient-physician communicative interaction process. In H. Werley, A. Zuzich, M. Zajkowski, & A. Zngornik (Eds.), *Health Research: The Systems Approach.* Springer Publishing Co., Inc., 1976.

Davitz, J. R. *The Communication of Emotional Meaning.* New York: McGraw-Hill, Inc., 1964.

DePaulo, B. M., Rosenthal, R., Eisenstat, R. A., Rogers, P. L., & Finkelstein, S. Decoding discrepant nonverbal cues. *Journal of Personality and Social Psychology,* 1978, 36, 313-323.

DiMatteo, M. R., A social-psychological analysis of physician-patient rapport: Toward a science of the art of medicine. *Journal of Social Issues,* 1979, 35 (1).

Duncan, D. S., Jr., & Rosenthal, R. Vocal emphasis in experimenters' introduction reading as unintended determinant of subjects' responses. *Language and Speech,* 1968, 11, 20-26.

Ekman, P., & Friesen, W. Nonverbal leakage and clues to deception. *Psychiatry,* 1969, 32, 88-105.

Ekman, P., & Friesen, W. *Unmasking the Face.* Englewood Cliffs, N.J.: Prentice-Hall, Inc., 1975.

Ekman, P., Friesen, W., & Ellsworth, P. *Emotion in the Human Face.* New York: Pergamon Press, Inc., 1972.

Ellsworth, P. Direct gaze as a social stimulus: the example of aggression. In P. Pliner, L. Krames, and T. Alloway (Eds.). *Nonverbal Communication of Aggression.* New York: Plenun Publishing, 1975.

Ellsworth, P., Friedman, H., Perlick, D., & Hoyt, M. Some effects of gaze on subjects motivated to seek or to avoid social comparison. *Journal of Experimental Social Psychology,* 1968, 14, 69-87.

Exline, R. V. Visual Interaction: The glance of power and preference. In J. Cole (Ed.), *Nebraska Symposium on Motivation* 1971. Lincoln: University of Nebraska Press, 1972.

Frank, J. D. The medical power of faith. *Human Nature*, 1978, 1, 40-47.

Friedman, 11. S. The interactive effects of facial expressions of emotion and verbal messages on perceptions of affective meaning. *Journal of Experimental Social Psychology,* in press.

Friedman, H. S., DiMatteo, M. R., & Taranta, A. A study of the relationship between individual differences in nonverbal expressiveness and factors of personality and social interaction. *Journal of Research in Personality,* in press.

Goffman, E. *Stigma.* Englewood Cliffs: Prentice-Hall, Inc., 1963.

Goodman, R., & Gorlin, R. *The Face in Genetic Disorders.* St. Louis: C. V. Mosby Co., 1970.

Hall, E. T. *The Hidden Dimension.* Garden City: Doubleday & Company, Inc., 1966.

Harlow, H. F., & Zimmermann, R. R. Affectional responses in the infant monkey. *Science, 1959,* 130, 421-432.

Henley, N. *M. Body Politics.* Englewood Cliffs: Prentice-Hall Inc., 1977.

Hippocrates. *The Medical Works of Hippocrates.* (J. Chadwick and W. N. Mann, trans.). Oxford: Blackwell Scientific Publications, 1950.

Howard, J. *Please Touch.* New York: Dell Publishing Co. Inc., 1970.

Izard, C. E. *Human Emotions.* New York: Plenum Press, 1977.

Johnson, B. S. The meaning of touch in nursing. *Nursing Outlook,* 1965, 13, 59-60.

Johnson, J. E. Effects-of accurate expectations about sensations on the sensory and distress components of pain. Journal of *Personality and Social Psychology* 1973, 27, 261-275.

Jones, R. A. *Self-fulfilling Prophecies.* New York: Lawrence Erlbaum Associates, Inc., 1977.

Jourard, S. M. An exploratory study of body-accessibility. *British Journal of Social and Clinical Psychology,* 1966, 5, 221-231.

Kleck, R. Physical stigma and nonverbal cues emitted in face-to-face interaction. *Human Relations, 1968,* 21, 119-128.

Knapp, M. L. *Nonverbal Communication in Human Interaction.* New York: Holt, Rinehart and Winston, 1978.

Knapp, M. L., Hart, R. P., & Dennis, H. S. An exploration of deception as a communication construct. *Human Communication Research, 1974,* 1, 15-29.

Korsch, B. M., Gozzi, E. K., & Francis, V. Gaps in doctor-patient communication. I: Doctor-patient interaction and patient satisfaction. *Pediatrics,* 1968, 42, 855-871.

Lanzetta, J. T., Cartwright-Smith, J., & Kleck, R. Effects of nonverbal dissimulation on emotional experience and autonomic arousal. *Journal of Personality and Social Psychology, 1976,* 33, 354-370.

Largey, G. P., & Watson, D. R. The sociology of odors. *American Journal of Sociology, 1972,* 77, 1021-1033.

Leverithal, H., & Sharp, E. Facial expressions as indicators of distress. In S. S. Tomkins & C. E. Izard (Eds.), *Affect, Cognition and Personality: Empirical Studies.* New York: Springer, 1965.

Liggett, J. *The Human Face.* New York: Stein and Day, 1974.

Making waves. *Newsweek,* March 24, 1975, page 91.

Meerloo, J. A. M. *Unobtrusive Communication.* Assen, The Netherlands: Koninklijke Van Gorcum & Comp. N. V., 1964.

Mehrabian, A. *Nonverbal Communication.* Chicago: Aldine-Atherton, 1972.

Milmoe, S., Rosenthal, R., Blane, H. T., Chafetz, M. E., & Wolf, I. The doctor's voice: postdictor of successful referral of alcoholic patients. *Journal of Abnormal Psychology, 1967,* 72, 78-84.

Montague, A. *Touching.* New York: Harper & Row, 1978.

O'Brien, M.J. *Communications and Relationships in Nursing.* St. Louis: The C. V. Mosby Company, 1974.

Riscalla, L. Healing by laying on of hands: myth or fact. *Ethics in Science and Medicine, 1975,* 2, 167-17 1.

Rosenthal, R. *Experimenter Effects in Behavioral Research.* New York: Irvington Publishers, Inc., 1976.

Schachter, S. *The Psychology of Affiliation.* Stanford: Stanford University Press, 1959.

Shapiro, A. K. A contribution to a history of the placebo effect. *Behavioral Science, 1960, V,* 109-135.

Shapiro, A. K. Placebo effects in medicine, psychotherapy, and psychoanalysis. In A. Bergin & S. Garfield (Eds.), *Handbook of Psychotherapy and Behavior Change.* N.Y.: John Wiley & Sons, Inc., 1971.

Slack, W. Computer-based interviewing system dealing with nonverbal behavior as well as keyboard responses. *Science, 1971,* 1 71, 84-87.

Stone, G. C. Patient compliance and the role of the expert. *Journal of Social Issues*, 1979, 35 (1).

Szasz, T. S. *Pain and Pleasure: A Study of Bodily Feelings.* New York: Basic Books, 1957.

Taylor, S. E. Hospital patient behavior: reactance, helplessness, or control? *Journal of Social Issues, 1979,* 35 (1).

Vine, I. Communication by facial-visual signals. In J. H. Crook (Eds.), *Social Behavior in Birds and Mammals.* London & New York: Academic Press, 1970.

Vortman, C. B. & Dunkel-Schetter, Co. Interpersonal relationships and cancer: a theoretical analysis. *Journal of Social Issues, 1979,* 33 (1).

Caregiver-Patient Interaction: Empirical Research and Implications

Doctor-Patient Communication: Clinical Implications of Social Scientific Research

Howard Waitzkin

The literature on doctor-patient communication was fairly uninformative until about ten years ago. Many generalities were written, most having little basis in research. During the last decade, however, there has been a growing interest in empirical studies of communication. From this research, we are getting a better idea about the nature of doctor-patient communication, its problems, and how we can try to improve it. My aim is to spell out some implications of recent social scientific research on doctor-patient communication and to emphasize those studies that have importance for clinical practice.

Medical Education

In 1977 and again in 1979, the American Board of Internal Medicine tried to specify the meaning of "clinical competence."[1, 2] Through position papers published in the *Annals of Internal Medicine* and elsewhere, the Board argued that ambulatory care should be a fundamental part of internal medicine training programs and that the development of interpersonal communication abilities should be emphasized. The Board asked that faculty members observe the interaction skills of trainees on a regular basis and that they evaluate these skills formally before a resident is declared eligible to take the Board's certification examinations.

Some training programs in internal medicine have used these mechanisms to collect data on residents' communication skills; sometimes this research also has examined faculty members' abilities, but not often. The results have not inspired confidence about doctor-patient communication. Based on more than 300 interviews that they observed, Platt and McMath[3] defined the syndrome of "clinical hypocompetence," by which they referred to poor interviewing skills. They found a variety of communication problems; I will return to one of these, the "high control style," when I consider the linguistic structure of the medical encounter. Duffy and his colleagues[4] studied their own interns and residents. They discovered major difficulties in that residents tended not to ask patients what they understood about their illnesses, often did not take a medical history, tended not to inquire about the patients' emotional responses to illness, and

---

Waitzkin, H. Doctor-patient Communication: Clinical Implications of Social Scientific Research. Journal of the American Medical Association, November 2, 1984, Volume 252, No. 17, pp. 2441-46.

1 Council on General Internal Medicine, American Board of Internal Medicine: Attributes of the general internist and recommendations for training. *Ann Intern Med* 1977:86:472-473.

2 American Board of Internal Medicine: Clinical competence in internal medicine. *Ann Intern Med* 1979;90:402-411.

3 Platt FW, McMath JC: Clinical hypocompetence: The interview. *Ann Intern Med* 1979; 91:898-902

4 Duffy DL, Hamerman D, Cohen MA: Communication skills of house officers: A study in a medical clinic. *Ann Intern Med* 1980;93:354-357.

frequently did not explain the nature of the patients' problems.

During recent years, leaders of the other primary-care specialties—family medicine and pediatrics—have designated communication skills a major goal of training programs.[5, 6, 7] Motivated partly by such official pronouncements, research also has begun in these clinical disciplines. Typically this research confirms the disconcerting misunderstanding, confusions, and barriers that often arise in doctor-patient communication.[8, 9, 10] The process of communication takes on added importance because it can affect the outcomes of medical care, such as satisfaction, compliance, and physiologic responses to treatment.[11, 12, 13] Educational efforts that aim to improve practitioners' communication skills can lead to encouraging results. [14, 15]

The next part of the discussion focuses on social structural barriers to effective communication in medical encounters. Such barriers have to do with the differing sex, race, and social class of patients and doctor, ethnicity, language differences, and age, although these are not the only barriers that arise in clinical practice. There also are some strictly psychological or personality issues that obviously play a part in communication skills. However, I am less concerned about how our personalities affect us practitioners than I am about the social structural issues that impede effective communication.

Information Giving and Withholding

How much information to give to patients, and how much to withhold, are questions of never-ending speculation in medicine. Hippocrates[16] set the tone for this debate by arguing that doctors have the subtle impossibility of deciding how much information is in patients' best interests. Textbooks of medicine, like *Harrison's*,[17] agree with this point of view and claim that doctors should decide how much information to convey, based on patients' educational background, age, prognosis, and other characteristics. Ethicists like Bok,[18] however, point out that doctors withhold information and even lie from time to time, perhaps more than they should.

---

5 *Special Requirements for Residency Training in Family Practice.* Kansas City, Mo, American Academy of Family Practice, 1978.

6 Hornsby JL, Payne FE: A model for communication skills development for family practice residents. *J Fam Pract* 1979;8:71-76.

7 Pantell RH, Stewart TJ, Diaz JK, et al: Physician communication with children and parents. *Pediatrics* 1982;70:396-402.

8 Catlin RJO: Does the doctor understand what I am asking? *Am J Pubic Health* 1981; 71:123-124.

9 Starfield B, Wray C, Hess K, et al: The influence of patient-practitioner agreement on outcome of care. *Am J Public Health* 1981; 71:127-131.

10 Byrne P, Long B: *Doctors Talking to Patients.* London, Her Majesty's Stationery Office, 1976.

11 Korsch BM, Gozzi EK, Francis V: Gaps in doctor-patient communication: Doctor-patient interaction and patient satisfaction. *Pediatrics* 1968;42:855-871.

12 Francis V, Korach BM, Morris MJ: Gaps in doctor-patient communication: Patients' response to medical advice. *N Eng J Med* 1969;280:535-540.

13 Waitzkin H, Stoeckle JD: The communication of information about illness: Clinical, sociological, and methodological considerations. *Adv Psychosom Med* 1972;8:180-215

14 Frankel RM, Becksmith HA: Impact: An interaction-based method, in *Explorations in Provider and Patient Interactions.* Clifton, NJ, Humana Press. 1982.

15 Goldberg DP, Steele JJ, Smith C., et al: Training family doctors to recognize psychiatric illness with increased accuracy. *Lancet* 1980; 2:521-523.

16 Hippocrates: *On Decorum and the Physician.* London, Heinemann Medical Books, 1923, vol 2.

17 Petersdorf RG, Adams RD, Braunwald E, et al (eds): *Harrison's Principles of Internal Medicine.* New York, McGraw-Hill Book Co, 1983, pp 4-5.

18 Bok S: *Lying: Moral Choice in Public and Private Life*, New York, Vintage Books, 1979, pp 232-255.

Patients' views of these questions are usually clear-cut and unequivocal. Patients almost always want as much information as possible, and doctors often do not realize this. The misattribution of the desire for information is one of the most common errors in clinical practice. Moreover, doctors and patients frequently frame their communication on the basis of their unspoken perceptions concerning each other's expectations in the situation.[19] In framing their remarks, doctors may make benign judgments about what patients want to know or should know, but the basis of such judgments may be problematic.

Misattributions and Misperceptions.

For example, several studies of dying patients during the 1960s and 1970s have shown that the majority of doctors—between 69% and 90%, depending on the study—tend to withhold information from patients with fatal disease. Studies of patients' attitudes show equally high numbers who want information from their doctors. The great majority of normal patients, patients suffering from cancer, and family members of these patients wish to receive accurate information about their illnesses.[13] This is a paradoxical finding when compared with doctors' behavior.

Although the problems of dying patients are somewhat unique, patients with more run-of-the-mill problems also have difficulty getting the information that they want from doctors. This frustration has been reported numerous times, so a few examples will suffice. A recent study investigated the disclosure of information by neurologists to patients with epilepsy.[20] The vast majority of patients with seizures and parents of children with seizures wanted to be informed about all benefits and risks associated with medication, including rare side effects. On the other hand, a very small proportion of neurologists responded in a questionnaire that they routinely discuss each benefit and risk of medication. In framing their communication, doctors and patients may take quite different views of the desirable state of affairs.

Our own study of communication in medicine reached similar conclusions[21, 22, 23, 24, 25] (also, unpublished data, 1984). We constructed a random sample of practicing internists in Massachusetts and California and tape-recorded 336 encounters in several clinical settings, including private practice and hospital outpatient departments. Regarding information giving and withholding, we asked the doctors to rate each patient's desire for information and the helpfulness of giving the information; patients completed a self-rating based on the same seven-point scale. According to their responses, patients wanted to know almost everything and thought that the information would be helpful, but doctors underestimated the patients' desire for information and, when compared with the patients, underrated the clinical usefulness of information giving. In 65% of the encounters, doctors underestimated their patients' desire for information; in 6%, they overestimated; and in 29%, they estimated correctly.

---

19 Goffman E: *Frame Analysis: An Essay on the Organization of Experience.* New York, Harper & Row Publishers Inc, 1974.

20 Faden RR, Becker C, Lewis C, et al: Disclosure of information to patients in medical care. *Med Care* 1981;19:718-733.

21 Waitzkin H, Stoeckle JD: Information control and the micropolitics of health care. *Soc Sci Med* 1976;10:263-276.

22 Waitzkin H, Stoeckle JD, Beller E, et al: The informative process in medical care. *Instr Sci* 1978;7:385-419.

23 Waitzkin H: Medicine, superstructure, and micropolities. *Soc Sci Med* 1979;13A:601-609.

24 Wallen J, Waitzkin H, Stoeckle JD: Physician stereotypes about female health and illness: A study of patient's sex and the informative process during medical interviews. *Women Health* 1979;4:135-146.

25 Waitzkin H: *The Second Sickness: Contradictions of Capitalist Health Care.* New York, Free Press/Macmillan Publishing Co Inc, 1983, pp 137-183.

Time Spent in Information Giving.

One way that we looked at the transmittal of information was simply the amount of time devoted to the process. We found that doctors spent very little time giving information to their patients—a little more than a minute on the average in encounters lasting about 20 minutes. After the recorded encounters, we asked the doctors how much time they thought they devoted to information giving, and then we compared this perception to the actual time that we measured from the tape recordings. On the average, doctors overestimated the time they spent giving information by about a factor of nine. Doctors thought that they spent much more time informing their patients than they actually did.

We tried to relate doctors' information giving to other variables that we thought might be important. In this analysis, we looked at the time doctors spent informing patients. We also studied the number of explanations and the level of technicality of the explanations. Considering the clinical process of information transmittal, we thought that a possibly effective type of communication might involve the doctor's giving a technical explanation and then translating it into simpler terms. This was what we meant by "multilevel" explanations. "Nondiscrepant" responses were answers by doctors at the same level of technicality as patients' questions; we thought that this measure would reflect doctors' tendency to respond at a similar linguistic level, rather than "talking up" or "talking down" to the patients. The following paragraphs present some highlights of our multivariate analysis.

Patients' Charteristics.

First, we assessed the relationships between information transmittal and patients' characteristics. We expected an association between information giving and *patients' sex*. Based on feminist critiques of medicine, we thought that doctors might give less information to women patients. The findings were just the reverse. Women received more doctor time, more total explanations, more multilevel explanations, and more nondiscrepant responses. This finding may reflect sexual differences in language use, as described in the sociolinguistic literature.[26, 27, 28, 29] Women also tended to ask more questions and generally to engage in more verbal behavior within the encounters that we studied.

Patients' education and *social class* (measured by occupation) also were predictors of doctors' tendency to give them information. College educated patients tended to receive more information, measured in each of the four ways, than patients who did not go to college. Patients from upper- or upper-middle positions received more doctor time, more total explanations, more multilevel explanations and more nondiscrepant responses than did patients from lower-middle or lower-class backgrounds. There was no difference between poorly educated, lower-class patients and better educated, upper-class patients in their desire for information. However, doctors misperceived this desire much more commonly for poorly educated or lower-class patients. This observation confirmed what other researchers already had observed—lower-class patients tend to be diffident, that is, they usually ask fewer questions.[13, 30, 31, 32] Partly as a result, doctors tend to

26 Lakoff R: *Language and Woman's Place*. New York, Harper & Row Publishers Inc, 1975.

27 Henley N: *Body Politics: Power, Sex and Nonverbal Communication*. Englewood Cliffs, NJ, Prentice-Hall Inc, 1977.

28 Thorne B, Henley N (eds): *Language and Sex: Difference and Dominance*. Rowley, Mass, Newbury House Publications Inc, 1975.

29 Fishman PM: Interaction: The work women do. *Soc Probl* 1978;25:397-406.

30 Cartwright A: *Human Relations and Hospital Care*. London, Routledge & Kegan Paul Ltd, 1964.

31 Bernstein B (ed): *Class, Codes and ControL: Applied Studies Towards a Sociology of Language*. London, Routledge & Kegan Paul Ltd, 1973.

misperceive their patients' desire for information and generally believe that they want or could use less information. This finding is clinically important; lower class patients want more information than we may think, and their diffedence reinforces a structural barrier to communication in doctor-patient encounters.

We also looked at the *certainty of patients' diagnoses*, their *prognoses*, and the *certainty of prognoses*. Many writers have emphasized uncertainty as a fundamental part of medical practice, and we wanted to see how uncertainty related to information giving. We found that high uncertainty, as determined by questionnaire, was positively related to information giving; the more uncertain doctors were about diagnosis and prognosis, the more information-giving behavior that they tended to show, although the relationship was weak statistically. On the other hand, patients' prognosis was a fairly strong predictor of information giving. Patients with an unfavorable prognosis tended to get more doctor time, more total explanations, more multilevel explanations, and more nondiscrepant responses. Only ten patients in our sample had cancer or other potentially fatal illnesses. Poor prognosis usually did not mean that patients were dying. For this reason, the results did not necessarily contradict the findings of previous studies that doctors tend to withhold information from patients with fatal diseases. The earlier pattern of information withholding also may be changing over time, as clinicians' concern with the problems of death and dying increases. In either case, poor prognosis in itself did not seem to impede doctors from giving information.

Doctors' Characteristics.

Regarding doctors' characteristics, there was an apparent association between doctors' information giving and their own *social-class backgrounds*. Doctors who came from an upper- or uppermiddle-class background tended to spend more time informing their patients, gave more explanations, and provided more nondiscrepant responses than doctors from a lower middle-class or lower-class background. This finding was noteworthy in view of the observed diffidence of lower-class people. More orientation to verbal behavior may be a class-linked phenomenon that affects doctors as well as patients. Doctors' verbal behavior seems to differ, associated in part with their varying class backgrounds.

The *income* of the internists in our sample was a strong predictor of their informative behavior. Doctors who earned less money tended to spend more time informing their patients, gave more explanations, offered more multilevel explanations, and gave more nondiscrepant responses. The inverse relationship between income and information giving probably had to do with wealthier doctors' seeing more *patients per day*. Doctors who saw more than 20 outpatients per day spent much less time giving information and also gave a smaller number of explanations. Although the differences were large, they were more or less what we would expect; doctors who had less time to spend because they were busy did spend less time. On the other hand, a busy practice also was related to the manner of communicating. Busier doctors gave fewer multilevel and nondiscrepant explanations. This finding also was pertinent for clinical practice. Information giving takes time. We cannot expect it to go well if we are too busy. Alternatively, individual practitioners or the institutions for which they work may be willing to make this sacrifice in the interest of patient census. If the sacrifice is made, however, it probably should be a more explicit decision than it has been until now.

---

32 Shapiro MC, Najman JM, Chang A, et al: Information control and the exercise of power in the obstetrical encounter. *Soc Sci Med* 1983: 17:139-146.

We also studied the association between doctors' *general attitudes* toward information giving, as measured by the questionnaire, and their actual behavior, as manifested in the tape recordings. There was little clear-cut relationship between attitudes and behavior; this was an important negative finding. Besides looking at general attitudes toward information giving, we asked doctors what their *specific perception* were of patients' desire for information and how helpful information giving would be for the patients' progress. Doctors' perceptions were good predictors of the time that they spent communicating and the multilevel explanations that they gave, but the relationship did not hold for number of explanations or for nondiscrepant responses. Although doctors' perceptions of their patients' concerns tended to predict doctors' actual behavior, we should remember that doctors' perceptions were inaccurate the majority of the time. One clinical implication is that we need to find a way to increase doctors' perceptual sensitivity to patients' needs for information, and to let doctors know that patients often want more information than doctors perceive that they do.

Nonverbal Communication

In making a transition from verbal to nonverbal communication, I will refer briefly to research methods that have been used for many years in the social sciences to study interaction. This approach, called "interaction process analysis," employs tape-recorded encounters between patients and doctors and asks judges to code the interaction into categories such "doctor gives orientation," "patient shows antagonism," "doctor shows tension release," and so forth. The researchers then obtain a statistical distribution of the categories of interaction for each encounter, and next they try to relate these findings to outcomes of medical care such compliance and satisfaction.[33, 34]

Tension and Anxiety.

Using these techniques, Carter and coworkers[35] found some results that were not intuitively obvious. Contrary to what might be expected, patients' satisfaction seemed to increase when patients themselves showed tension, anxiety, and nervousness, and also when doctors showed tension or antagonism. The researchers noted that doctors' tension-laden statements complaining about the organization (or, one might say, disorganization) of the Veterans Administration clinic where the study was done were associate with patients' dissatisfaction. But tension-laden statements that occurred when the doctor were conveying sensitive information about the patients' conditions were associated with patients' satisfaction. The findings indicated that patients appreciated the chance to express tension themselves (this might have been part of the cathartic function of the encounter) and that they also were satisfied by doctors' expression of tension in combination with the information that doctors conveyed. Therefore, patients often may not want their doctors to say that everything is all right with a carefree statement ignoring the tension that is present.

Other studies of nonverbal communication support this inference. Research in this area has employed an electronic device that filters out the words that are said in tape-recorded interaction but leaves the nonverbal tone of voice. Judges

---

33 Roter DL: Patient participation in the patient-provider interaction: The effects of patient question making on the quality of interaction, satisfaction, and compliance. *Health Educ Monogr* 1977;5:281-315.

34 Wasserman RC, Inui TS: Systematic analysis of clinician-patient interactions: Recent approaches with suggestions for future research. *Med Care* 1983;21:279-293.

35 Carter WB, Inui TS, Kukull WA, et al: Outcome-based doctor-patient interaction analysis: II. Identifying effective provider and patient behavior. *Med Care* 1982;W.550-566.

then can rate this filtered speech for the emotions that are conveyed in the conversation, separately from the verbal content.

Using this technique, Hall and Rosenthal and their colleagues[36, 37] produced some provocative observations. They audiotaped doctor-patient encounters, prepared written transcripts of the sessions, and also created filtered speech for each encounter. They asked judges to rate each transcript, each unfiltered encounter, and each filtered encounter for a number of emotions. Then they tried to see if there was an association between the ratings and outcomes such as satisfaction and compliance. They found that doctors' anxiety as rated in the transcripts (that is, from the verbal content only) was negatively associated with patients' satisfaction, that doctors' sympathetic qualities in the transcripts were positively associated, and that doctors' anger and anxiety in the filtered speech were positively associated. The researchers also found that doctors' anger and anxiety as rated from the original audiotapes were positively associated with patients' subsequent compliance.

Hall and Rosenthal and colleagues argue that patients' satisfaction and possibly compliance seem related to both reassuring words by doctors and to an angry or anxious tone of voice. The investigators claim that the unsaid message conveyed by positive words and negative tone is a strong task orientation toward patients' concerns; patients appear to respond favorably to this orientation. They also point out that patients' perceptions of doctors' seriousness about the importance of patients' concerns may be at odds with the perception of doctors' friendliness, and that perceived seriousness apparently is a stronger predictor of patients' satisfaction.

Nonverbal Communication Skills.

Doctor's nonverbal abilities, both to recognize nonverbal cues from patients and successfully to convey nonverbal messages, also affect satisfaction. A study by DiMatteo and Friedman and their colleagues[38, 39, 40] made this point by testing the nonverbal abilities of residents in internal medicine through the Profile of Nonverbal Sensitivity (PONS) test. This test had been developed previously and determined to be both valid and reliable. In this study, the residents were requested to state what kinds of emotions were conveyed in a film that they observed. In addition to the PONS test, the residents were given a test of nonverbal encoding ability. They were asked to record sentences conveying the emotions of happiness, sadness, anger, and surprise; these recordings then were given to judges, who rated them blindly according to the emotion that they thought was being communicated. The researchers also assessed the satisfaction of patients whom the residents were seeing in their practices, by a completely different questionnaire.

DiMatteo and Friedman and coworkers found that patients tended to be satisfied if their residents were skilled at decoding body movement and postural cues to emotion (that is, if they scored high on the "body channel" portion of the PONS test). The researchers also learned that residents who could successfully encode emotions themselves had patients who were more

---

36 Hall JA, Rotor DL, Rand CS: Communication of affect between patient and physician. *J Health Soc Behav* 1981;22:18-30.

37 Rosenthal R, Hall JA, DiMatteo MR, et al: *Sensitivity of Nonverbal Communication: The PONS Test*, Baltimore, Johns Hopkins University Press, 1979.

38 DiMatteo MR, Taranta A, Friedman HS, et al: Predicting patient satisfaction from physicians' nonverbal communication skills. *Med Care* 1980;18:376-387.

39 DiMatteo, MR: A social-psychological analysis of physician-patient rapport: Toward a science of the art of medicine. *J Soc Issues* 1979;35;12-33.

40 Friedman HS: Nonverbal communication between patients and medical practitioners. *J Soc Issues* 1979;35:82-99.

satisfied; if residents could not communicate emotions well, their patients tended to be less satisfied. These findings were replicated in two separate research protocols, conducted about one year apart. DiMatteo has subsequently found, in preliminary research still in progress, that residents can be taught these nonverbal skills and that their interaction with patients changes accordingly. That training can improve the subtleties of nonverbal communication is one of the most hopeful findings to emerge from this difficult field of research, which DiMatteo has called the "science of the art of medicine."[39]

Sociolinguistic Structure of Medical Communication

In medical school and residency training, practitioners learn the many questions that they presumably need to ask in taking a medical history. Some doctors later continue to ask these many questions throughout their careers, but others find themselves asking fewer and fewer questions as time goes on. As research in sociolinguistics has shown, the interrogative mode is a subtly dominating format.[41] Asking many questions usually is the prerogative of a person in power, just as interrupting is.

High-Control Style

The "high-control style" is one of Platt and McMath's[3] examples of "clinical hypocompetence" in internal medicine. The doctor asks many questions, keeping tight control over the interaction, but not letting the patient speak at any length. The patient's subsequent complaint, that the doctor "doesn't listen to me," corresponds closely to the reality of the encounter. Usually there is no need for this degree of control, and open-ended questions often lead to more suitable information, as well " the patient's sense that he or she is being heard. In similar research, Coulthard and Ashby[42] have confirmed the detrimental impact of frequent interruptions and the high-control style. Sociolinguistic studies by Frankel[43, 44] and West[45] have shown that the vast majority of questions within doctor-patient encounters (between 80% and 95% in the encounters studied) are doctor initiated. Doctors pose questions frequently. Usually, but not always, these questions pertain to the medical history. Doctors rarely explain the questions' rationale to patients, who often become confused or mystified about the purpose of the questions. These investigators have concluded that in doctor-patient encounters there is a "dispreference" for patient-initiated questions; this dispreference persists despite doctors' formal query, usually as the interview concludes, "Are there any questions?"

Interruptions and Sex.

One other important study of sociolinguistic structure focused on sexual differences between male and female doctors. West[46] looked at doctors' interruption behavior and found that doctors

---

41 Mishler EG: Studies in dialogue and discourse: II. Types of discourse initiated and sustained throughout questioning. *J Psycholinguist Res* 1975;4:99-121.

42 Coulthard M, Ashby M: Talking with the doctor. *J Commun* 1975;25:140-147.

43 Frankel RM: Talking in interviews: A dispreference for patient-initiated questions in physician-patient encounters, in Psathas G (ed): *Interaction Competence*. New York, Irvington Publications Inc. 1983.

44 Frankel RM: The laying on of hands: Aspects of the organization of gaze, touch, and talk in a medical encounter, in Fisher S, Todd AD (eds): *The Social Organization of Doctor-Patient Communication*, Washington, DC, Center for Applied Linguistics, 1983.

45 West C: 'Ask me no questions. . . .: An analysis of queries and replies in physician-patient dialogues, in Fisher S, Todd AD (eds): *The Social Organization of Doctor-Patient Communication*. Washington, DC, Center for Applied Linguistics, 1983.

interrupted patients a great deal. Studying physicians in family medicine, West noted that male doctors, an expected, interrupted patients much more than patients interrupted them. Male doctors initiated more than two thirds of the interruptions that were observed, and the only exception, when a patient interrupted more, involved a mentally retarded patient. Remarkably, female doctors interrupted their patients to a much lesser degree—between 8% and 50% of the time. Male patients of female doctors interrupted more than the doctors interrupted; interruptions were almost evenly divided in encounters when both patients and doctors were women.

Many studies in sociolinguistics have shown that interruptions are dominance gestures. They tend to be initiated by whatever party in a conversation holds a dominant position (for example, a teacher tends to interrupt a student, a parent tends to interrupt a child).[47, 48] Although West's findings deserve replication, it appears that doctors tend to interrupt patients, except when the doctor is a woman. This observation may have some interesting implications for future changes in doctor-patient communication as the proportion of female doctors increases.

Voices in the Medical Encounter.

From a similar viewpoint, Mishler[49] has used audiotapes from our own research on doctor-patient encounters to study their sociolinguistic structure. Mishler theorizes that there are typically two voices in the medical encounter. One is the "voice of medicine." In this voice, the doctor tries to get the patient to give a history that meets the technical requirements of diagnosis, treatment, and record keeping. The voice of medicine is involved in repetitive questioning, getting the patient back on track during the medical history, and maintaining the high-control style. On the other hand, the "voice of the life world" has to do with the patient's concerns about everyday life. These concerns do not always fit neatly into the format of history taking. At various points in medical encounters, the voice of the life world interrupts the voice of medicine, but often not very successfully.

Learning the standards of medical history taking involves a set of cognitive processes in the practitioner that are different from those the patient brings to the medical encounter. The drive for thoroughness and technical comprehension that is internalized during medial education may interfere with practitioners' sensitivity to patients' needs. This difficulty may express itself through the sociolinguistic structure of doctor-patient communication. Sometimes, then, a practitioner might want to forget about the voice of medicine when he or she hears the voice of the life world trying to make itself heard.

Conclusion

From the last decade of social scientific research, we have learned that doctor-patient communication is neither as smooth as practitioners sometimes assume nor as disastrous as critics commonly portray. A variety of studies have reported the dismal side of communication in medicine. Improvement is not only desirable but also possible, and training programs should emphasize these potentialities.

In the first place, it is important to enhance practitioners' perception of patients' need for effective communication and to promote a con-

46 West C: When the doctor is a 'lady': Power, status and gender in physician-patient dialogues, in Stromberg A (ed): *Women, Health and Medicine.* Palo Alto, Calif, Mayfield Publishing Co, in press.

47 West C, Zimmerman DH: Women's place in everyday talk: Reflections on parent-child interaction. *Soc Probl* 1977;24:521-529.

48 West C: Against our will: Male interruptions of females in cross-sex conversation. *Ann NY Acad Sci* 1979,327:81-97.

49 Mishler EG: *The Discourse of Medicine: Dialects of Medical Interviews*, Norwood, NJ. Ablex Publishing Co, in press.

sciousness about the communicative process. Many studies have clearly shown that doctors tend to underestimate their patients' desire for full information about illness and treatment. Practitioners also tend to misperceive the time that they spend informing patients and the nature of the information that they do transmit. Educational programs should teach that patients frequently want more information than practitioners perceive that they do. In training and probably at regular intervals during subsequent practice, doctors also should accept the opportunity of hearing and seeing themselves in recorded interaction with their patients. Through this technique, practitioners can sharpen their perceptions of their own communicative skills and can observe the discrepancy between perceptions and reality.

In seeking to improve communication, medical practitioners should become more aware of sociolinguistic differences in language use. Specific research findings have clarified the social-class differences in communication within medical encounters. In general, upper-class and upper-middle-class patients tend to be more verbal in their interactions with physicians than are patients from lower-middle-class and lower-class positions. The latter patients tend to be diffidence in asking direct questions to obtain information. Because of such differences in language use, practitioners may assume that lower-middle-class and lower-class patients want less information. Several studies have demonstrated, however, that there are no major social-class differences in the desire for full information communicated in comprehensible terms. Sociolinguistic research outside the field of medicine has confirmed the profound associations between social class and language use.[50, 51] The diffidence of lower-middle-class and lower-class patients in asking questions is only one manifestation of sociolinguistic barriers to communication. Practitioners should be knowledgeable about the reluctance to ask questions among patients from lower-middle-class and lower-class positions and should increase the information that they provide spontaneously to the patients.

Sexual differences in language use also create certain problems in doctor-patient interaction. Women patients tend to receive more information than men, probably because of a greater tendency to ask direct questions. In addition, both as practitioners and as patients, women tend to receive more interruptions during medical encounters than men do. Women's tendency to ask more questions yet to receive more interruptions may be partially responsible for frustration in medical encounters that involve male practitioners and female patients. As the sexual composition of the medical profession changes, the nature of doctor-patient communication also may change, and it will be interesting to assess this possibility in subsequent research.

Nonverbal communication skills in medical encounters are as important as verbal skills, if not more so. Some of the most innovative research on doctor-patient communication has disclosed unexpected and occasionally counterintuitive findings. Practitioners' expression of tension and an anxious tone of voice appear to be positively associated with patients' satisfaction and possibly compliance. The reasons for these preliminary findings need further clarification, but may reflect patients' perception that their concerns are taken seriously. Practitioners who are skillful in understanding and transmitting emotions nonverbally are more successful in satisfying their patients. There is evidence that then nonverbal communication skills can be taught, so that practitioners' capabilities can be improved.

---

50 Bernstein B: *Class, Codes and Control: Towards a Theory of Educational Transmission.* London, Routledge and Kegan Paul Ltd, 1977.

51 Dittmar N: *A Critical Survey of Sociolinguistics.* New York, St Martin's Press Inc, 1976.

The sociolinguistic structure of medical communication needs rethinking. Standards of thoroughness in clinical history taking encourage a style of high control, frequent interruptions initiated by practitioners, and deemphasis of patients' concerns that do not contribute to diagnosis and treatment. As shown in research outside medicine, the interrogative mode is a format that is subtly dominating.[41] In medical encounters, this format can interfere with a mutual exchange of information and can create dissatisfaction as patients' concerns are overlooked. To the extent that it impedes adequate communication, the traditional medical history deserves reconsideration.

Communicating well is an important part of practicing medicine. Previously, practitioners often have paid lip service to doctor-patient communication, have felt that it is someone else's problem, and have immersed themselves in the technical challenges of practice. The common assumption has been that communication is either too obvious or too mysterious to justify much detailed attention. Communication, as well as trying to improve it, requires time. Conditions of practice may interfere with taking this time, and it is doubtful that these constraints will disappear in the future. On the other hand, patients have become more articulate in their expectations of effective communication with doctors. The social sciences have provided some useful techniques and discoveries. Improvement of doctor-patient communication demands a combination of humility and courage, in short, the best qualities of medical work.

Evaluating the Patient's Primary Problem(s)

Richard Frankel and Howard Beckman

Introduction

Despite the technological advances of the past 20 years, many consumers are dissatisfied with the health care they receive. This dissatisfaction manifests itself as noncompliance with treatment recommendations, malpractice litigation, the use of nontraditional health care providers, anger over waiting time, and frustration with the quality of interactions with physicians. Medical educators and practitioners have become aware that the physician-patient relationship in general, and the office consultation in particular, require improvement. This chapter reviews research on patient-centered interviewing and describes the tasks and skills necessary to identify and evaluate the patient's primary problems.

The American Board of Internal Medicine (1983) issued a statement describing the humanistic qualities required of the internist and guidelines for their evaluation in practice. Similarly, Lipkin, et al. (1984), representing the SGIM Task Force on the Medical Interview, published a model curriculum for teaching interviewing skills to internal medicine residents.

As interest in patient-centered interviewing and patient involvement in care has grown, so too has criticism of the classical biomedical model of disease. Barsky (1981) has observed, for instance, that patients seek the care of a physician for many reasons, only one of which is disease. Patients also seek physician consultation for life stress, psychiatric illness, social isolation, and, increasingly, education. Often the physician is perceived as the only person available to listen to and comfort distressed patients of all ages.

In 1977, George Engel [see in this volume] proposed the biopsychosocial model of care, which identifies psychological and sociological factors that accompany and contribute to the expression of disease and to the patient's decision to seek medical care. The model gives equal weight to biomedical and psychosocial factors in the presentation of a problem and distinguishes between disease (a pathological condition of the organism) and illness (the individual's social or psychological response to disease).

Besides recognizing the interrelationship of biological, psychological, and sociological factors, the biopsychosocial model contrasts with the physician-centered interviewing style that dominates the delivery of most medical care in the United States today. Specifically, the model challenges the assumption that the patient is merely a conduit for the extraction of clinical information, regardless of the physician's interviewing style. Current research demonstrates that the quantity, quality, and impact of information obtained during the medical encounter is related to the interviewer's style, interest, and involvement (Beckman and Frankel, 1984; Greenfield,

Frankel and Beckman (1989) Evaluating the patient's primary problem(s). M. Steward and D. Roter, COMMUNICATING WITH MEDICAL PATIENTS (p. 86-98). Reprinted by permission of Sage Publications, Inc.

et al., 1985; Headache Study Group, 1986; Roter, et al., 1987; Suchman and Matthews, 1988).

The type of interviewing that best facilitates use of the biopsychosocial model has been variously termed mutual participation (Morgan, and Engel, 1969), co-participation (Quill, 1983), and patient-centered interviewing (Stewart, 1984). These approaches are unique in viewing patients and physicians as individuals who mutually participate and influence one another during the medical encounter. The physician brings technical knowledge and clinical experience to the relationship; the patient brings his or her life experiences, health beliefs, and goals for service. The success of the encounter depends largely on the skill of clinical negotiation and the development of mutual respect and trust (Benarde and Mayerson, 1978; Brody, 1980; Lazare, et al., 1975a; Siegler, 1982). This discussion focuses on skills and methods that use negotiation as a primary strategy for opening the medical encounter.

We define the opening of the interview—one of its most important components—as the initial greeting, solicitation, and evaluation of the patient's primary concern(s). Whether a new or return visit, this portion of the interview should focus on those problems and concerns that both provider and patient agree are important. The accurate recognition of the primary concern(s) or problems(s) is central to providing care that will be relevant, satisfying, and medically sound.

The tasks of the opening segment of the interview are to:

1. define the specific concern(s) or problem(s) for which the patient seeks professional guidance;
2. understand the concerns in the context of the patient's life circumstances;
3. develop rapport with the patient, paving the way for a successful therapeutic outcome;
4. satisfy both participants by creating a therapeutic alliance;
5. utilize time efficiently.

Determining the Primary Problem(s)

One of the most complex tasks in evaluating the patient's primary problem(s) is accurate determination of the reason or reasons that the patient seeks medical care. Traditional medical education teaches that there is a single chief complaint. This assumption appears to cause tremendous difficulty in medical interviewing. In reviewing hundreds of transcripts, simulated patient interviews, and videotapes, we have observed several problems with the chief complaint model. The most common problem is that the provider assumes the first concern voiced by the patient is the chief complaint.

In a recently published study of opening moments in physician-patient encounters, Beckman and Frankel (1984) observed that patient responses to the physician's opening solicitation were completed in only 23% of 74 visits studied. In 6 return visits, no solicitation for concerns was made, and the provider began the encounter by focusing on identified problems from earlier visits. In 51 (69%) of the visits, the physician interrupted the patient's opening statement—after a mean time of only 18 seconds—and directed questions toward a specific concern. Importantly, in only one of these 51 visits was the patient afforded the opportunity to return to, and complete, his or her opening statement, i.e., the concerns for which they sought care.

Since 34 of the 51 visits were interrupted after the patient's initial concern, we hypothesized that the interrupting physicians assumed that the patient's first complaint was the chief one and began, at that point, to obtain the history of the present illness. To test this hypothesis, a group of internists, blinded to the nature of our study, were asked to rate the clinical importance of an abstracted list of all the concerns expressed in the 74 visits. They rated concerns that occurred first, second, and third in the patient statements as equally important clinically. We concluded that serial order is not related to the clinical importance of patient concerns, rejecting the hypothesis that the patient's first stated concern is more important than subsequent concerns.

These data also explain why Burack and Carpenter (1983) found that patients typically wait to share psychosocial concerns until late in the visit and that patients and doctors agree on the chief complaint in only 76% of somatic problems and 6% of psychosocial problems. In summary, physicians, both in training and in practice, often make implicit assumptions about the patient's chief complaint, most often without soliciting the patient's full range of concerns or priorities for treatment.

These findings are also consistent with the recommendations of Lipkin et al. (1984), who suggested that listening helps to elicit the full range and priority of patient concerns, and Nardone, et al. (1980), who suggested symptom lists rather than a chief complaint, to avoid premature and limited hypothesis testing. Several other investigators report findings showing that patients often have more than one concern to discuss (Good and Good, 1982; Greenfield, et al., 1985; Starfield et al., 1981; Wasserman, et al., 1984). The mean number of concerns in these studies ranges from 1.2 to 3.9 in both new and return office visits.

Platt and McMath (1979) have observed that one cause of "clinical hypocompetence" in interviewing is the failure to consider more than a single problem, and suggest asking "Anything else?" or "What else?" after each item in the patient's opening statement. We find that completion can be facilitated by either remaining silent or employing acknowledgment tokens such as "mmh hmh," "okay, or "I see" until the patient indicates the end of the statement of concerns. The following example shows that, given sufficient time and opportunity, the patient will mark the conclusion of his or her opening statement of concerns.

Physician: What problems are you having?

Patient: My back has been hurting me, I've had headaches for three weeks, and recently I have been having a hurting in my chest which causes me to have to sit down after I've walked only half a block.

(1.0 second pause)

Physician: Go on.

Patient: That's all I wanted to talk about today.

Barriers to completion of patients' statements of concerns have also been identified. Beckman and Frankel (1984), for example, found that recompleters, defined as repetition of the content or sense of the patient's previous statement, interrupted the patient's full enumeration of concerns. For example, if a physician responds, "You have chest pain?" to a patient's initial statement, "I have chest pain," this will usually lead to a series of closed-ended questions that terminate the solicitation of the presenting complaint and begin the history of present illness segment. In our study, recompleters accounted for 35% of the interruptions of patients' opening statements. Other causes of interruption were closed-ended questions (46%), elaborators (10%), and statements (10%). Although recompleters are regarded as generic facilitators in most interviewing texts, our findings suggest that their benefit depends on their location in the encounter.

Concern over the time required to permit patients to fully express their concerns is frequently cited as a barrier to more open-ended facilitation. In fact, we found (Beckman and Frankel, 1984) that no completed opening statement took more than 150 seconds. Although physicians may believe that patients will discuss their problems indefinitely if given the opportunity, there is evidence to the contrary, as the following example of an actual completed opening statement shows:

Physician: How have you been doing?

Patient: Oh, well, I've been doing okay, except for Saturday, well, Sunday night. You know I've been kinda nervous off and on but I had a little incident in my house Saturday and it kinda shook me up a bit.

➡Physician: Okay.

Patient: And my ulcer has been burning me off and on like when I eat something if it don't agree with me then I'll find out about it.

➡Physician: Mmh hmh.

Patient: But lately I've been getting this funny, like I'll lay down on my back and my heart will go "brrr," you know like that like it's skipping a beat or something and then it will just start on back off beating like when I get upset it will just start beating boom, boom, boom and it will just go back to its normal beat.

➡Physician: Okay.

Patient: Is that normal?

Physician: That's a lot of things. Anything else bothering you?

Patient: No.

This exchange took less than 60 seconds. It required three acknowledgment statements (indicated by arrows in the transcript) and a question by the physician to confirm that the patient was finished. In that short period of time the patient provided a cohesive and uninterrupted statement of concerns and, in so doing, stated her agenda for the day's visit. Interrupting the patient before she had completed her statement would have given the physician an incomplete picture of the patient's needs, preventing him from effectively using the time allotted for the visit. With a complete statement of concerns the physician could understand the range of patient concerns, develop a short- and long-run plan, and negotiate which problems were of primary importance so that time could be appropriately allotted to deal first with those issues that required the most attention.

In addition to more effectively organizing the visit, there is evidence that eliciting the full range of concerns early in the visit reduces the occurrence of late concerns that Barsky (1981) has termed "hidden" agendas. Although some patients may hesitate in sharing concerns they perceive as psychosocially sensitive early in the visit, Beckman, et al. (1985) found that patients who completed their statement of concern in the opening moments of the encounter were significantly less likely to raise concerns toward the end of the visit.

At the conclusion of a successful opening, the physician should have determined the spectrum of available concerns that the patient chose to offer and defined the concerns so that an agenda may be established. Rapport is facilitated by politeness, mutuality, and positive regard for the patient's input and point of view. Achieving rapport early in a relationship is useful in treatment planning and negotiation, and may actually influence the outcome of care. At the conclusion of a successful opening, the physician is ideally situated to begin the evaluation of the concern or concerns that both participants believe are most important.

Evaluation of Primary Concerns(s)

Nardone et al. (1980) have conceptualized the information necessary to evaluate the patient's primary concern(s). They view this portion of the interview as having three overlapping components: content, context, and conduct.

Content

In 1969, Morgan and Engel described seven logical dimensions for evaluating symptoms: chronology, bodily location, quality, quantity, setting, aggravating and alleviating, factors and associated symptoms. Reiser and Schroder (1980) in their text, *Patient Interviewing: The Human Dimension,* described the order in which dimensions of the symptom should be evaluated. While useful for structuring written histories and case presentations, rigid adherence to logical structure may be a barrier to data collection. Nardone et al. (1980) and Beckman and Frankel

(1984) noted that the logic of clinical decision making is often stressed in texts on interviewing without regard for context or logic of social interaction within which information is gathered. Many interviews are flawed by inattention to patients' signals of concern about a particular aspect of their problem. When interviewers use sequences of closed-ended questions organized exclusively around the seven dimensions of a symptom, they often prevent the patient from elaborating, questioning the meaning of an aspect of a problem, or providing their own attribution for the problem.

Teachers of interviewing must recognize the organization of the seven dimensions of a symptom as relevant to post interview activities such as presentations and written history taking, but that in the elicitation of the history, the interview should flow from the patient's descriptions of these dimensions. As an example, a physician begins the evaluation segment of the interview by asking, "When did your chest pain begin?' The patient responds, "Three days ago." The physician then asks, "Can you show me where the chest pain bothers you most?" By overdirecting the questioning, an important component of chronology has been ignored. In the following example, encouraging the patient to elaborate on the question of chronology produces a clinically important piece of information.

> Physician: When did this chest pain begin?
>
> Patient: About three days ago.
>
> Physician: Go on.
>
> Patient: That was when I was working in the backyard. I lifted five 100-pound bags of concrete and developed this pulling in my chest.

We consider all patient responses as potentially complex rather than simple. In soliciting information about aggravating factors, for example, we suggest that the interviewer resolicit (indicated by arrows in the transcript) after the patient offers one or more aggravators. For example:

> Physician: What have you found that makes your headaches worse?
>
> Patient: Lack of sleep.
>
> ➡Physician: Anything else?
>
> Patient: Now that you mention it, I believe that stress seems to be related also because by the end of the work day I usually have a headache.
>
> ➡Physician:Anything else?
>
> Patient: No.
>
> Physician: Is them anything that relieves your headaches?

Elaboration of the initial description produces clinically relevant information about the context of the symptom.

Lazare et al. (1975) suggested two additional components: the patient's goal for seeking care and the patient's request to the provider. Lazare defined the goal for care as the outcome the patient would like to achieve as a result of treatment, and the request as the method or means by which the patient would like the provider to be of help. Lazare hypothesized that eliciting and fulfilling the patient's goal(s) and request(s) will produce increased satisfaction, compliance, and ultimately clinical improvement. Starfield et al. (1979) found that patients reported improvement in problems in 49.4% of visits where there was agreement between physician and patient, and only 26.7% improvement in cases where the physician alone identified the problem as important.

Good and Good (1982) evaluated 460 office visits to four different practices and found 13 major request categories. Although requests varied depending on the practice site, 61% to 96% of patients wanted an explanation for their symptoms and results of laboratory tests, and had requests for symptomatic treatment, medical advice, and/or a diagnosis. In a subgroup from a holistic health center, the most commonly expressed patient goal was to share their experience of a problem with, and to receive a sense of being cared for from, a responsive physician. In fact, soliciting the patient's request often simplifies the physician's job because the patient's desire for help is more limited than the physician assumes.

Context

All problems, whether scientific or superstitious, exist within a system of beliefs, attitudes, and theories. The second component for evaluating a problem is identifying the emotional, social, and cultural milieu in which a problem occurs. Kleinman, et al. (1978) suggested that eliciting patient attitudes and beliefs about disease and treatment substantially increases therapeutic success. Snow (1974) counseled that understanding a patient's beliefs about a problem can help to generate for treatment, educate the patient, and prospectively identify potential therapeutic problems. Snow's description of the beliefs of southern rural blacks about hypertension has been instrumental in explaining why treatment often fails in urban areas where southern rural blacks have migrated (Snow, 1983). Kleinman et al. (1978) asserted that the consequences of neglecting the patient's view of the illness are noncompliance, dissatisfaction, litigation, criticism of the medical profession, and increased use of alternate health care providers. Their approach is especially important in determining the meaning of an illness to the patient and soliciting expectations for care. They suggested several useful questions to determine the impact of a problem on the patient's social and emotional context:

1. What do you think caused your problem?
2. Why do you think it started when it did?
3. How severe is your sickness?
4. What are the most important results you hope to achieve?
5. What do you fear most about your sickness?

We have found the solicitation of patients' attributions so important and useful in our own practice that we now teach it as the eighth major dimension of a symptom. We have also found that eliciting patient attributions increases participation in the process of care, demonstrates respect for the patient by including his or her perceptions of the problem, and helps to create a therapeutic alliance, one of the major goals of the consultation.

For example, a 46-year-old male presented in our clinic high blood pressure. A traditional evaluation was performed; he was diagnosed as having essential hypertension and was given hydrochlorothiazide and clonidine. He returned to the clinic monthly but his blood pressure continued to be elevated on each occasion. After three visits we asked the patient why his blood pressure was still elevated. He stated that he wasn't taking his medicine because it had nothing to do with the cause of his blood pressure. When asked what caused his high blood pressure, he said that a person had put a hex on him and that he was currently seeking its removal through a faith healer. We discussed the risks of sustained, uncontrolled hypertension and negotiated an interim treatment plan. The plan consisted of taking the medication until the healer had completed his healing program. When the healer concluded that the hex was removed, we would discontinue therapy for one month. If the high blood pressure was resolved, no further medical treatment would be considered. However, if his blood pressure continued to be elevated, he would agree to reinstitute his medical therapy. The patient was pleased with the plan and expressed relief at being able to share his explanation for his problem without being ridiculed. At the conclusion of the healer's intervention, we discontinued his medication. His blood pressure rose and, as agreed, he reinstated his medication. His blood pressure has been controlled for the past 18 months.

Seeing the problem in the patient's context often results in a major shift in the provider's conceptualization of the problem. In the evaluation of headache, for example, failure to address the complete context of the patient's concern often creates a barrier to successful communication. A patient who attributes headaches to a brain tumor, threatened stroke, or a subarachnoid hemorrhage, is unlikely to be satisfied by simple reassurance. Instead, some patients' fears are heightened by the fact that the physician did *not* explicitly refer to, or exclude, their particular theory or attribution.

Determining attribution, health beliefs, and expectations is best accomplished after the content of the problem has been established; otherwise many patients will conclude that the physician is unable to diagnose the problem. Equally important is the wording of the attribution question. Bass and Cohen (1982) found, for example, that when patients were asked "What *worries* you about this problem?," the majority of patients responded with, "I'm not worried." When the same patients were asked, "What *concerns* you about the problem?," more than a third (33.8%, N= 125) voiced previously unrecognized concerns.

The major challenge of added responsibility for exploring belief structures is, of course, time. Common sense and experience suggest, however, that time-intensive activities such as eliciting a complete data base, elaborating patient descriptions, and exploring attributions are far more efficient as predictors of effective long-term treatment and overall quality of care than a narrow, symptom-specific approach.

Conduct

Perhaps the most frequently investigated portion of the interview to date has been its conduct or dynamics. Investigators have studied behaviors that increase satisfaction, foster participation, and encourage honest open-ended interaction between physician and patient. In virtually all cases, patient satisfaction and physician "interest" have been positively related.

Carter et al. (1982) and Inui and Carter (1985), for instance, reviewed studies of behaviors associated with positive and negative outcomes. To summarize a few of the most widely recognized associations, Wasserman et al. (1984) found a highly significant association between empathy and patient satisfaction. They also found that encouraging statements were associated with increased patient satisfaction, and that use of these statements increased the perception of providers as a source of information and advice.

In terms of empathy, Francis et al. (1969) found that provider warmth was associated with increased patient satisfaction. Similarly, Stewart (1984) found an association between patient satisfaction and the opportunity to share opinions during the interview. In addition, Benarde et al. (1978) found a positive association between patient-provider respect, eye contact, question answering, and the physician's emotional sensitivity. Carter et al. (1982) also found a positive relationship between opinion sharing and patient knowledge about illness, and compliance with medical recommendations. They further found that patient satisfaction was correlated with the opportunity to give an orientation to the problem(s). Finally, Carter et al. (1982) found an association between the patient's understanding of the problem(s) and release of tension.

Although the literature supports these physician behaviors, a comprehensive model of the interview process has not yet been tested. As a result, systematic application of the research findings has been slow in coming. For example, in 1977, Roter, found a positive association between patient satisfaction and the opportunity to ask questions. Almost a decade later, West (1983) and Frankel (1987), in reviewing transcripts and tapes of primary care visits, observed that patient opportunities to ask questions were infrequent at best.

The skills of being patient-centered and interested in building rapport fundamentally challenge the notion of emotional neutrality in routine practice. Interviewers new to behaviors that demonstrate encouragement, empathy, transfer of control to the patient, and support may initially feel uncomfortable using the biopsychosocial model. Teachers of interviewing need to encourage and support learners as they explore new feelings and approaches to interviewing. There must also be positive reinforcement of behaviors that promote *interactional* rather than *individual* competence. Mutuality, respect, and compassion are dynamic concepts achievable only in the context of social interaction and social exchange.

Summary

In this chapter, we have addressed a relatively small, and specific, aspect of the medical encounter. Research is beginning to accumulate on other aspects of the encounter, such as compliance and the delivery of diagnostic information to patients, that depend on interactional skills and social context for their success. We have made great strides in developing theoretical frameworks for health care that are currently being adopted and taught in medical schools and postgraduate programs in primary care and family medicine. We are just beginning to understand the implications of the biopsychosocial model and its impact on the delivery of coordinated, comprehensive health care. The initial results are very encouraging, suggesting that enhanced communication between physicians and patients, and expanded understanding of the role of psychosocial factors in disease and illness will lead to better, more comprehensive, and mutually satisfying care in the future.

References

American Board of Internal Medicine (1983). *Annals of Internal Medicine*, 99, 720-724,

Barsky, A.J. (1981). Hidden reasons why some patients visit doctors. *Annals of Internal Medicine*, 94, 492-498.

Bass, L.W. & Cohen, R.L (1982). Ostensible versus actual reasons for seeking pediatric attention: another look at the parental ticket of admission. *Pediatrics*, 6, 870-874.

Beckman, H.B., & Frankel, R.M. (1984). The effect of physician behavior on the collection of data. *Annals of Internal Medicine*, 101, 692-696.

Beckman, H.B., Frankel, R.M., & Darnley, J. (1985). Soliciting the patients' complete agenda: A relationship to the distribution of concerns. *Clinical Research, 33,* 714A.

Benarade, M.A., & Mayerson, E.W. (1978). Patient-physician negotiations. *Journal of the American Medical Association*, 239, 1413-1415.

Brody, D.S. (1980). The patient's role in clinical decision-making. *Annals of Internal Medicine*, 93(5), 718-722.

Burack R.C. & Carpenter, R.R. (1983). The predictive value of the presenting complain. *Journal of Family Practice, 16,* 749-754.

Carter, W.B., Inui, T.S., Kukull, W., & Haigh, V. (1982). Outcome-based doctor-patient interaction analysis: II. Identifying effective provider and patient behavior. *Medical Care*, 20, 550-566.

Francis, V., Korsch, B.M., & Morris, N.J. (1969). Gaps in doctor-patient communication: Patients' response to medical advice. *New England Journal of Medicine*, 280, 535-540.

Frankel, R.M. (1987). Talking in interviews: A dispreference for patient initiated questions in physician-patient encounters. In G. Psathas (Ed.), *Interactional Competence*. New York: Irvingron.

Good, M.J.D., & Good, B.J. (1982). Patients requests in primary care clinics. In N.J. Crisnan & T.W. Maritzia (Eds.). *Clinically applied anthropology*. Boston: D. Reidel.

Greenfield S, Kaplan S, Ware Jr. (1985). Expanding patient involvement in care: effects on patient outcomes. *Annals of Internal Medicine*, 102, 520-528.

Headache Study Group of the University of Western Ontario. (1986). Prediction of outcome in headache patients presenting to family physicians - A one year prospective study. *Headache Journal*, 26(6), 285-294.

Inui, T.S. & Carter, W.R. (1985). Problems and prospects for health services research on provider-patient communication. *Medical Care, 23,* 521-538.

Kleinman, A., Eisenberg, L., & Good, B. (1978). Culture, illness and care: Clinical lessons from anthropologic and cross-cultural research. *Annals of Internal Medicine*, 88, 251-258.

Lazare, A., Eisenthal, E., & Wasserman, L. (1975). The customer approach to patienthood. *Archives of General Psychiatry, 32,* 553-558.

Lipkin, M., Jr., Quill, T.E., & Napodano, R.J. (1984). The medical interview: A core curriculum for residencies in internal medicine. *Annals of internal Medicine,* 100, 277-284.

Morgan, W.L., & Engel, G.L. (1969). *The clinical approach to the patient.* Philadelphia: W.B. Saunders.

Nardone, D.A., Reuler, J.B., & Girard, D.E. (1980). Teaching history-taking: Where are we? *Yale Journal of Biology and Medicine*, 53, 233-250.

Platt, F.W., & McMath, J.C. (1979). Clinical hypocompotence: The interview. *Annals of Internal Medicine,* 91, 898-902.

Quill, T.E. (1983). Partnerships in patient care: A contractual approach. *Annals of Internal Medicine*, 98, 228-234.

Roter, D.L., Hall, J.A., & Katz, N.R. (1987). Relations between physicians' behaviors and analogue patients satisfaction, recall, and impressions. *Medical Care*, 25; 135-154.

Siegler, M. (1982). The patient-physician accommodation: A central event in clinical medicine. *Annals of Internal Medicine*, 142, 1899-1902.

Snow, L.F. (1974). Folk medical beliefs and implications for care of patients. *Annals of Internal Medicine*, 81, 82-96.

Starfield, B., Wray, C., Hess, K. Gross, R., Birk, P.S., D'Lugoff, B.C. (1981). The influence of patient-practitioner agreement on outcome of care. *American Journal of Public Health*, 71(2), 127-132.

Stewart, M.A. (1984). What is a successful doctor-patient interview? A study of interactions and outcomes. *Social Science & Medicine*, 19, 167-175.

Suchman, A., & Mathews, D.A. (1988). What makes the patient-doctor relationship therapeutic? Exploring the connexional dimension of medical care. *Annals of Internal Medicine*, 108, 125-130.

Wasserman, R.C., Inui, T.S., Barriatua, R.D., Carter, W.B., & Lippencott, P. (1984). Pediatric clinician-patient interaction. *Pediatrics,* 74, 1047-1053.

West, C. (1983). "Ask me no questions..": An analysis of queries in physician-patient dialogues. In S. Fisher and A.D. Todd (Eds.), *The Social organization of Doctor-Patient Communication*, (pp. 75-106). Washington, DC: Center for Applied Linguistics.

Doctor Talk/Patient Talk: How Treatment Decisions Are Negotiated in Doctor-Patient Communication

Sue Fisher

Hysterectomies are performed at a higher rate than any other surgical procedure. The National Center for Health Statistics estimates that 794,000 women had hysterectomies in 1976, which represents a 15 % increase over the three previous years. In 1976, 10 out of every 1,000 women underwent this surgery. At the current rate, the Center notes, more than half the women in the U.S. will have their uteruses removed before they are 65 years old (National Center for Health Statistics 1976).

The increase in hysterectomies is a major problem. A 1976 congressional subcommittee estimated that in 1974, there were 2.4 2.4 million unnecessary surgeries at a high cost to the American public. The costs were more than monetary. Unnecessary surgery caused 11,900 deaths in 1975 ("Cost and Quality of Health Care" 1976). The death rate for hysterectomies is higher than the reported death rate for uterine/cervical cancer (Larned 1977). The American Cancer Society estimates that of the 46,000 cases of uterine or cervical cancer reported every year, 12,000 are fatal (Virginia Health Bulletin 1977). For hysterectomies, the fatality rate is 1,000 out of every one million. In addition the Cancer Society claims that the majority of these cancer deaths could be prevented with regular Pap smears and gynecological examinations (Larned 1977; Virginia Health Bulletin 1977).

Yet, these figures do not represent the psychosocial costs of hysterectomies. A 1973 English study found that within three years of having hysterectomies, one-third of the women studied were treated for depression (Caress 1977). Psychiatrists agree that a hysterectomy can often damage a woman's sense of identity. Larned reports Dr. Peter Barglow's findings that

> the hysterectomy is clearly and immediately visualized [by the patient] as an irreversible drastic procedure which removes an organ with high value in the ego's image of the body, as well as with considerable conscious value in the woman's sense of self and identity. Surely, the loss of an organ whose presence was reaffirmed monthly cannot be so easily denied. (Larned 1977:206)

Physicians believe that with adequate counseling, "well-adjusted" women can cope with hysterectomies (Larned 1977).

How are treatment decisions negotiated in practitioner-patient communication? How is the exchange of information in medical interviews organized, and how does that organization produce and constrain the negotiation of treatment

Fisher, S. (1983). Doctor talk/patient talk: How treatment decisions are negotiated in doctor-patient communication. In S. Fisher and A. D. Todd, (Eds.). THE SOCIAL ORGANIZATION OF DOCTOR PATIENT COMMUNICATION (pp. 135-157). Washington, D. C. Center for Applied Linguistics.

decisions? Given the asymmetry inherent in the doctor-patient relationship, medical practitioners not only have technical skills and medical knowledge that patients lack, but they also have the potential to control patients' access to and understanding of the information on which they will make their treatment decisions. This power imbalance increases when practitioners, especially residents, perceive patients as poor and powerless.

This discussion shows how medical practitioners act as gatekeepers, providing options to some that are denied to others. It suggests that medical interviews are social events in which the asymmetry in the practitioner-patient relationship combines with the practical concerns each brings to the examining room or consulting office, which influences therapeutic discourse and the treatment decisions.

The Background Context

The research discussed here was done in a university teaching hospital. Like most teaching hospitals, the delivery of health care was organized into inpatient and outpatient services. The outpatient services were further divided into two clinical systems. These clinical systems were organized around medical specialties. My research was done in a paired set of clinics in the Department of Reproductive Medicine and the specialty of oncology (cancer).

Because of the organization and staffing of each clinic, I have called them the Faculty Clinic and the Community Clinic. The Faculty Clinic was staffed by professors of reproductive oncology and, for the most part, accepted patients referred by other medical practitioners in the community. The Community Clinic was staffed by residents under the supervision of staff physicians and primarily accepted patients referred by social agencies of other clinics in the hospital's system of community clinics.

Over the course of a nearly two-year period, I followed 21 women with abnormal Pap smears referred to, diagnosed, and treated in the Faculty and Community Clinics. I found, among other things, that women with abnormal Pap smears referred to the Community Clinic were more likely to receive nonconservative treatment (i.e., to have hysterectomies) than were women referred to the Faculty Clinic (see Fisher 1979a).

The sample population was assembled largely for practical reasons. My entry into the hospital had been gained with the help of a staff physician who was a gynecological oncologist. As a consequence, the population was defined as women with cancerous or precancerous problems in their reproductive systems.

As I was interested in patients' careers as well as the negotiation of treatment decisions, I followed patients longitudinally through the diagnosis/treatment/recovery process. Doctor-patient interactions were captured on audiotape. Early in my involvement with patients, I found that I was not prepared to deal with death on a daily basis; thus, no patients with invasive disease were part of the sample population.

To document the organization of doctor-patient communication, I spent nearly two years as a participant-observer. For the first 13 months, I conducted informal interviews with staff physicians, attending physicians, residents, medical students, nursing staff, and other support personnel. I attended lectures for residents, read patients' files, observed in consulting offices and examining rooms, and visited patients in the hospital to talk informally about what they were feeling. For the next eight months, I audiotaped the exchange of information between practitioners and patients.

The analysis in this chapter is drawn from verbatim transcripts of audiotaped practitioner-patient communication, information gathered from medical files, and other ethnographic materials. My background knowledge grew from impromptu interviews with practitioners and was heightened by attending lectures with residents, studying the residents' training manual, and reading appropriate sections of their gynecological textbooks.

To display how medical decisions were negotiated in practitioner-patient communications, I extended the analysis beyond the linguistic boundaries of the transcripts and blended verbatim linguistic data with more impressionistic ethnographic data. Neither practitioners nor patients say aloud all that contributes to their decision making.

For example, patients rarely say aloud that they do not trust their medical practitioners or that they suspect them of trying to manipulate the situation. Similarly, neither staff doctors nor residents say aloud that a patient looks like a poor woman, of that she talks like an uneducated woman. They do not say that how patients talk, look, of dress leads them to believe that the patients are not responsible,and will not return for necessary follow-up care. They do not say that these factors contribute to their recommending a less conservative treatment. Neither doctors nor residents say aloud that a particular patient has all of the children she needs or should have because she is on welfare and cannot afford the children she already has. They do not say that hairy underarms and legs, asking too many questions or being too quiet, acting too passive or too aggressive, or wanting children (or more children) contributes to the treatment they recommend. Residents do not say aloud that they need surgery experience or that a particular patient is a good candidate for a hysterectomy (even though a hysterectomy is not absolutely necessary on medical grounds). Although not said aloud, my observations suggest that these factors (and others like them) contribute to the negotiation of treatment decisions.

The Medical Context

Women with abnormal Pap smears provided an ideal population to study the negotiation of differential decision making. Pap smears are preventive health measures. They are recommended for most women once a year as a screen for cervical cancer.

The results of Pap smears traditionally come in five classes. Class 1 is normal, and class 5 is the most abnormal and may indicate invasive disease. Classes 2, 3, and 4 represent a gray area between normal cells and invasive disease. They often indicate dysplasia, of abnormal changes in cells that, although not cancerous, may be precursors to cervical cancer.

Pap smears in the gray area give medical practitioners the widest latitude in their decision making. When a Pap smear is abnormal, the medical task is to ensure that the whole area of abnormal cells can be visualized to rule out the possibility of invasive disease. Once the extent of the lesion and the degree of abnormality have been determined, treatment decisions are based on two separate but interrelated goals: *(a)* to protect the patient from developing more extensive disease (cancer), and *(b)* to preserve, where possible, the patent's reproductive functions.

During my study, I observed three treatment options routinely used to treat women with Pap smears in the range between normal and invasive disease: cryosurgery (freezing), cone biopsy or conization, and hysterectomy.

Cryosurgery is an office procedure that retains a woman's reproductive capacity. Cone biopsy or conization is a hospital procedure done under anesthetic. A thin, cone-shaped slice is cored out of the endocervical canal and examined. Cone biopsies can be either diagnostic or therapeutic. If the upper limits of the cone sample are free of abnormal cells, then this diagnostic procedure becomes an effective therapeutic one. It threatens, but does not terminate, reproductive capacity and his been demonstrated to be as effective in treating dysplasia as has the hysterectomy. Hysterectomy is the surgical removal of the uterus.

The manual prepared for residents further stipulates how treatment decisions are to be made. It says that when the limits of the lesion are seen and there is no evidence of invasive disease, treatment should be based on the patient's wish.

If she wishes to retain her reproductive capacity, conservative measures like cryosurgery may be used. If she requests sterilization, hysterectomy is the treatment of choice. According to the manual, hysterectomies are indicated only when conservative techniques fail, when there is evidence of invasive disease, or when a patient requests a hysterectomy for sterilization.

These seem rather clear criteria for medical decision making. Yet, based on my observations, treatment decisions are not as clear as they seem. On purely medical grounds, it is hard to explain why no patients in the Faculty Clinic received hysterectomies. Or, even though there was no evidence of invasive disease, why 7 out of 13 women in the Community Clinic were given hysterectomies.

Given the parameters just outlined, we could speculate that perhaps the women in the Community Clinic requested hysterectomies for sterilization. However, I was in the examining room while treatment decisions were reached; and during the two years of my research, these patients never requested sterilization.

The Social Context

If treatment decisions are not made on medical grounds alone, how, then, are they made? Much of the literature of medical sociology (cf. Ehrenreich and Ehrenreich 1970; Freidson 1970; Mechanic 1968; Navarro 1973; Stevens 1966; Waitzkin and Waterman 1974) suggests that medical decisions are made using social criteria.

Still, the medical decisions made in the study cannot be justified solely on social grounds. Social criteria like referral patterns, organization of the setting, and such demographic factors as age, ethnicity, number of children, and social class did not completely account for the distribution of treatment decisions. When social criteria were considered, a trend emerged. Young, Caucasian, single or divorced women with few or no children who are referred by private physicians or social agencies to the Faculty Clinic are more likely to receive conservative treatment. Older, Mexican, or Mexican-American women, married or divorced with multiple children, referred from within the system of Community Clinics or by social agencies to the Community Clinic are more likely to receive less conservative treatment (i.e., to receive hysterectomies).

These social factors are important, yet they are not explanatory. An analysis of the medical and social factors that underlie treatment decisions focuses on the product of a decision. Once products, or treatment decisions, are tabulated and grouped together, all instances of a given treatment are treated the same. This kind of analysis leaves several questions unexplored. Chief among them are as follows: How do practitioners and patients gather information from each other to reach decisions? What input do practitioners and patients make into the decision-making process? Given the practitioners' specialized medical knowledge and technical skill and the asymmetry inherent in the relationship, how do practitioners decide what treatment to recommend? Once they have decided, how do they convey that information to patients, and what are the consequences, in terms of treatment outcomes, of how information is exchanged?

These questions shift the focus from an exclusive concern with products to an analysis of process as it occurs in organization contexts. It displays treatment decisions as produced and constrained by the exchange of information in medical interviews.

The Analytic Context

When listening to conversation, one is impressed with the variety of ways that information is exchanged. When analyzing discourse, one is equally impressed with its organized character. Theory and research in several disciplines suggest that language is a social production in which different linguistic arrangements are visible in different situations and in which there is a relationship between the words spoken, the actions performed, and the structure of talk. More recently, language has been analyzed as discourse—a naturally occurring, locally organized, social production.

Hymes (1962) states that one of the goals of an "ethnography of speaking" is to capture naturally occurring talk, do a detailed analysis of it, and display it as socially produced. The sociolinguistic concepts of "communicative competence" and its methodological counterpart, an "ethnography of speaking," (Hymes 1962, 1972, 1974) have been the foundation of many studies that examine the properties of natural language use (cf. Bernstein 1971; Ervin-Tripp and Mitchell-Kernan 1977; Halliday and Hasan 1976; Labov 1972; Philips 1972; Shatz 1975; Shatz and Gelman 1973; Shuy 1983).

Labov and Fanshel (1977) demonstrate Hymes's (1962) claim that discourse is a social or speech event organized around an exchange of information. As a speech event, therapeutic discourse is a routinized form of behavior with well-defined boundaries. It is an interview structured by who initiates the event and who is helped by it.

Labov and Fanshel found the speech event in therapeutic discourse to be asymmetrical. The participant who initiates the event and is helped by it (the client/patient) is in a subordinant position. In addition, they demonstrated that the asymmetry is socially produced and structures the exchange information between participants.

The asymmetry Labov and Fanshel discuss is similar to Waitzkin and Waterman's (1974) "competence gap." Waitzkin and Waterman claim that socioeconomic factors cause doctors and patients to enter a therapeutic interview with different resources. This produces an inherent asymmetry, which affects health care delivery.

In a discussion of medical interviews, Shuy (1982) suggests that a great deal hinges on small features of the interview that are normally taken for granted by medical practitioners and only recently have come under investigation by social scientists. He points out that medical interviews are like other conversations in that they are structured, predictable, and organized around topics. He also demonstrates that medical interviews are different from normal conversation.

In normal conversation, there is an expectation of balanced participation. Participants talk, introduce topics, and respond to topics in about the same quantities. Not so in medical interviews. Shuy further claims that the differences in medical interviews have an impact on patient's participation and understanding. Others also have argued that how information is exchanged his an impact on how it is understood (cf. Chafe 1976; Cicourel 1974, 1975; Keenan and Schieffelin 1976; Kuno 1976).

The Decision-making Context: The Medical Interview

An analysis of the practitioner-patient communication through which treatment decisions are negotiated provides information not available when only the medical and social criteria underlying medical decision making are considered. These criteria are, in many ways, external and constraining "social facts" that produce and inhibit the decision-making process. Yet, treatment decisions are also affected by the participants' interactional activities and, as such, are socially produced in the setting. An analysis of the strategic use of language in medical interviews displays how treatment decisions are accomplished within the contextual framework provided by medical and social factors.

Medical interviews are social events oriented toward the specific end of a treatment decision. In this event, practitioners have, and use, quite a wide latitude of choice in recommending treatment options. In analyzing how language is strategically used to accomplish treatment decisions, I do not intend to characterize the field of medicine as a whole or to praise or criticize particular medical practitioners. Rather, it is my intention to demonstrate that medical practitioners and patients have different practical concerns that organize how they exchange information. This organization has consequences in terms of the decisions reached.

Patients enter medical interactions from a position of relative weakness. For example, they have an abnormal Pap smear and feel threatened by the possibility of a cancer-related medical problem. They enter unfamiliar surroundings in which all of the other participants seem to share a common language. This language is, for the most part, unintelligible and frightening to them.

Medical practitioners, on the other hand, are in their "home court" in the medical setting. They understand and have some control over the workings of the hospital and clinic bureaucracies. The special medical jargon is their professional lexicon. They have knowledge and skills that are usually mysterious to patients. It is from this position of relative strength that practitioners greet patients and the medical interview begins.

Medical practitioners, in addition, are very busy. Their time is budgeted and oriented toward making a diagnosis and recommending treatments. For practitioners, the diagnostic/treatment process is a general concern. Their focus is on how, within certain parameters, to treat a specific medical problem. The patient is one among many with similar problems,

For residents, the diagnostic/treatment process includes an additional concern. They need surgical experience if they are to become competent practitioners. This creates a dual focus for them: (a) providing adequate medical care, and (b) producing maximum opportunities for surgery experience.

In addition, medical practitioners are not as able to separate themselves from death as I had been. The relationship between abnormal Pap smears, cancer, and the kind of death most cancer causes may contribute to the practitioners' treatment recommendations. This may be especially true when they treat lower-class, minority women, who practitioners may view as immature, irresponsible, and unlikely to return for the necessary follow-up care.

The practical concerns are not the same for patients. Patients are not interested in making a diagnosis. They cannot recommend treatments, do not need surgery experience, and have not faced death on a daily basis. Their time is not measured into equal increments to be divided among a maximum number of patients. For patients, the focus is on the meaning of their medical problem and how it will affect their everyday lives. Time is measured as time away from school, job, or family; time until they find out the results of laboratory tests or treatments to be recommended; time as a bomb ticking away precious moments before the suspected cancer explodes and takes over their lives. Patients are interested in finding out what their abnormal Pap smears mean, whether they indicate cancer, and what needs to be done. They are afraid of the unknown, worried about the possibility of having cancer, and fearful that their lives, reproductive capacities, and value as women may be at risk (Fisher 1979b).

Both the practitioner and patient have information that is necessary to the decision-making process of the other. To gain access to this information, they exchange information organized around topics by requesting and providing information to each other. During the exchange, language functions strategically to move the decision-making process closer to a treatment decision. On some occasions, requests for information function as "questioning strategies." Both the practitioner and patient request specific information and provide access to less specific information. For example the question, "What did Karen tell you about your Pap smear?" is a request for specific information. It is also a way to gain less specific information about the woman's competence as a patient.

Both practitioners and patients use questioning strategies. They are used by medical practitioners during talk about reproduction to gain access to information that only patients can supply. Patients use questioning strategies during talk about treatment options to gather information about the necessity of a recommended treatment. When used by residents and staff physicians, they are used differently and these differences impact upon the decision-making process.

On other occasions, information is provided in ways that function as "presentational" and "persuasional" strategies. Both strategies are negotiating mechanisms. They provide information while *suggesting or specifying* how the information should be understood.

Presentational strategies are "soft sells." They provide information while *suggesting* how patients should make sense out of it. For example, a practitioner would say, "We usually treat this by freezing." This presentation provides the patient with information about a treatment option while suggesting that it is the "usual" of "normal" way to treat her condition.

Persuasional strategies are harder sells. They provide information while *specifying* how it should be understood. For example, a practitioner might say, "What you should do if you don't want any more children is have a hysterectomy. No more uterus, no more cancer, no more babies, no more birth control, and no more periods." This presentation provides the patient with information about what treatment she should have while specifying why she should have it (no more uterus, no more cancer, etc.).

Only practitioners use presentational and persuasional strategies. And, again, the strategies are used differently by residents and staff physicians. They are used when talking about cancer and treatment options to provide information about what treatment decision the patient should make.

Questioning, presentational, and persuasional strategies are interactional mechanisms that accomplish treatment decisions. They are the strategies through which the information necessary to negotiate treatment decisions is exchanged.

The Communication Context: Negotiation Mechanisms

An analysis of the strategic use of language suggests that practitioners have power that patients lack, a power manifested and reflected in how practitioners present information to patients. Although patients do not have the same kind of power practitioners do, they too have input into the decision-making process. They can ask questions that can redirect talk about treatment options and that can affect how the treatment decision is reached.

The discussion of how language is strategically used takes the analysis beyond the linguistic bounds of the transcript and embeds it in its ethnographic context. A comparison across settings, participants, and treatment decisions provides a view of how treatment decisions are negotiated and accomplished in the situated actions of the participants and in specific organizational contexts.

Medical Practitioners' Use of Questioning Strategies

Questioning strategies provide a slot for patients to display their competence.[1] Marrianna, for example, was diagnosed and treated in the Faculty Clinic. She was a 21 -year-old Anglo woman; a student at a local university; had never married; and had been pregnant once and had an abortion. She was referred to the union oncologist in the Faculty Clinic by a women's health care specialist. A routine Pap smear taken in this clinic was returned with the notation that it contained abnormal cells; and because of the professional relationship between the women's health care specialist and the new doctor in the hospital (the junior staff oncologist), she was referred to the Faculty Clinic.

1 In this discussion *competence* is not intended to index the patient's overall ability, but rather it indexes the patient's ability to display herself as appropriate within the doctor's medical framework.

On her first visit, the doctor twice requested information in a strategic manner. He said, "Now did Karen explain to you the abnormal, what this abnormal Pap smear business is?"

The patient answered, "She [the women's health care specialist] explained that the cells looked abnormal. . . the cells are in a dysplastic condition."

The doctor continued by asking, "Dysplasia, what's your understanding of that?"

To which she responded, "Well, what's anyone's understanding of it? They're abnormal and you don't know why and they don't know if it leads to cancer."

In both of these requests for information, Marrianna responded by providing the information requested, and in so doing, presented herself as a competent young woman.

In the next case, the same doctor asked similar questions, but the patient did not display herself as competent. The patient, Anelen, was a 30-year-old Anglo woman. She had been married once, divorced, been pregnant once, and given the child up for adoption. She was referred by the same women's health care specialist.

During the interview the doctor asked a question that functioned strategically. He said, "Do you know that the Pap smear, do you understand what the Pap smear means? What it does?"

The patient responded by saying, "Uhmm, Karen explained a little, but I'm not sure of the possibilities. I don't even know what all those are but she told me not to worry yet."

Anelen's response neither provided the information requested nor made her appear as a competent woman. To be sure that Anelen had the necessary information to understand her medical problem and reach a decision, the doctor followed this exchange by providing information about her Pap smear and about the diagnostic and therapeutic procedures used to manage it.

In the third example, no slot was provided for the patient to display her competence. Marvi, a 23-year-old Mexican-American woman, was married, the mother of three small children, and was referred to the Community Clinic from the Primary Care Clinic where a postpartum checkup and routine Pap smear disclosed abnormal cervical cells. At the time of Marvi's visit to the Community Clinic, she was pregnant with an unwanted pregnancy, which led to an abortion. Although this was her first abortion, it was not the first time her birth control had failed. Given these factors, it is not surprising that the practitioner had recommended a hysterectomy. What is more surprising is that she did not have a hysterectomy. Marvi is the only woman in the sample population with multiple children who was treated with cryosurgery.

The bureaucratic organization of the Community Clinic contributed to Marvi's treatment with cryosurgery. At the Community Clinic, Marvi was discouraged from having a tubal ligation for sterilization. Instead, a hysterectomy was recommended to treat her medical problem and for sterilization. When the patient was referred to another clinic for abortion counseling, that clinic did not discourage a tubal ligation. Marvi, then, had an abortion and a tubal. When she returned to the Community Clinic, there were no longer any medical grounds on which a hysterectomy could be performed, and so she was treated with cryosurgery.

The exchange of information in Marvi's case took place differently from the exchange in Marrianna and Anelen's case. Marrianna and Anelen were treated in the Faculty Clinic by a professor of medicine—a staff physician. In each case, the physician asked questions that functioned strategically. These questions provided a slot into which patients could respond—displaying their competence in the process.

On the other hand, Marvi was treated in the Community Clinic by a resident who did not use questions in a strategic manner. Thus, Marvi did not have an opportunity to show herself to be a competent patient. When the resident questioned her, he used very specific questions about her birth control practices. Because she had come to the clinic with an unwanted pregnancy, it was quite clear that Marvi had not been a competent user of birth control. It is interesting to speculate on why the resident did not use more general questions, which might have allowed Marvi to display her competence as a patient. I suspect that he had already judged her to be incompetent on grounds that are not displayed in the verbal communication between them. These assumptions structured the exchange of information that followed and had an impact on the treatment recommended.

Patient Use of Questioning Strategies

Patients also ask questions. They ask them in response to information provided by medical professionals during a discussion of treatment options. When asked by patients, questions have the potential to change the direction of the treatment decision, as shown in the following examples.

When Anelen returned to the Faculty Clinic to discuss the results of her tests and make a treatment decision, she asked a question during a discussion of treatment options. On her previous visit Anelen provided the information that she did not want to have any more children. The doctor responded by recommending a hysterectomy as a permanent method of sterilization and to treat her abnormal Pap smear.

On the second visit, the exchange opened with a discussion that reviews what had transpired on the previous visit and during a previous phone conversation. The doctor reminded Anelen that he has recommended a hysterectomy, and Anelen asked a question that redirected the talk about treatment options and affected the final treatment. She said "Have a hysterectomy and that, I'm that, if there's an alternative. I'm terrified of operations." The doctor responded, "Uh, okay, well, there certainly is an alternative, yeah, we can treat this by just freezing it here in the office and that usually will take care of it about 90% of the time." The discussion of options and the treatment performed was redirected after the patient raised a question. She was treated with cryosurgery.

The next patient, Lucy, was diagnosed and treated in the Faculty Clinic after being referred from a social agency staffed by native Spanish-speaking workers. Lucy was a 42-year-old, bilingual, Mexican-American woman. She was married and had three children. Her diagnosis and treatment in the Faculty Clinic was related to her being a poor, bilingual Mexican-American woman, and to my participation as both a researcher and translator.

The patient had a medical problem for which she went to her private physician. He recommended surgery, and she did not have the money to pay for it. In her search for less expensive medical care, a friend referred her to the outreach clinic staffed by native Spanish-speakers. At the clinic, Lucy received advice about how to apply for MediCal (the California equivalent of Medicaid) and was referred to the junior staff oncologist at the Faculty Clinic.

When the doctor and patient met to discuss treatment options, he informed her that the extent of her lesion had not been visualized, told her that she needed to have a conization biopsy as the next diagnostic step, and talked about a hysterectomy. Lucy was concerned about how she would pay for hospital care and confused by the letter she had received from MediCal. She asked the doctor to clarify the letter and he was unable to do so (which does not speak well for MediCal's style of communication).

To provide the information Lucy requested, the doctor called the billing office. While he was on the phone, Lucy turned to me and asked, in Spanish, if the doctor had said he was going to take out her uterus. I explained, in Spanish, the difference between conization biopsy and hysterectomy and confirmed that the doctor had been talking about removing her uterus. She asked if that would be necessary and I suggested that she ask the doctor.

Two things particularly struck me about our exchange. First, because Lucy spoke English so well, both the doctor and I assumed she understood it equally well. She did not. After reviewing the transcript, I was not surprised. When talking about treatments, the doctor had used several words interchangeably: *womb, uterus, cervix, and hysterectomy.* I was also struck by the consequences of out exchange. At the next opportunity, which occurred during a discussion of treatment options, the patient requested information that functioned strategically, changed the direction of the discussion of options, and affected the treatment performed.

While talking about how long the patient would have to be in the hospital, the doctor explained that the longer stay was because they would be taking out her uterus. The patient then asked, "Is that necessary?" The doctor responded, "Well, it isn't absolutely necessary; it may or may not be. . ." For much of the remaining exchange of information, the doctor worked to move the patient toward a treatment decision of hysterectomy. In each instance, the patient responded by asking if it was necessary or by saying that if it was not necessary, she did not want it. She was treated with a conization biopsy.

Another patient, Pat, asked questions, but did not change the direction of the discussion of options or the treatment performed. Pat, a 32-year-old Anglo woman, had been married, divorced, pregnant five times, and had three children. Although she was an American citizen, she married and had lived most of her adult life in Ireland. Her children still lived there with their father. When she returned to the Community Clinic to discuss her treatment options, she was told that the extent of the lesion had not been visualized, asked if she wanted more children, and told that a conization biopsy followed by a hysterectomy was the best treatment for her.

During the discussion of treatment options and in response to information that the resident was presenting, she made a request for information, a request that functioned strategically. She said,

> Well, for this way now would you say, for instance, you're talking about there could be surgery, if, uh, there is an advancement of cancer there, a sign of cancer. Well, also the fact that you asked me did I want any more children, there's another way of doing it too, but it also means that it could travel, is that it, the cancer could spread, say for instance, if I don't have a hysterectomy, is that the idea?

The doctor responded, "Well, if you have cancer, then it has to be treated because it can spread, right?" The talk about treatment options did not change the direction of the discussion of options or the treatment performed. This patient was treated with a vaginal hysterectomy.

The communication in this case between practitioner and patient is different from that with the two previous patients (Anelen and Lucy). Pat is the only patient who added information to the "facts" provided by the medical practitioner. She added the notion that cancer could spread if not treated with a hysterectomy. It was this information the resident picked up and used to justify his treatment recommendation. Pat's question is also not as clear or as strong as those used by the other two patients. She did not ask if there were alternatives or if a hysterectomy was necessary. In addition, she asked two questions during the same utterance. The resident avoided discussing alternatives entirely. And he answered only part of the second question. He did not address whether the abnormal cells would spread if she did not have a hysterectomy. Instead, he answered a hypothetical question that she had not really asked. He answered the question, If it is cancer, would it spread without a hysterectomy? He did not tell her that if she did not have cancer, there were other alternatives.

In Anelen's, Lucy's, and Pat's cases the medical professional's presentation of information provided a slot into which the patient could request information that functioned strategically. In each case, the medical professional's response to the question was different. In addition, the medical professionals themselves elicited information from patients differently in each case. With Anelen, the doctor asked questions to request specific information and to provide a slot for her to display her competence. In response, she neither provided the information he asked for nor displayed her competence. In Lucy and Pat's cases, no questions were asked. Neither patient was given an opportunity to display her understanding of her medical problem or her competence as a patient. It is interesting to speculate why Lucy and Pat were not given the opportunity to display their competence, as Anelen was; or why neither Lucy nor Anelen were given a hysterectomy, as Pat was. On closer inspection, Lucy shares features with both Anelen and Pat. Although Lucy and Anelen were both treated in the Faculty Clinic by the same staff physician, their referral patterns had been quite different. Anelen had been referred by a women's health care specialist with whom she had a long-standing relationship. This relationship provided an outside advocate who could hold the medical practitioner in the hospital accountable. Neither Lucy nor Pat had an outside advocate. Lucy had been referred from an outreach clinic staffed by native Spanish-speakers, and Pat had ben referred from within the system of community clinics. In each case, neither the interest of the referring medical practitioner nor the organization of the bureaucracy provided the kind of support Anelen had developed with the women's health care specialist.

It seems reasonable to speculate that both Lucy and Pat were judged as less powerful than Anelen on grounds that are not immediately apparent in their verbal communication. This judgment structured the exchange of information between practitioner and patient and had an impact on the treatment decision reached. Although in each case the medical practitioner provided a slot for the patient to request information that functioned strategically, he responded to the questions patients inserted into these slots differently.

At first glance, then, it would be reasonable to assume that Lucy and Pat, denied the opportunity to display their competence and perceived as less powerful, would be treated with hysterectomies and Anelen would not. My observations suggest two reasons this was not the outcome. First, Lucy was treated in the Faculty Clinic by a staff physician and Pat was treated in the Community Clinic by a resident. Staff physicians do not have the same "need" to perform hysterectomies as do residents, who must have the surgical experience to become fully qualified doctors. Second, Lucy, unlike Pat, used a strong questioning strategy and kept returning to it each time the doctor suggested a hysterectomy. Pat used a weaker questioning strategy and did not return to it, even when her questions were not fully answered. Thus, Pat's impact on the decision-making process was weak, and she was treated with a hysterectomy.

Medical Practitioners' Use of Presentational and Persuasional Strategies

Although both practitioners and patients ask questions, doctors do so during exchanges of general information to gather the details of patients' reproductive history and desire. Patients, by contrast, ask questions during discussions about treatment options. In addition, there are differences in how medical practitioners present information to patients when discussing cancer and treatment options. They use presentational and persuasional strategies to provide patients with the information necessary to reach treatment decisions and with ways of understanding or making sense out of that information.

In each of the previous three cases, the medical professional's response to patients' questions provided specific information and suggested how that information should be understood. In Anelen's case, the doctor responded by saying, "There certainly is an alternative. . ." and by providing the information that cryosurgery is an alternative that is 90% effective. He provided specific information, and by the tone of his presentation, made the choice of cryosurgery perfectly acceptable.

In Lucy's case, the doctor responded by saying, "Well, it isn't absolutely necessary. . . ." The statement that "it isn't absolutely necessary" frames the medical information to suggest a preference: Although a hysterectomy is not absolutely necessary, it certainly is preferable.

In Pat's case, the resident avoided directly answering the patient's question. By answering only a small part of what was asked, he suggested that the answer to the whole was contained within the part; that is, that a hysterectomy was a necessary procedure.

In Anelen's, Lucy's, and Pat's cases the medical practitioners used presentational strategies to suggest how information should be understood. In the next case, information is presented in a way that does more than suggest how to make sense out of it. Persuasional strategies are used to specify the grounds on which understanding is to be based. In presenting the options to Marvi the resident said the following:

> What I was going to tell you is that there are two ways this can be treated. Okay? One is for dysplasia that we could do a hysterectomy and just remove the uterus. That means no more babies in the future and so you know, as a form of contraception also,

okay? The second is to freeze the cervix and then follow you with the understanding that that should cure it, but that you need to be followed in the future and that you could have children in the future if that's what your plans include.

The resident presented information about a hysterectomy as the means to have no more babies and as a method of contraception. To a woman who is pregnant with an unwanted pregnancy and who has had repeated birth control failures, this is a particularly persuasive presentation. He continues by saying that she could be treated by freezing the cervix but she could still have children and would have to be followed. Again, a very persuasive presentation. This is a poor woman who does not want more children and does not have either the time or the money to return to the hospital for frequent follow-up cafe. In addition, the resident presented the hysterectomy option first, and then presented cryosurgery as an option. This order suggested that the less conservative treatment (hysterectomy) was somehow preferable. Later in the exchange, the resident summed up his position using another persuasional strategy. He said, "Absent uterus, no periods, no cancer, no babies."

Similarly, in Pat's case, when the resident presented her with an informed consent form to sign, he said,

> Even though with this form that I have before me that the government requires you to sign, it's a request for a hysterectomy for sterilization, even though it says here that you have no problems which require a hysterectomy and we know that you do, the hospital and state require me to ask you to sign this so that you understand that what we're talking about is permanent sterilization with no possibilities of future pregnancies.

This, again, is a particularly persuasive presentation. The patient in no way requested a hysterectomy for sterilization. She had been referred to the clinic with a class 5 Pap smear. During a discussion about treatment options, a hysterectomy was recommended as the most appropriate treatment. The grounds for this recommendation were specified as follows: "It [cancer] could come back, and for somebody your age, that's had your family, you're sure that you don't want children, I'd recommend a hysterectomy." To a woman who has had a class 5 Pap smear and is already afraid that she has a life-threatening medical problem, this is a particularly persuasive presentation. It heightens the emotional impact of the abnormal Pap smear by stressing that "it" could come back. The "it" being referred to is, of course, cancer. In addition, it is the resident, not the patient, who links the need for a hysterectomy with the patient's age, her childbearing history, and her lack of desire for additional children. To a woman who lived many of her childbearing years in a Catholic country and has had three children and two abortions, this again is a very persuasive presentation.

The persuasive overtones were strengthened when the resident gave her the informed consent to sign and told her that although the form said that she had no problems requiring a hysterectomy, "We know that you do." He brings all of the authority of his medical role to bear in this statement. As a man, as a medical practitioner, and as her physician, he is telling her what to do and implying dire consequences if she does not comply.

There is an additional issue involved in this presentation. The resident told the patient what he was required to by law and then suggested that she ignore it. This amplifies the power and authority of his medical role and his use of it to manipulate her decision-making process. One might ask, What kind of informed consent procedure does this represent?

Accomplishing The Treatment Event

Caress (1975, 1977) suggests several reasons for the explosion of hysterectomies in recent years. First, she argues, gynecologists and obstetricians are surgeons. As the birth rate continues to level out, these doctors face reduced opportunities to practice their surgical skills. Second, many physicians have united their professional skills and their political ideals. As a result, poor, minority women are bearing the brunt of unnecessary hysterectomies. Finally, she claims, hysterectomies are good money makers.

Other reasons for increased hysterectomies have also been discussed. Once reproduction is over, many doctors agree that the uterus is a useless organ. John Morris, M.D., told a congressional subcommittee that, "An arm is a useful structure. Breasts have cosmetic advantages. However, there are certain organs that are absolutely useless. One such is your appendix, another is the uterus after childbearing" ("Important Cost and Quality Issues" 1977:354).

The uterus, seen as a useless organ past childbearing, is also depicted as a potentially dangerous organ. As Dr. R.C. Wright wrote in a 1969 issue of *Obstetrics and Gynecology:* "The uterus has but one function: reproduction. After the last planned pregnancy the uterus becomes a useless, bleeding, symptom-producing, potentially cancer-bearing organ and therefore should be removed" (Larned 1977:199).

Ninety-seven per cent of all gynecologists in the U.S. are men. As men, to some extent their attitudes toward women reflect current views of women in society (Larned 1977). As Scully and Bart (1973) point out, these attitudes are magnified and reinforced in medical school. Medical students and residents learn to view the uterus and the women who have them negatively.

To quote from a widely used gynecological textbook:

> No drastic results are found following the removal of the uterus. . . . Indeed, it should be not construed as callous if many gynecologists feel that, in the woman who has completed her family, the uterus is a rather worthless organ. (Novak et al. 1970:26)

This attitude has been described as quite common: "This is indeed the attitude of most gynecologists. While it may seem harsh and ill-phrased, it is a logical viewpoint and one with which I personally agree" (Paulshock 1976:26). Scully (1980) points out, and the data in this article supports, that these attitudes provide the basis on which residents learn and use a regular sales pitch" for hysterectomies.

Summary

As I pointed out, no patients in the Faculty Clink received hysterectomies, while 7 out of 13 women in the Community Clinic did receive hysterectomies. It is logical to deduce, as Caress (1975, 1977) and Larned (1977) suggest, that if doctors believe that hysterectomies are in women's best interest, the number of hysterectomies will continue to increase.

It is likely that staff physicians and residents bring different sets of practical concerns into the examining room that affect how language is used and how treatment decisions are reached. It is also reasonable that patients referred from the private sector to professors of medicine in the Faculty Clinic are less likely to be treated with hysterectomies than are patients referred from the public sector to residents in the Community Clinic. The Faculty and Community Clinics provide very different settings in which to deliver and receive medical care.

Faculty and Community Clinics were organized in different ways, to serve a different population of patients and were staffed in a different manner. The Faculty Clinic was staffed by gynecological oncologists who were professors of medicine. There were no residents following in and out of the clinic; thus, there was a kind of continuity of care not normally found in teaching settings. The physical layout honored the humanness of patients. There was a separation of public and private space. The waiting room was separated from the backstage medical area. Examining rooms were separated from consulting offices.

The Community Clinic, on the other hand, was staffed in a rotating fashion. Everybody rotated-residents, support personnel, and supervising staff; thus heightening the lack of continuity of care. Assignment to the Community Clinic, the narrow definition of the medical problem under their care and the constant rotation also increased the fragmentation of the care delivered. In addition, the physical layout of the clinic did not honor the humanness of patients. There was no separation of public and private space. There was no waiting room. Patients sat in the hall outside of the examining room overhearing medical talk that frightened them. There were also no consulting offices. All talk with patients occurred either in the halls (in the presence of other patients) or in the examining rooms. I suspect that it is a very different experience to sit across the desk from a doctor, fully clothed, discussing your medical problem from having a similar discussion with a resident while you are sitting undressed on the examining table.

The data discussed in this chapter support the view that although the doctor-patient relationship is an asymmetrical one, the asymmetry increases when patients are perceived as poor and powerless and medical practitioners are residents rather than staff physicians. It seems that the need for surgery experience and the lack of an outside advocate plus internal norms of medical adequacy contribute to the differential outcomes in the Faculty Clinic and Community Clinic. It follows, quite naturally, that these structural and organizational features of the delivery of health care are manifested during medical interviews in the "change of information between participants, negotiated through the use of linguistic strategies, and have consequences for the treatment decision reached.

The linguistic and ethnographic data discussed here further suggest that the medical interview is organized in predictable ways. A detailed examination of how language is used and treatment decisions are negotiated provides information not available in an analysis of the medical and social facts underlying medical decision making. It displays the processes through which treatment decisions are jointly accomplished. First, medical practitioners and patients, exchanging the information necessary to reach treatment decisions, use language strategically, thus doing communicational work. In addition to specifying how treatment decisions are negotiated in the activities of participants, this kind of an analysis suggests that the communicational work of the participants is oriented toward the specific end of a treatment decision, thus linking interaction (or communication) to outcomes (or treatment decisions). Finally, this kind of analysis places the decision-making process in a specific organizational context.

By placing linguistic phenomena in their social context and analyzing how that context organizes linguistic structures, three levels of analysis (structural, organizational, and interactional) that are normally treated separately are linked. The detailed analysis of the communicational process through which treatment decisions are negotiated displays how the negotiation of hysterectomies is produced and constrained by structural, organizational, and interactional contexts and accomplished through the communication between participants.

There are theoretical, methodological, and practical ramifications inherent in the documentation of the communicational work through which treatment decisions are reached. Theoretically and methodologically, a systematic analysis of the communicational strategies used to accomplish treatment decisions provides insights not normally available when the subtleties of the practitioner-patient relationship are not examined. These insights can have practical consequences for medical education, resident training, and the creation of informed consumers.

In an era in which both medical practitioners and patients are displaying increasing dissatisfaction with the way things are—the high costs of medical care, the increasing performance of unnecessary medical procedures, the difficulties with patient compliance, the problems with informed consent, and the use and possible abuse of medical malpractice procedures—awareness of the processes used to communicate hold the potential for improving communication and improving the delivery of health care.

References Cited

Bernstein, Basil
1971 *Class, Codes and Control.* London: Routledge & Kegan Paul.

Caress, Barbara
1975 *Sterilization.* Health/PAC Bulletin #62, January/February, pp. 1-13.
1977 *Womb-boom.* Health/PAC Bulletin, July / August.

Chafe, Wallace L.
1976 Givenness, contrastiveness, definiteness, subjects, topics and point of view. In *Subject and Topic*, Charles H. Li, Ed., pp. 25-56. New York: Academic Press.

Cicourel, Aaron V.
1974 Interviewing and memory. In *Pragmatic Aspects of Human Communication*, Colin Cherry, Ed., pp. 51-82. Dordrecht: Reidel.

_____.
1975 Discourse and text: Cognitive and linguistic processes in studies of social structure. To appear in *Versus*. (Portions presented at 1975 American Sociological Association Meetings.)

Cost and Quality of Health Care: Unnecessary Surgery Report by the Committee on Oversight and Investigations of the Committee on Interstate and Foreign Commerce, House of Representatives, Ninth Congress Second Session, January, 1976. YN.IN 8/4 H 34/35.

Ehrenreich, Barbara, and John Ehrenreich
1970 *The American Health Empire.* Health-PAC Book. New York: Vintage.

Ervin-Tripp, Susan, and Claudia Mitchell-Kernan
1977 *Child Discourse.* New York: Academic Press.

Fisher, Sue Carole
1979a The Negotiation of Treatment Decisions in Doctor/Patient Communications and Their Impact on Identity of Women Patients. Doctoral dissertation, University of California, San Diego, California.

_____.
1979b Mirror, mirror on the wall; Women's identities and women's role. Paper presented at annual meetings of the Mid-South Sociological Association, Memphis, Tennessee, November 1979.

Freidson, Eliot
1970 *Profession of Medicine.* New York: Dodd, Mead.

Halliday, Michael A., and Ruqaiya Hasan
1976 *Cohesion in English.* London: Longmans.

Hymes, Dell
1962 The ethnography of speaking. In *Anthropology and Human Behavior*. Washington, D.C.: Anthropological Society of Washington.

_____.
1972 Models of the interaction of language and social life. In *Directions in Sociolinguistics: The Ethnography of Communication*, John J. Gumperz and Dell Hymes, Eds., pp. 38-71. New York: Holt, Rinehart and Winston.

_____.
1974 *Foundations of Sociolinguistics*. Philadelphia: University of Pennsylvania Press.

Important Cost and Quality Issues of Health Care Hearings before the Subcommittee on Oversight and Investigations of the Committee on Interstate and Foreign Commerce, House of Representatives, 95 Congress/First Session, April 25 and 29, May 2 and 9, 1977. V/4. IN8/4:95-32.

Keenan, Elinor Ochs and Bambi B. Schieffelin
1976 Topics as a discourse notion: A study of topic in the conversations of children and adults. In *Subject and Topic,* Charles N. Li, Ed., pp. 335-384. New York: Academic Press.

Kuno, Susumu
1976 Subject, theme, and the speaker's empathy—a reexamination of relativization in phenomena. In *Subject and Topic,* Charles N. Li, Ed., pp. 417-444. New York: Academic Press.

Labov, William
1972 *Sociolinguistic Patterns*. Philadelphia: University of Pennsylvania Press.

Labov, William and David Fanshel
1977 *Therapeutic Discourse: Psychotherapy as Conversation.* New York: Academic Press.

Larned, D.
1977 The epidemic in unnecessary hysterectomy. In *Seizing Our Bodies.* The Politics of Women's Health, Claudia Dreifus, Ed. New York: Vintage Books.

Mechanic, David
1968 *Medical Sociology.* New York: The Free Press.

National Center for Health Statistics
1976 Surgical operation in short-stay hospitals, US, 1973. *In Vital and Health Statistics,* Series 13, No. 21. Washington, D.C.: Author.

Navarro, Vincente
1973 *Health and Medical Care in the US.: A Critical Analysis.* Farmingdale, N.Y.: Baywood Publishing Co.

Novak, E. R. et al.
1970 *Novak's Textbook of Gynecology.* Baltimore: Williams and Wilkeses.

Paulshock, B. Z.
1976 What every woman should know about hysterectomy. *Today's Health* 54(2) (February):23-26.

Philips, Susan
1972 Participant structures and communicative competence: Warm Springs children in community and classroom. In *Functions of Language in the Classroom,* Courtney Cazden, Vera John, and Dell Hymes, Eds., pp. 370-394. New York: Teachers College Press.

Scully, Diana
1980 *Men Who Control Women's Health: The Misedication of Obstetricians-Gynecologists.* Boston: Houghton Mifflin.

Scully, Diana, and P. Bart
1973 A funny thing happened on the way to the orifice: Women in gynecological textbooks. *American Journal of Sociology* 78(4):1045-1050.

Shatz, Marilyn
1975 Towards a Developmental Theory of Communicative Competence. Doctoral dissertation, University of Pennsylvania.

Sharz, Marilyn, and Rochel Gelman
1973 The Development of Communication Skills; Modifications in the Speech of Young Children as a Function of Listener. *Monographs of the Society for Research in Child Development 38.*

Shuy, Roger W.
1983 Three types of interference to an effective exchange of information in the medical interview. In *The Social Organization of Doctor-Patient Communication.* Sue Fisher and Alexandra Dundas Todd, Eds., pp. 189-202. Washington, D.C.: The Center for Applied Linguistics.

Stevens, Rosemary
1966 *Medical Practice in Modern England: The Impact of Specialization and State Medicine.* New Haven: Yale University Press.

Virginia Department of Health
1977 Uterine cancer and the Pap test. *Virginia Health Bulletin* 29, Series 2, Number 3. Richmond, Va: Author.

Waitzkin, Howard B. and Barbara Waterman
1974 *The Evolution of Illness in Capitalist Society.* Indianapolis: Bobbs-Merrill.

Acknowledgment and thanks for providing helpful comments in the *preparation of this manuscript go to Hugh Mehan, Sam Wallace, Irving Kenneth Zola, and Donna Eder. This paper was presented as the Society for the Study of Social Problems Annual Meeting, New York, New York, August 1980. An earlier version appeared in* Linguistics and the Professions, *edited by Robert J. Di Pietro, Norwood, N.J.: Ablex, 1982.*

Medical Mortality Review: A Cordial Affair

Marcia Millman

A mortality and morbidity conference for doctors bears some resemblance to a wedding or a funeral for members of a family. In all these ceremonies there is some feeling among those who attend that tact and restraint must be exercised if everyone is to leave on friendly terms. But steering a mortality meeting along on a pleasant and even course is occasionally difficult, for as in weddings and funerals, the very nature of the event often prompts participants to come dangerously close to saying to one another those upsetting things that are usually left unsaid.

Mortality meetings are regularly scheduled conferences at Lakeside HospitaL; they are held in a large auditorium to accommodate the entire medical staff (private attending physicians, house officers, and teaching staff). Their avowed purpose is to review, in fine detail, those medical cages that ended in an in-hospital patient death. and in which there is some question of error, failure, or general mismanagement on the part of the physicians involved. One of the implicit if unspoken concerns that always underlies the review is the question of whether the patient's death might have been avoided had the medical judgment been more sound for what is usually involved in these cases is a question of misdiagnosis or of appropriate medical action taken too late.

In consideration of the delicacy of the occasion, the meetings are restricted to the medical staff of the hospital. Even the surgical staff is generally not invited. The surgical service has its own mortality meetings, and a surgeon would be considered meddlesome for attending a medical mortality conference simply out of curiosity. Only those surgeons who were directly involved in a particular case under consideration will be asked to attend a medical mortality meeting. Families are not informed that their deceased relative's case has been chosen for review. Although the meetings may be considerably embarrassing for the doctors involved, the Medical Mortality Conference is, at least on the surface, treated as an *educational* rather than a punitive, affair. At Lakeside, the conferences are not investigations or formal hearings held to consider the competence of particular doctors, although they are often presented this way on television medical dramas. There are no formal sanctions applied to doctors at the end of these conferences. Rather, Mortality Review Conferences are .,educational" sessions organized around reviewing particular cases rather than individual doctors, even though the cases are selected because there is disagreement over the appropriate treatment and often a question of physician error involved.

The Mortality Review Conference has a special quality of high tension, and the meetings are better attended than are those of the other regular teaching conferences. At Lakeside Hospital, the Chief of Medicine stands on the stage and presides over the Mortality Review Conference as a master of ceremonies. As the case is reviewed in chronological order, starting with the time of the patient ad. mission to the hospital, and proceeding to the autopsy report, the chief calls on the various doctors who were involved in the case, asks them to step to the front of the auditorium, and instructs them to recall and explain what they did and what they thought at each moment in time. He counsels them not to jump ahead of the chronological order, nor to divulge information gained at a later time, in order not to spoil the final diagnosis for the members of the audience. As one after another of the staff testifies about how they were led to the same mistaken diagnosis, a convincing case for the justifiability of the error is implicitly presented and the responsibility for the mistake is spread so that no one doctor is made to look guilty of a mistake that anyone else wouldn't have made, and in fact, didn't make. As in a good detective story, the case is reconstructed to show that there was evidence for suspecting an outcome different from the one that turns out to be the true circumstance. Responsibility for the error is also neutralized by making much of unusual or misleading features of the case, or showing how the patient was himself to blame, because of uncooperative or neurotic behavior. Furthermore, by reviewing the case in fine detail the doctors restore their images as careful, methodical practitioners and thereby neutralize the actual sloppiness and carelessness made obvious by the mistake. The doctors' discomfort is further minimized by treating the review as an educational occasion rather than an investigatory event.

In order to appreciate the special atmosphere and significance of the Mortality Review, it is important to understand that doctors who work together ordinarily live by a gentlemen's agreement to overlook each other's mistakes. The aim is not merely to hide errors and incompetence from the patients and the public, but also to avoid interfering in one another's work and to avoid acknowledgment of the injury that has been done to patients. Such a conspiracy to look the other way regarding the failures of one's colleagues is not always recognized by the doctors for what it is, for blindness to injury done to patients and a convincing set of justifications and excuses for medical mistakes are carefully built into their training and professional etiquette. Most doctors are therefore capable of comfortably viewing themselves as altruistic and highly responsible practitioners all the while they engage in collective rationalizations for ignoring and condoning each other's errors and incompetence.

Still, there are special occasions in the hospital routine, such as the Mortality Meeting, when doctors are gathered together to examine the sorts of unpleasant facts they would otherwise ignore. At these times a great deal of effort is expended to make the embarrassing facts seem less damaging. For if such medical incompetence or error were fully and publicly (among themselves) acknowledged. physician-colleagues might feel forced to take measures against one another, and this is one of the things they least like to do.

As the Chief of Medicine at Lakeside explained, "Eighty percent of the mistakes made around here are ignored or swept under the rug. I can only pick *certain* cases for mortality review—it's got to be a cordial affair."

Perhaps that description of the selection procedures for mortality review accounts for the curious fact that at Lakeside, most of the medical situations presented at these conferences conveniently seem to involve an illness that would have ended in the patient's death in any case, even if the correct diagnosis had been made immediately. There is a strange absence of cases review in those meetings in which the patient would clearly have lived had it not been for the medical mismanagement. By selecting only those cases in which the physician's error was not fateful in an ultimate sense the discussion of mistakes largely becomes an academic affair.

Practicality rather than sentiment is the key to in the tact and with which doctors respond to each other's errors. A doctor's reluctance to criticize a colleague's mistakes to his face at a large meeting is not motivated out of respect or affection. Indeed, many doctors are willing, in small groups, to say that another physician (not present) is a menace or a terrible doctor. And even at the mortality review conferences, those doctors who are not involved in a case may sit back and enjoy the gentle roasting of a disliked work associate. The reluctance to point out and criticize another doctor's mistakes at an official meeting comes rather out of a fear of reprisal and a recognition of common interests. For each doctor knows that he has made some more or less terrible mistakes in his career, and that he is likely to make others—mistakes, moreover, which will be obvious to his colleagues. That is why, in matters of peer regulation, doctors observe the Golden Rule.

So it is that mortality meetings are built upon a simultaneous admission and coverup of mistakes. For although the avowed purpose of those meetings is to review mistakes and prevent their recurrence, in actuality the meetings are organized and conducted in ways that absolve the doctors from responsibility and guilt and provide the self-assuring but somewhat false appearance that physicians are monitoring each other and their standards of work. In case after case physician errors are systematically excused and justified, and their consequences made to look unimportant.

Before turning to some actual cases, it should be noted that despite the tact and sensitivity with which doctors treat each other's errors, a mortality meeting is not an entirely comfortable situation. Like a family trying collectively to ignore that the father is having an affair, or that the daughter is a drug addict, the doctors at a mortality meeting are often pushed to extreme displays of courtesy to overlook the worst and find good excuses for regrettable behavior.

Case No. 1: Jonathan Thomas

Jonathan Thomas was a 34-year-old insurance salesman who had complained of abdominal pain and black stool (indicating gastrointestinal bleeding). His problem was diagnosed as gastric ulcer and he was placed on a regimen of tranquilizers and an ulcer diet. His subsequent complaints were explained as being consistent with an ulcer and a neurotic personality. Ten months later Jonathan Thomas died of cancer spread throughout his abdominal cavity.

This was to be a particularly uncomfortable case for the staff to consider in Mortality Review because of a number of factors. First of all, the patient was a young man with a large family, and this made his life more valuable in the eyes of the doctors. Second, mistakes in diagnosis had been made repeatedly, and important information overlooked more than once. Third, a large number of people had been involved in this case, and while this offered the consolation of spreading out the responsibility, it also pointed out the weaknesses of the hospital consulting system. For if not one of a dozen physicians had caught the obvious errors, it was probably because each of the consultants involved in the case had been too accepting of each other's erroneous assumptions instead of carefully doing the diagnostic jobs they were supposed to be doing.

Notices about the mortality meeting had been distributed days beforehand and signs posted around the hospital. The chief's secretary had made sure that all the doctors involved in the case would be there for the review. As always, the meeting was held in the large theater-like auditorium and members of the staff seated themselves in the rows of seats facing the stage in a steep incline.

The meeting was called to order by the Chief of Medicine, who welcomed everyone and made brief announcements of unrelated matters. Next, an intern described the hospital's mortality profile for the preceding month: he described how many patients had died in the hospital in each major disease category. Finally, the Chief of Medicine, Dr. Tanner, returned to the stage and introduced the Thomas case. As usual the patient's history was reviewed in chronological order, each doctor being called to the front of the room to recall his thoughts and describe his participation at that moment in time in the case.

The early history was reviewed by Dr. Backman, the specialist in gastrointestinal disorders who had managed the case. Backman was highly respected and well liked by most of the staff, and so there were no undertones of questioning his competence but rather friendly empathy for the usually careful physician who had made an uncharacteristic mistake. From the beginning, Backman explained, he had assumed that the gastrointestinal bleeding indicated by the black stool was caused by a stress-induced gastric ulcer: "What led us down the garden path last October was the fact that he was taking on added responsibility for his family's business. The sudden pain seemed to coincide with that, so we put him on an ulcer regimen and gave him tranquilizers and released him in satisfactory condition. After discharge, a GI series was negative, but epigastric pain reappeared and in April he reported severe upper left quadrant pains which became persistent."

Dr. Jenkins, one of the supervisors of the teaching program, interrupted: "Was this severe upper left quadrant pain different from the epigastric pain? Was it something new?"

Dr. Backman: "He described it as different. He had it at night, and it wasn't relieved with antacids."

Dr. Jenkins: "Well, didn't that make you uncomfortable with the diagnosis of gastric ulcer?"

Dr. Backman: "No. because he had resumed smoking and drinking now, and we suspected alcoholic hepatitis, because of his abnormal liver function test. He reported clay-colored stools and we readmitted him to the hospital. From the start of his readmission he was quite agitated and needed more sedation, so we called in Dr. Sheingold [the Chief of Psychiatry]."

Dr. Sheingold had considered saying something about Dr. Backman's description of the patient as "drinking again." In fact, he knew the patient drank very little, only a few beers when he went bowling once a week, and it seemed unfair to imply that the man was drinking enough to justify a diagnosis of alcoholic hepatitis. The trouble, Sheingold felt, was that once the doctors decided to bring a psychiatrist into the case most of them no longer believed anything the patient said. And so it had been easy for the doctors to regard this patient as an alcoholic. Still, Dr. Sheingold had observed that Backman was one of the few doctors in the hospital who thought that psychiatry had anything to offer them in their treatment of medical patients, so he had refrained from objecting to the imputation of alcoholism.

Sheingold was motioned to the stage to report on his participation in the case. He began: "Yes, I was invited to walk down the garden path with the others. I talked with the patient on his fourth day of admission. His father-in-law had just retired and appointed the patient as director of the family insurance business. Mr. Thomas had never liked the business and found it morbid. Indeed, he had complicated feelings about his business exacerbated by a long history of depression. Ten years ago he had been responsible for an automobile accident in which his oldest daughter, then three years old, had died. So I was quite sure along with Dr. Backman that this was gastric ulcer disease, and I wrote that in my notes. I also noted that there was an unlikely chance of pancreatic carcinoma [cancer] because I knew that would be considered at some time, but I was quite sure that it was an ulcer."

Dr. Stevens, one of the department chiefs in medicine, had been upset with the reasoning in this case. As he explained, one of his pet peeves was the stupid use of psychiatry, especially by the GI doctors, and he had noticed that Backman was one of the frequent offenders in this regard because as a GI specialist Backman also considered himself something of an expert in the field of psychiatry. As Stevens described the situation, every time one of the GI doctors heard a patient complaint that couldn't be explained he called in a psychiatrist.

Stevens wished they would instead just admit to the patient that they didn't know what was wrong, and explain that they would have to wait or do more tests. Instead, complained Stevens, a psychiatrist came in and spoke to the patient and *always* found a psychiatric complication. " And," concluded Stevens, "what did that tell you? That everyone has problems?"

Dr. Rosen, another internist on the hospital staff, was questioning Backman. "Why weren't the clay-colored stools considered? Didn't you believe him?"

Backman replied: "Well, the clay-colored stools could have been caused by the antacids he was taking, but to be perfectly frank, I didn't know how much credence I could give to his report. He was quite upset and had gone into a rage about having to pay for the use of the television in his room. I should also add that he was now complaining about leg pain as well. He was re-endoscoped and a liver scan was taken. It showed an enlarged liver without focal abnormalities and the liver function was not impaired. A liver biopsy was normal,which surprised us. We expected to find alcoholic hepatitis. After the biopsy there was hemoptysis (coughing up blood). We were concerned because that had never happened and we thought that bleeding from the liver biopsy might have gone into the lung area. We did a cholangiogram and it was normal but we noted that he had an elevated alkaphosphotase level. We released him from the hospital once again on a bland diet with tranquilizers, and his discharge diagnosis was peptic ulcer."

Dr. Davis, one of the younger internist, directed more questions to Backman: "Why wasn't a surgical exploration done at this time?"

Backman smiled, shaking his head. "I'm not sure. I guess we weren't smart enough." Davis continued: "Why was no attention paid to the calf pain?" Backman answered. "The reason we ignored his complaints of leg pain was that his roommate in the hospital had thrombophlebitis in the leg. So when Thomas complained of it, it just seemed too coincidental and we figured it was just a hysterical reaction."

Dr. Sheingold was afraid that this case was certainly not going to encourage the doctors in the hospital to turn to the psychiatry department for help. It made him angry that the only situation in which most of the doctors considered psychiatry to be useful was for the management of what they considered a "crazy" patient, and once a patient in the hospital was seen by a psychiatrist the doctors would attribute to the patient all sorts of psychological mechanisms that had nothing to do with the patient's personality (in this case they were imputing "hysterical" behavior to a nonhysterical patient) and they wouldn't even read the notes that Sheingold wrote in the patient's chart about which psychological mechanisms were relevant. Also, since they didn't regard psychiatric illness as real, they always disliked patients with psychiatric symptoms. As Sheingold later explained, all the doctors had disliked this patient when they thought that he suffered only from an ulcer, and they had only decided that he was likable after they realized that he was "really" sick with cancer.

Backman was still explaining why he had released the patient despite abnormal laboratory findings. "Oh, and to finish your question about surgery—his abdominal pain went away after three days so we didn't consider it any more." He leafed through the pages of the chart and continued "He was readmitted the following week with a swollen foot, and enlarged liver, extensive thrombophlebitis." Backman nodded to Cohen, the cardiologist who had been consulted at this point. Cohen stood up and briefly spoke from his place in the audience. " I was asked to say whether the problem was due to pulmonary emboli or from hemoptysis to the lung from the liver biopsy. I thought he had pulmonary emboli."

Attention was now directed to the Chief of Surgery. who described his part in the case. "I saw him at this point and I knew something terrible was going on. He was going downhill rapidly. It looked like an abdominal mass. The plan was now to deal with his phlebitis—so here we were in a bind. We had a GI bleeder who had to be anticoagulated for his emboli [a treatment that would increase bleeding], and now he had shortness of breath. The problem in dealing with this patient was that he was dead opposed to surgery. He had been in the life insurance business all his life, and every time we talked about surgery he would say, 'Now my family's gonna be collecting on my policy.'" The surgeon turned to Davis, who had earlier criticized Backman for not calling in a surgeon sooner. "I'll tell you why we didn't do an exploratory laparotomy [surgical investigation] earlier. He was so frantic and had been sick so long. He had abdominal pain and calf pain and GI bleeding. He dreaded surgery, and frankly I dreaded going in there. His wife kept yelling at me, asking what was wrong, and when I said I didn't know she called me stupid. I guess maybe we *were* stupid. Anyway that's why we didn't do an exploratory earlier." In the back of the auditorium, some of the medical residents were smiling and mumbling that the reason the Chief had delayed surgery was that he hated to operate. Douglas had a reputation among the younger aggressive doctors in the hospital of being too cautious and slow to act. It was not clear whether Douglas noticed their remarks, and he continued, "So we did a venous clip and when we later did an exploratory we saw that there was cancer all over. The patient died three days later, and I just want to add here that according to the chart he was in severe anguish on the last day of his life, and not given the painkillers we had prescribed, so we can thank our nurses for the making the last day of his life as miserable as possible." The surgeon nodded to the pathologist and the lights were switched off. Color slides of the patient's affected organs were flashed on the screen. Each one showed gross abnormalities from the spread of the cancer. Throughout the auditorium murmurs could be heard at the extensiveness of the cancer, as if to emphasize that with so dramatic and pervasive a disease they as doctors could hardly have been expected to stop such an invasion.

When the lights were turned on the surgeon drew the meeting to a close, explaining how at that very moment the patient's brother was waiting in his office; the brother had come to show him an article about a so-called wonder drug, which was illegal, for curing cancer. Douglas added that he had given the brother an appointment so that the man could yell at him for having refused to try this illegal drug. Several doctors in the audience laughed and shook their heads sympathetically, breaking into small groups as they moved into the adjoining room for coffee and doughnut.

The Thomas case, described above, illustrates how doctors often justify their errors by pointing to misleading or unusual features of the case. By demonstrating that they had good reason (though later shown to be mistaken) for doing what they did, they may avoid censure and discomfort, and save face before their colleagues. Physical symptoms inconsistent with the final diagnosis are the misleading cues which provide the most comforting and persuasive type of excuse for making the wrong diagnosis. However, when physical justifications are unavailable, doctors often resort to psychological and social evidence as the factors which misguided them and justified their behavior. In these cases. the nonphysical evidence is represented as being so convincing as to justify overlooking even physical evidence which should have alerted doctors to the correct diagnosis. In the Thomas case, for example, the doctors overlooked clear symptoms of organic disorder (such as the elevated alkaphosphotase level) because they were so convinced that the patient was neurotic and that his complaints and symptoms could be explained psychologically.

In other cases where physical findings are overlooked, or erroneously discounted, the physician will often excuse his embarrassing error by blaming the patient. If the patient can be "discredited" as crazy, alcoholic, obnoxious, uncooperative, or otherwise difficult or undeserving, then the responsibility for the medical error can be shifted away from the doctor to the patient's own doing. The following case illustrates this process.

Case No. 2: Alice McDonald

Mrs. McDonald was a 50 year-old woman who died in the Emergency Room of a perforated duodenal ulcer which the staff failed to diagnose, despite her complaints of severe abdominal pain.

The case was introduced in the meeting by the intern who had seen her in the Emergency Room. He opened the discussion by describing her as "An obese, alcoholic woman of Irish extraction who was very uncooperative and used very abusive language" thereby fixing her in the minds of the physicians in the audience as the type of patient who is difficult to treat.

In explaining why they had not paid much attention to her complaints of abdominal pain, the doctors involved in the case made much of her appearance of being "mentally disconnected."

Asked to be more specific about her mental state, both the intern and the medical doctor covering the Emergency Room that night stated that they remembered noting the smell of alcohol on her breath, and therefore felt they could dismiss her complaints as the ravings of a drunken woman.

Toward the end of the meeting someone in the audience offhandedly asked what the alcohol level in the blood had been at the time of the incident. Now the Chief of Medicine sheepishly admitted a fact that had been previously left unmentioned: although much had been made of this woman's drunkenness, the fact was that the alcohol level in the blood had been zero at the time of her examination.

This embarrassing fact was passed over quickly. No longer able to use her drunkenness as an excuse for their failure to take her complaints seriously, the doctors now turned more exclusively to emphasizing her angry, "disconnected" and uncooperative behavior toward them as the factor responsible for the poor treatment she received.

The power of the doctor's self-justification is highlighted in this case. For even after implicitly acknowledging that drunkenness was falsely attributed to the patient, the doctors continued to blame this woman's death on her own anger and abusive language, and ignored the possibility that such behavior was appropriate for a woman dying in great pain while the doctors around her treated her complaints as the fabrications of a hysterical alcoholic.

The case also illustrates how doctors may overlook important physical findings (which should indicate a serious illness) if they have already discounted the complaints by viewing the patient as a certain kind of neurotic individual. For a "neurotic" individual is viewed by doctors as an unreliable reporter, and once characterized this way, a patient's remarks are likely to be ignored. Indeed, these patients are commonly known among many doctors as "crocks" or "turkeys" and are considered undeserving of serious attention.

It is a complicated problem, for certainly doctors will occasionally meet with an anxious patient who will refuse to believe that he is in good health. But serious errors are often made as a result of characterizing patients as "crocks" for doctors are usually not in a position to correctly guess who is really sick and who isn't, from behavior alone.

Furthermore, doctors appear to assign the label "crock" quite often on grounds of personal or prejudiced responses. They are more likely, for example, to dismiss a patient as neurotic and not really sick if the patient seems angry. mistrustful, or disrespectful to the doctor. The label "crock" also seems to be applied erroneously more often to women.

Assessing the Effects of Physician-Patient Interactions on the Outcomes of Chronic Disease

Sherrie H. Kaplan, Sheldon Greenfield, and John E. Ware, Jr.

Physician-patient communication has traditionally been recognized as important to the practice of clinical medicine. Methods for eliciting an accurate history from and establishing rapport with the patient have been the subject of a substantial body of literature [1-4] and are featured in major medical texts.[5] Separate texts have been written on effective interviewing skills[6-8]; the elements of good patient interviewing techniques have been incorporated into many residency training programs[9-14]; professional societies are calling for more "humanism" in the physician-patient relationship, including more effective communication[15]; patients appear to value information from their doctors highly[6-18]; and third-party payers and health maintenance organizations are using the physician-patient relationship as a marketing strategy.

Contrasted with the bioscientific technologies in medicine, physician-patient communication has not attracted the scientific attention needed to identify its general effectiveness, or lack thereof, in achieving the goals of patient care. More specifically, information about the nature of the elements of communication that "work" in clinical terms is absent. Which are the appropriate outcomes against which the effectiveness of physician-patient communication should be evaluated? Are there discrete, identifiable, and mutable elements of physician-patient communication that lead to better outcomes?

In the current era, there are several compelling reasons to measure the effectiveness of (and to identify ways to improve) physician-patient communication, especially in the management of chronic disease. First, the nature of chronic disease requires substantial responsibility by the patient for implementing treatment regimens settled on during the physician-patient visit. Tasks of effective physician-patient communication must include transfer of sufficient information to chronically ill patients to permit them to implement the treatment regimen correctly and, equally importantly, to persuade them that the regimen, as agreed upon, should be carried out. Second, research evidence suggests that patients want a more active role in their medical care[19,20] and specifically want more information from their physicians.[17,18] Finally, if current interest in reimbursing physicians for "cognitive services" becomes policy, then it is unreasonable to ask less of the assessment of the quality of physician-patient communication than of the assessment of quality of technical care.

The purposes of this paper are to advance the salience of generic measures of health status as appropriate outcomes for assessing the effectiveness of physician-patient communication and to present empirical evidence that specific aspects

Kaplan, S. H. Greenfield, S. and Ware, J. E. (1989). Assessing the effects of physician-patient interactions on the outcomes of chronic disease. MEDICAL CARE, 27 (3) S110-S127.

of physician-patient communication can influence health outcomes. We describe here the results of three randomized controlled trials among patients with chronic diseases and a fourth non-equivalent controlled trial of breast cancer patients in which we audiotaped physician-patient conversations, coded these conversations using a modification of Bales' interaction analysis,[21] and compared measures of patients' functional status, subjective health evaluations, and physiologic health to conversational behaviors of physicians and patients during office visits at baseline and following the experiment.

Choice of Outcome Measures

Patient satisfaction is by far the most recognized and widely used measure for gauging the effectiveness of physician-patient communication. The logical and intuitive appeal of this measure as an appropriate indicator of effective physician-patient communication, in addition to the relative ease with which it can be administered, makes it an attractive candidate for one of the best outcome measures for assessing the quality of physician-patient communication. If, as research evidence suggests,[19,20] patients want more involvement in their care, then they should be happier when such involvement is realized. Moreover, dissatisfied patients have been shown to disenroll from health plans,[22] to engage in "doctor-shopping,"[23] to initiate complaints about physicians, [24] and to be noncompliant with medical recommendations.[25,26]

Several things should be considered in determining the appropriateness of patient satisfaction as the sole indicator of effective physician-patient communication, as it has typically been treated in empirical studies to date. Patients might be satisfied with less than optimal health care [27,28] or outcomes.[29] Satisfaction may not necessarily lead to the self-care activities required for improved health, particularly in chronic disease. In one of the few studies of the relationship of patient satisfaction to patient health status, more satisfied patients were found to be less healthy.[29] Satisfaction may also be in part an attribute of the patient[30] rather than an objective reflection of physician behavior. For these reasons and because patient satisfaction has shown a relatively consistent positive relationship to certain elements of physician-patient communication, [31-41] satisfaction should be included among but not be the only indicator of effective physician-patient communication. It should be used to supply information that is complementary to health status in assessing the quality of physician-patient communication.

Compliance has also been used as an indicator of effectiveness of physician-patient communication. Unlike those of patient satisfaction, the research findings do not show a clear relationship between physician-patient communication and subsequent patient compliance. Intuitively, patients who are provided with sufficient information to implement treatment regimens and persuaded effectively to carry out those regimens should comply. However, patients may or may not comply with recommendations for reasons unrelated to the quality of physician-patient communication (such as financial problems, transportation or other difficulties with access to care). In addition, compliance with medical care itself is necessary but insufficient to produce optimal health outcomes. Particularly in the case of chronic disease, passive adherence to medical regimens may be incompatible with the active monitoring and regimen adjustment needed to control the disease effectively. Compliance is useful, therefore, but limited as an indicator of effective physician-patient communication.

Optimally, effective physician-patient communication should lead to better health outcomes for the patient. Why? Beyond the obvious—the transfer of the information patients need to manage their disease effectively—the communication between physicians and patients can be a source of motivation, incentive, reassurance, and support as well as an opportunity for revision of expectations of both patient and physician. For many, if not most, patients the physician represents a formidable source of power and influence.[42] As such, the physician may be in a unique position not only to influence the patient's technical care and to persuade the patient to follow the dictates of that care, but also to change patients' perceptions of their health status and beliefs about and self-confidence regarding their ability to influence their health status and to provide motivation and incentives for engaging in health promotion. Physician behaviors that reinforce patients' self-confidence, motivation, and positive view of their health status may therefore indirectly influence patients' health outcomes.

Which outcomes? Clinically, the best understood outcomes are physiologic. A major disadvantage in using physiologic outcomes to assess the effectiveness of physician-patient communication is their lack of availability for many chronic illnesses, such as rheumatoid arthritis. Further, and perhaps most importantly, these outcomes are also highly specific and may contribute minimally to the understanding of the patient's overall health at any point in time.

Physician-patient communication occurs in the context of a dynamic, reciprocal, emergent relationship. If effective physician-patient communication works more narrowly, affecting patients' health status by increasing patient adherence to treatment regimen, then, to the extent that such adherence improves disease status, physiologic measures may be the most sensitive indicators of quality physician-patient communication. If, however, the communication between physician and patient works more broadly, affecting patients' health status by increasing patient self-confidence, motivation, and perceptions of their general health status, then any physiologic indicators of the status of an individual disease may be too focused to detect the effect of high quality physician-patient communication.

Although there is a rather widely shared belief in medicine that the communication between physicians and patients is less about the sterile transfer of information and more about the emotional context of reassurance, support, and understanding in which the information is exchanged,[11-14] there is little empirical support for this notion. Table 1 displays findings from studies in which specific behaviors of physicians and patients during office visits have been compared with patients' health status measured at some point following the visit. In six of the eight studies reviewed, an association was observed between physician-patient communication and health outcome.

Generic measures of health status[51,52] provide a comprehensive scope and tap the target that best fits the espoused goals of effective physician-patient communication, namely, patients' sense of their ability to perform usual daily routines and their overall sense of well-being. Accordingly, we have chosen functional status[51] and patients' subjective evaluations of their health status, along with traditional physiologic outcome measures, both to assess the effectiveness of physician-patient communication and to evaluate the impact of an intervention designed to improve this communication.

Methods

Our data came from three separately conducted randomized controlled trials among patients with ulcer disease,[53] hypertension,[50] and diabetes[49] along with a fourth nonequivalent controlled trial among patients with breast cancer. The purpose of the intervention evaluated was to improve physician-patient communication by providing patients with individualized information about their medical care in the form of their medical record, along with an algorithm describing disease management with which to interpret this information, and coaching in behavioral strategies for increasing their participation in care during the office visit. These behavioral strategies included techniques for improving question asking, negotiating skills, and medical care "focus" during the conversation, along with techniques for decreasing barriers such as

TABLE 1. Studies Relating Physician-Patient Communication to Patients' Health Outcomes

Investigator	Data Source	Health Outcome	Effect
Orth et al.[43]	Audiotapes	Blood pressure control	Observed
Starfield et al.[44]	Questionnaire	Problem resolution	Observed
Stewart et al.[45]	Questionnaire	Perceived recovery	Observed
Bass et al.[46]	Questionnaire	Problem resolution	Observed
The Headache Study[47]	Questionnaire	Problem resolution	Observed
Woolley et al.[28]	Questionnaire	Functional status	Not observed
Hulka et al.[48]	Questionnaire	Blood sugar control	Not observed
Kaplan and Greenfield, et al.[49,50]	Audiotapes	Blood pressure control; blood sugar control	Observed

embarrassment, anxiety, and intimidation likely to reduce patients' effectiveness during the visit. The goal of this experimental program was to change the behavior of physicians as well as that of patients by training patients to take a more active role in their care.

This program was compared with a control intervention in which patients were provided general information regarding the etiology, prevalence, and nature and necessity of self-monitoring and self-care (compliance) activities. Control group patients were given copies of standardized materials documenting this information, but unlike experimental patients they were neither shown nor given copies of their medical records nor encouraged to ask questions. These interventions are well documented elsewhere.[49,50,53]

Description of the Study Samples

Patients participating in these studies came from four very different health care settings and vary considerably in sociodemographic characteristics. Participating patients with ulcer disease were chosen from clinical rosters of a local Veterans Administration hospital outpatient clinic; hypertensive patients were sampled from the hypertension clinic of a local free clinic; diabetic patients were randomly selected from the roster of patients attending an endocrinology clinic at a university teaching hospital; and breast cancer patients were chosen from postmastectomy patients scheduled to receive adjuvant chemotherapy at several local private office practices. There were statistically significant differences in years of education completed ($F_{(1,247)} = 9.18$, $P < .01$), proportion of females, and ethnic composition of the study samples (Table 2). The replication of our findings across trials is impressive in light of these differences in settings and sample characteristics.

Study Designs

At enrollment, audiotape recordings of the physician-patient visit were obtained for patients in all study samples to serve as baseline data. At this visit, patients also completed a self-administered questionnaire measuring health status, preference for active involvement in medical decision making knowledge of disease, and satisfaction with care. This questionnaire was returned by mail. Baseline physiologic measures were also collected at this visit for patients in the diabetes and hypertension samples. At the time of their next regularly scheduled clinic visit, patients in the randomized controlled trials were assigned to experimental or control group and the appropriate intervention was administered. Patients in the

TABLE 2. Sociodemographic Characteristics of Study Samples

Patient Characteristics	Ulcers (N = 45)	Hypertension (N = 105)	Diabetes (N = 59)	Breast Cancer (N = 43)
Age (years)[a]	55 (12)	54 (13)	50 (14)	47 (10)
Education (years)[a]	13 (3)	8 (5)	13 (3)	14 (2)
Percent female	2	68	49	100
Percent Spanish speaking[b]	0	62	0	0

[a] Data are means with standard deviations in parentheses.

[b] Exclusively Spanish speaking; patients in the ulcer, diabetes, and breast cancer samples were selected

breast cancer sample were enrolled in the experimental group until the quota for that sample had been reached; patients enrolled after that time were assigned to the control group. Physicians saw patients in both experimental and control groups in all study samples but were blind to group membership. The physician-patient visit immediately after each intervention session (experimental and control) was again tape recorded.

At the next regularly scheduled visit, the third after study enrollment, patients were seen for a second time by the research assistants who administered the appropriate intervention just before the patient saw his or her physician. This physician-patient visit was also tape recorded. From 8 to 12 weeks after the last intervention session, patients in all study samples were mailed a second questionnaire measuring functional and subjectively evaluated health status, preference for involvement in medical decision making, satisfaction with care, and knowledge of disease. Physiologic measures were also obtained at this visit for the diabetic and hypertensive patients.

Description of Measures

Measurement of Doctor-Patient Communication

Audiotape recordings of the physician-patient office visits before and after the intervention were analyzed using a coding scheme that classified each utterance by patient or physician into one of thirty codes, only one of which could be assigned to each utterance. These codes were grouped into three categories—control, communication, or affect—based on whether the utterance was aimed at controlling the behavior of the other party, communicating information, or conveying emotion.[54,55] For example, a statement by the doctor to "see the dietician for a diabetic weight reduction diet" would be coded as a "direction" and classified as a controlling behavior; "ulcer disease occurs more frequently among smokers" would be coded as "information" and classified as communication; "congratulations on your weight loss!" would be coded as "support" and classified as positive affect. Because of the importance of affect or emotion and the relative infrequency with which it occurs during physician-patient interviews, expressions of emotion were given precedence over all other codes.

We derived several indicators of the style of physician-patient communication that combined these codes within speaker, including physician control, patient control, information giving, and expression of positive and negative affect by physician and patient. Each of these indicators was a sum of the conversational codes for physicians and for patients within each of the three categories (control, communication, and affect).

In addition, we grouped the conversational codes into empirically derived combinations of both physician and patient behaviors during the visit including: an index of patient effectiveness (numbers of factual statements by the physician divided by the sum of all controlling utterances by the patient; communication ratio (proportion of patient to physician utterances during the visit); and one of three patterns describing all conversation during the visit, including physician direction (characterized by questions, interruptions, etc., by the doctor and responses by the patient), patient direction (characterized by questions, interruptions, etc. by the patient and responses by the physician), and affect/opinion exchange (combining any display of emotion with statements of personal opinions by either physician or patient). More complete descriptions of these measures appear in Table 3. All conversational codes were divided by the length of the interview to control for differences in lengths of office visits across patients.

Measurement of Heath Outcomes

To determine the effects of physician-patient communication on health outcomes, we compared data from the analyzed tape recordings of office visits with patients' functional status and self-reported evaluations of their health (including number of health problems, days lost from work, and overall health rating) obtained from questionnaires. In addition, for diabetic and hypertensive patients we compared tape data with blood sugar and blood pressure, respectively. For breast cancer patients, we obtained a summary index of their experience of chemotherapy-related symptoms gathered from monthly diaries.

Table 3 summarizes these health status measures. Blood sugar among diabetic patients was measured as the level of glycosylated hemoglobin ($HbAl_c$)[56]; sitting diastolic blood pressure readings were used to measure hypertension control. We also used a 13-item shortened version of the RAND Functional Status Questionnaire (including such items as "Are you unable to do certain kinds or amounts of work, housework, or schoolwork because of your health?" and "Do you have trouble either walking several blocks or climbing a few flights of stairs because of your health?") to measure patients' functional status. This scale was coded such that a high score meant more limitations in functioning due to illness. Three single-item measures were used to obtain patients' subjective health evaluations: number of self-reported health problems; number of days lost from work because of illness; and overall health rating. The summarized symptom-experience index obtained for breast cancer patients derived from a symptom checklist completed during the interim between each chemotherapy cycle (approximately 1 month) for the 6-month course of adjuvant chemotherapy by each patient in the study.

All multi-item scales including derived indicators of physician-patient communication were tested for internal consistency reliability using Cronbach's alpha formula[57] and were shown to be satisfactory (alpha > .65) for group comparisons.

Results

Doctor-Patient Communication and Functional Status: Patient Evaluations of Health Status

Tables 4 through 6 present the correlations between each of the derived indicators of physician and patient conversational behavior during the baseline office visit and survey measures of patients' health status at follow-up (measured as functional status and subjective evaluations of health 8 to 12 weeks after the last intervention session). We observed similar results when this correlational analysis was performed separately for each of the four study samples; accordingly, data presented in these tables represent a combined sample (N = 252).

"Good health," whether reported behaviorally as functional status or perceptually as more subjective health status evaluations, was consistently related to patient conversational behavior during the office visit. Specifically, as seen in Table 4, patients who were more controlling (asked more questions, made more attempts to direct the flow of conversation and their physicians' behavior)

TABLE 3. Description of Measures

Measure	No. of Items	Meaning of High Score	When Measured	Definition	Data Source	Scoring
I. Physician-patient interation indicators	NA	More patient control	Baseline	Control attempts by patient during interaction	Tapes	Sum of all controlling utterances made by patient (that is, those intended to influence behavior of the physician or to control the nature of the conversation, such as interruptions, suggestions, assertions)
Level of patient participation		More patient involvemen	Baseline	Ratio of patient to physician utterances	Tapes	Sum of all patient uttereances during the encounter divided by all physician utterances; an indicator of patient assertiveness relative to the physician
Effectiveness of patient information seeking	NA	More effective information seeking	Baseline	Ratio of physicians' information-conveying statments of patients' control attempts	Tapes	Sum of all factual statements made by the physician divided by the sum of all patient controlling utterance; an indicator of patients' ability to elicit information effectively from the physician
Interaction pattern	NA	More doctor direction	Baseline	Physician direction of interaction	Tapes	Sum of all physician controlling utterances and all patient factual statments divided by length of encounter in minutes; portion of the encounter directed by the physician
		More patient direction	Baseline	Patient direction of interaction	Tapes	Sum of all patient controlling utterances and all patient factual statments divided by length of encounter in minutes; portion of the encounter directed by the physician
		More affect and opinions	Baseline	Affect-opinion sharing between physician and patient	Tapes	Sum of all affect (emotion) expressed by physicians and patients, plus all non-factual opinion statments of physicians and patients divided by length of the encounter reflecting personal involvement

TABLE 3. Description of Measures (continued)

Measure	No. of Items	Meaning of High Score	When Measured	Definition	Data Source	Scoring
II. Physiologic measures of health						
Blood sugar	1	Poorer control of diabetes	Baseline	Level of glycosylated hemoglobin, measured using boronate affinity colum kit (Endocrine Sciences, Tarzana, CA)	Lab reports	Continuous; range : $6 \leq 15$
Blood pressure	1	Poorer control of hypertension	Baseline	Level of diastolic pressure; average of three consecutive seated readings	Medical record	Continuous; range : $60 \leq 125$
III. Survey measures of health						
Overall health ratings	1	Better health	Baseline and follow-up	Patients' rating of their present health status	Questionaire sample item: "How would you rate your overall health?"	1 = excellent 2 = good 3 = fair 4 = poor
Number of health problems	1	More health problems	Baseline and follow-up	Sum of current health problems or illnesses listed by patient (including study condition)	Questionnairesample item: "What health problems do you now have?"	Continuous; range : 0-6
Days lost from work	1	More days lost	Baseline and follow-up	Number of days lost from work in the previous month due to illness	Questionnaire	Continuous
Functional limitations index	13	More limitation	Enrollment and follow-up	Limitations imposed by illness on physical, rol, social, mobility	Questionnaire sample item: "Are you unable to drive a car because of your health?" (mobility	1 = yes 2 = no range = 0-10

TABLE 4. Relationship of Patients' Conversational Behaviors to Health Status

Survey Measures Health[c]	Patient Conversation Indicatorsb			
	Control	Positive Affect	Negative Affect	Information Sharing
Overall health ratings	.30*	.38	.31*	-.43*
Days lost from work	-.22*	.20*	-.35*	-.32*
Number of health problems	-.44*	-.09	-.32*	-.26*
Functional limitations	-.41*	-.36	-.26*	.49*

TABLE 5. Relationship of Patients' Conversational Behaviors to Health Status[a]

Survey Measures Health[c]	Patient Conversation Indicatorsb			
	Control	Positive Affect	Negative Affect	Information Sharing
Overall health ratings	.17	-.16	.30*	.30*
Days lost from work	.36*	-.10	-.23*	-.13
Number of health problems	.41*	-.12	-.39*	-.37*
Functional limitations	.37*	-.03	-.45*	-.29*

[a] Data presented are Pearson product-moment correlations.

[b] Measures of doctor-patient communication were obtained at baseline.

[c] Health status was measured approximately 1 month after last follow-up visit.

* $P < .05$.

TABLE 6. Relationship of Combined Physician-Patient Conversational Behaviors to Health Status[a]

Measures of Health[c]	Doctor-Patient Interaction Indicatorsb: Patient Effectiveness Index	Communication Ratio	Affect-Opinion Sharing
Overall health ratings	.42*	.21*	.22*
Days lost from work	-.16	-.30*	-.29*
Number of health problems	-.31*	.13	.12
Functional limitations	-.47*	-.36*	-.46*

[a] Data presented are Pearson product-moment correlations.
[b] Measures of physician-patient communication were obtained at baseline.
[c] Health status was measured approximately 1 month after last follow-up visit.
*P < .05.

during the baseline office visit reported fewer days lost from work, health problems, and functional limitations because of illness and rated their health more favorably at follow-up. Similarly, expression of affect by the patient (both positive and negative) was consistently associated with better health at follow-up. The amount of factual information given by the patient, however, was inversely related to health status at follow-up.

Physicians' conversational behavior during the baseline office visit was also related to patients' health status at follow-up (see Table 5), although less consistently so than conversational behaviors by the patient. More control by the physician (asking questions, giving directions, interrupting) was associated with poorer reported health for three of the four indicators of patients' health status at follow-up—days lost from work, health problems, and functional limitations. In contrast to the results for patient conversational behaviors, positive affect expressed by the physician during the baseline visit was not related to any indicator of patients' health status at follow-up. Conversely, expression of negative affect by the physician (tension, anxiety, strain, self-consciousness, frustration, impatience) during the baseline visit was associated with better health status at follow-up according to all four health status indicators. In contrast to the relationship of patient information giving to health status, information giving by the physician during the baseline visit was related to better health status at follow-up.

Table 6 presents associations between the health status measures and interaction indicators that combine physician and patient conversational behaviors. Patients who were more effective in information seeking (the ratio of factual statements by the physician to controlling behaviors by the patient) at baseline reported better health at follow-up according to three indicators. Similarly, patient involvement in the interaction (the ratio of patient to physician conventional behaviors) was related to better health follow-up according to three indicators.

Of the three interaction pattern measures defined in Table 3, only affect/opinion exchange (combining all emotion expressed by physician and patient during the visit plus all non-factual opinion statements) was significantly related to patients' health status at follow-up (results for the

TABLE 7. Correlations Between Measures of Physician-Patient Communication and Physiologic Measures of Health[a]

DYAD Indices[b]	Blood Glucose[c]	Blood Pressure[d]
Patient control	-.49*	-.29*
Patient positive affect	-.15	-.22*
Patient negative affect	-.31*	-.49*
Patient information sharing	.22*	.06
Physician control	.29*	.30*
Physician positive affect	.10	.18
Physician negative affect	-.42*	-.53*
Physician information sharing	-.27*	-.27*
Effectiveness index	-.43*	-.36*
Communication ratio	-.29*	-.41*
Physician-directed pattern	.08	.15
Patient-directed pattern	-.20	-.28*
Affect-opinion exchange pattern	-.26*	-.39*

[a] Data presented are Pearson product-moment correlations.
[b] DYAD indices pertain to baseline visits.
[c] Hemoglobin A1 was used to measure blood glucose; values were obtained at follow-up.
[d] Average of three seated diastolic blood pressure readings; values were obtained at follow-up.
*$P < .05$.

latter are presented in the last column of Table 6). Patients with baseline encounters having more emotion (positive and negative) expressed along with more opinion exchange during the baseline visit had better health at follow-up according to three of the four health measures.

Relationship Between Doctor-Patient Communication and Physiologic Measures of Health

Disaggregated indicators of physicians' and patients' conversational behaviors during baseline office visits (e.g., physician control, physician and patient positive and negative affect, and information giving by physician and patient) showed significant patterns of association with health at follow-up as measured by physiologic indicators, although the associations tended to be weaker for the physiologic than for the survey measures of patients' health. Of the disaggregated conversational indicators, patient control during the baseline visit was most substantially related to lower follow-up blood glucose and blood pressure readings (see Table 7). Two of the three interaction patterns (physician direction and patient direction) were unrelated to either of the follow-up physiologic health measures. As for the survey measures of patients' health status, the affect-opinion exchange pattern was significantly related to both follow-up blood glucose and follow-up blood pressure.

In summary, poorer control of diabetes and hypertension at follow-up was associated with less patient control, less effective information seeking by and less involvement of the patient, and less emotion/exchange of opinions by physician and patient during the baseline office visit.

The effects of physician-patient communication on aggregated treatment-related symptom

TABLE 8. Effects of the Intervention on Physician-Patient Communications: Patient Controlling Behavior

Study Group	Study Period	Experimental[a]	Control[a]	t[b]
Diabetes (n = 59)	Postintervention	2.72 (.82)	.55 (.54)	2.25*
Hypertension (n = 105)	Postintervention	1.45 (.76)	.75 (.90)	2.15*
Ulcers (n = 45)	Postintervention	1.17 (.64)	.58 (.71)	2.09*
Breast Cancer (n = 43)	Postintervention	2.99 (.59)	.82 (.65)	2.41*

[a] Data reported in the table are means with standard deviations in parentheses.
[b] t-test values are reported for analysis of covariance comparing group means for each study group at follow-up,
controlling for baseline measures.
*P < .05.

experience reported by patients in the breast cancer study sample paralleled the observed relationship between number of health problems reported and indicators of physician-patient communication in the chronically ill study populations (data not presented). Symptom experience over the course of chemotherapy was less with greater patient control (Pearson's r = -.47, P < .05), patient negative affect (r = -.39, P < .05), and information giving by the patient (r = .41, P < .05). Symptom experience was also greater with more physician control (r = .47, P < .05), and more information giving by the physician (r = .55, P < .05), and was lower with more negative affect expressed by the doctor (r = -.50, P < .05). Symptom experience showed no relationship to positive affect expressed by physician or patient. Of the three combined indicators of physician-patient communication, two (patient effectiveness and affect-opinion exchange) were significantly negatively correlated with symptom experience (r = -.47, P < .05, and r = -.38, P < .05, respectively).

Effects of the Intervention on Doctor-Patient Communication

The data presented in Tables 4 through 7 combined both experimental and control groups for the purpose of analyzing the association between physician and patient conversational behaviors during the office visit and subsequent health status of the patient. Tables 8 through 10 summarize comparisons between these groups designed to test the effects of a change in physician-patient communication on patients' health status. Selected indicators have been chosen to represent effects observed across the conversational behaviors of the patient, those of the doctor, and their interaction. We first examine the effects of the intervention on conversational behavior and then link one of them to change in health status.

The intervention had a substantial effect on patient controlling behavior during the office visit (see Table 8). For all study samples, we observed no statistically significant differences between groups at baseline. Postintervention, we found that patients in the experimental group exerted more control during the visit after the intervention that did controls; these differences remained statistically significant when adjusted for baseline values in an analysis of covariance.

TABLE 9. Effects of the Intervention on Physician-Patient Communications: Effectiveness of Patient Information Seeking

Study Sample	Study Period	Experimental[a]	Control[a]	t[b]
Diabetes (n = 59)	Preintervention	.82 (.98)	.76 (1.31)	2.31*
	Postintervention	1.38 (.79)	.80 (1.09)	2.31*
Hypertension (n = 105)	Preintervention	.96 (.75)	1.11 (.66)	2.67*
	Postintervention	2.41 (1.70)	1.00 (.79)	2.67*
Ulcers (n = 45)	Preintervention	.49 (.38)	.44 (.25)	2.64*
	Postintervention	.93 (.52)	.49 (.34)	
Breast cancer (n = 43)	Preintervention	.99 (1.00)	.87 (1.11)	2.64*
	Postintervention	2.76 (1.95)	1.01 (.92)	2.46*

[a] Data in the table are means with standard deviations in parentheses.

[b] t-test values are reported for analysis of covariance by study group comparing experimental and control group means, controlling for baseline measures.

*$P < .05$.

TABLE 10. Effects of the Intervention and Changes in Physician-Patient Communication Patterns on Changes in Health Status

	Change in Functional Limitations[a]		
Dependent Variable	Zero-order Correlation Coefficients	Regression Estimates[b] Beta	t
Treatment group[c]	.69*	-.53	4.12*
Change in HbA[d]	.54*	.32	3.01*
Diabetes complications	.33*	.26	2.21*
Affect-opinion exchange	-.36*	-.29	2.65*
Age	-.23*	-.20	-1.87
Education	.25*	.12	1.02

[a] Change in health measured by subtracting score at baseline from follow-up score.

[b] Regression equation: multiple $R = .69$, $R^2 = .47$; $F(6,52) = 6.96$, P .01.

[c] Treatment group scored 1 = experimental; 0 = control.

[d] Sum of complications related to diabetes abstracted from medical record at baseline.

*$P < .05$.

Patients in the experimental group were more effective in obtaining information from their physicians after the intervention than controls across all four study samples, controlling for baseline differences (see Table 9). These similarities remained when adjusted for age, sex and education, variables that differed between study samples.

The combined physician-patient interaction patterns were affected similarly by the intervention for the four study samples. As reported elsewhere,[49,53] the physician-direction pattern was significantly reduced and the affect-opinion exchange pattern significantly increased after the intervention, adjusted for baseline differences.

Table 10 presents the relative contribution of the intervention, changes in physiologic health ($HbA1_c$), number of diabetic complications, patient sociodemographic characteristics of the patient and physician-patient communication behaviors to changes from baseline in patients' functional limitations between baseline and follow-up. Because many physician and patient verbal behaviors were highly intercorrelated, only the aggregated patterns of communication behaviors were included in this regression analysis to avoid multicolinearity problems. Among these patterns, only affect-opinion exchange was statistically significant in predicting functional limitations at follow-up. The other patterns were excluded in subsequent analyses. The results of the ordinary least squares regression presented in Table 10, therefore, include only the affect-opinion exchange conversational pattern. As evident, treatment group, change in the physiologic measure of health ($HbAl_c$), severity of diabetes (as measured by the number of complications reported in the patient's medical record), and the affect-opinion exchange conversational pattern were statistically significant predictors of change in the number of functional limitations reported between baseline and follow-up.

A similar pattern was observed for the hypertensive study sample. Favorable changes in functional limitations were predicted by treatment group (experimental), change in diastolic blood pressure, severity of hypertension, the affect-opinion exchange conversational pattern, the patient-direction conversational pattern, and education and native (vs. immigrant) status (data presented elsewhere).[50]

Discussion

The findings from our studies suggest that, consistent with theory about the impact of patient involvement in care on health,[58] a relationship exists between the way in which physicians and patient behave during an office visit and patients' subsequent health status. Of the individual behaviors of patients and physicians, we observed that more patient control, more affect, especially negative affect expressed by physicians and patients, and more information provided by physicians during office visits were associated with better health status reported at follow-up, measured both by functional status and subjective evaluations of health. Of the combined patterns of physician-patient communication, we observed that more effective information gathering by patients, and more conversation by patients relative to the physician during the visit, were related to better health status reported at follow-up, especially functional status. Expression of affect or emotion, both positive and negative, by physicians and patients was related to reporting of better functional status and subjective evaluations of health by patients at follow-up.

The relationship of the physiologic measures of patients' health status at follow-up to these measures of physician-patient communication followed a pattern similar to that for functional status and subjective evaluations of health. More control by patients, less control by physicians, more negative affect expressed by both, more effective information seeking by patients, and greater overall patient conversation relative to the physician were consistently related to better control of diabetes and hypertension as measured by hemoglobin Al^c and diastolic blood pressure, respectively. We can thus assert with some confidence that the effects we observed represent a real impact on patients' health-that patients "aren't just saying" that their health is improved.

In summary, with respect to the three broad categories represented in our coding scheme—control, communication, and affect—more patient and less physician control, more affect, particularly negative affect expressed by physician and patient, and more information provided by the physician in response to effective patient information seeking were related to better patient health status.

The relationship of negative affect to outcome is noteworthy both because it parallels findings from other studies relating patient satisfaction to physician-patient communication (more negative affect was associated with greater patient satisfaction[59]), and because it is strikingly consistent across all four study samples. We should note that the classic definition of "negative affect" originated by Bales[51] and used in this[54,55] and similar coding schemes[25,60] includes a broad spectrum of behaviors such as tension, impatience, strain, misgivings, stammering, nervous laughter, frustration, anxiety, and self-consciousness in addition to anger. These behaviors are rare in typical physician-patient communication, and the most frequently occurring among them is tension. Because they are so rare, we could not examine the relationship between each negative emotion and patients' health status meaningfully in these study samples. On the surface counterintuitive, the positive relationship between negative affect and patients' health status might very well be evidence of "healthy friction" or role tension between physicians and patients, in which patients' assertions of control compete with physicians' normal role-related dominance of the visit and creates some role strain for both. In support of this interpretation, the intervention designed to alter the patient's usual role during the visit changed the affect-opinion exchange pattern of interaction across all four study samples. Also, expression of frustration or impatience with a patient who, for example, has not lost weight, taken medication as recommended, stopped smoking, may be interpreted by the patient as an expression of caring on the part of the physician. It is interesting that the originators of the conversational coding scheme used in these studies defined an index of engagement, representing a higher quality interview between physician and patient, that included positive and negative affect.[54] The further understanding of the relationship between negative affect and patients' health status requires larger study samples and longitudinal observation of both physician-patient office visits and patient health outcomes.

Several explanations for our results are plausible. It could be that the relationship between physician-patient communication and patients' health status is not causal but associational—that sicker patients behave more passively during the visit with the physician and physicians are more controlling with sicker patients than with those who are healthier. Because of the known stability of health status, and because the interval between our baseline and follow-up measures ranged from 4 to 18 months among patients with chronic illnesses, it is certainly possible that we were not observing changes in health status but merely concurrent association. The relationship between greater physician control of the conversation during the visit and poor subsequent health status of the patient, for example, might reflect more intense questioning by physicians of sicker patients, rather than an adverse effect of physician domination on patient health. Similarly, more effective information seeking by patients during the visit might not have produced better health outcomes but might instead reflect the greater effectiveness of healthier patients in communicating with their physicians.

This simple associational interpretation of our data can be rejected for several reasons. First, although patients in our studies had a range of health states, both generic and physiologic, at baseline and at follow-up, only a few patients were so seriously ill that they would behave passively solely as a function of severe illness. Second, we experimentally manipulated patients' behavior during the visit and observed changes in patients' health status. The average change exceeded what would be expected by chance for each health status measure. Further, these changes were related to changes in physician-patient communication during the visit (controlling for patients' previous health state), suggesting a causal rather than an associational relationship. The design of these studies allowed us to compare experimentally manipulated patient behaviors to those that would occur after a more standard educational program. With no preintervention differences, we observed substantial differences' between these two groups after the interventions in both conversational behavior and in health outcomes, also suggesting a causal link.

Another plausible explanation for our findings is that greater participation by patients during the office visit, augmented by the active "engagement" of the physician, reinforced patients' confidence in their abilities to manage their disease. Recent studies have linked the exercise of control, even in modest amounts and limited situations, directly with improvements in health status.[61-63] Other studies have demonstrated that a sense of control over a situation, even if the individual actually has no actual control, has a positive effect on health.[64,65] Some investigators are now exploring the direct effects of control on the body's biochemical processes.[58,66] This evidence suggests a direct effect of control exercised in conversation with physicians during an office visit on the patient's health.

Perhaps a more conventional explanation of our findings would include an intervening step. Increased patient confidence generated by greater participation during the office visit might lead to closer adherence to treatment regimens that in turn leads to improved health status. Studies suggest that individuals are more likely to follow through on commitments in which they feel they had some say, compared with those in which they were passive.[67] We did not measure adherence in our studies. Further research is needed to explore the relationships between physician and patient behaviors during the visit and the steps patients take (or fail to take) to improve their health after the visit.

Our studies underscore the importance of the physician-patient relationship for patients' health outcomes. After our experimental interventions, patients changed their behavior during the office visit in several ways as reflected in varied conversational indicators. This rather generalized effect suggests that a more global change, even if temporary, was made in the manner in which patients treated their physicians. That these changes were related to improvements in a comprehensive array of health status indicators highlights the significance of the office visit for affecting the health outcomes of patients with chronic disease. Physicians may influence the outcomes of those patients not only through the medical care process, but also by shaping how patients feel about the disease and their ability to control or contain its impact on their lives. The notion that the physician has an influence on illness independent of diagnostic and therapeutic activities is not new. Hippocrates suggested that the physician might influence patients' health.[68] Most recently, the American Board of Internal Medicine recognized the importance of physician behaviors other than those related to the technical process of care for patient management.[15]

To create meaningful training programs for changing the behavior of both physicians and patients during the office visit, we need to conduct research that will increase the understanding of the specific behaviors that are both mutable and lead to improvements in health outcomes, measured comprehensively. This research could be done by tracking the effects of "naturally occurring" physician-patient behaviors on health outcomes. Recent research by Orth and Stiles,[43] showing an association between patients' expression of their complaints in their own words and physicians' provision of information during a visit, on the one hand, and reduction of diastolic blood pressure, on the other, is an excellent example of such research. Another path for such studies involved observing the effects of manipulations or interventions on physician-patient behavior and on patient health outcomes. Our studies have shown that an increase in emotion, particularly negative emotion, is related to improvement in health status. Other studies[38] have shown a similar relationship between negative emotions or feelings expressed by physicians during office visits and greater patient satisfaction with the visit.

It should not be concluded from our findings or those from any existing studies that physician anger or hostility leads to better patient health outcomes. All studies to date in which a positive relationship between negative physician affect and positive patient outcomes has been observed have relied on coding schemes that combine various feeling states (tension, sadness, anxiety, impatience, strain, misgivings, self-consciousness, frustration) each of which might have different meanings and implications for health status. Studies tracking large groups of physicians and patients over time with comprehensive health status assessment measures are needed.

We conclude that the physician-patient relationship is a primary bond that may act as a form of social support[69] to influence patients' health status. We assert that generic measures of patients' health, in addition to available physiologic measures, are the logical outcomes against which to assess effective physician-patient communication. The recognition of the salience of the physician-patient relationship and of communication between physicians and patients is particularly important at a time when the health care delivery system is undergoing changes that may place this relationship at risk.

References

1. West C. Ask me no questions ... : an analysis of queries and replies in physician-patient dialogues. In: Fisher S, Todd AD, eds. *The social organization of doctor-patient communication*. Washington, DC: Center for Applied Linguistics, 1983:75.
2. Wolf GA. *Collecting data from patients*. Baltimore, MD: University Park Press, 1977.
3. Kraytman M. *The complete patient history*. New York: McGraw-Hill Book Co, 1979.
4. Beckman HB, Frankel RM. The effect of physician behavior on the collection of data. *Ann Intern Med*, 1984;101:692.
5. Braunwald E, et al., eds. *Harrison's principles of internal medicine*. New York: McGraw-Hill Book Co, 1987.
6. Reiser DE, Schroeder AK. *Patient interviewing: the human dimension*. Baltimore: Williams and Wilkins, 1980.
7. Bernstein L, Bernstein RS. *Interviewing, a guide for health professionals*, 3rd ed. New York: Appleton-Century-Crofts, 1980.
8. Gordon RL. *Interviewing, strategy, techniques and tactics*. Homewood, IL: Dorsey Press, 1980.
9. Kahn GS, Cohen B, Jason H. The teaching of interpersonal skills in US medical schools. *J Med Educ*, 1979;54:29.
10. Engler CM, Saltzman GA, Walker ML et al. Medical student acquisition and retention of communication and interviewing skills. *J Med Educ*, 1981;56:572.
11. Lipkin M, Quill TE, Napodano RJ, et al. The medical interview: a core curriculum for residencies in internal medicine. *Ann Intern Med*, 1984;100:277.
12. Werner A, Schneider JM. Teaching medical students interactional skills: a research-based course in the doctor-patient relationship. *N Engl J Med*, 1974;290:1232.

13. Kauss DR, Robbins AS, Abrass I, et al. Long-term effectiveness of interpersonal skills training in medical schools. *J Med Educ*, 1980;55:595.
14. Barbee RA, Feldman SE. A three-year longitudinal study of the medical interview and its relationship to student performance in clinical medicine. *J Med Educ*, 1970;45:770.
15. Benson JA Jr., Blank LL, Frenkel EP, et al. Evaluation of humanistics qualities in the internist. *Ann Intern Med*, 1983;99:720.
16. Seeman M, Evans J. Alienation and learning in a hospital setting. *Am Sociol Rev*, 1962;27:772.
17. McIntosh J. Processes of communication, information seeking and control associated with cancer: a selective review of the literature. *Soc Sci Med*, 1974;8:167.
18. Cassileth BR, Zupkis RV, Sutton-Smith K, et al. Information and participation preferences among cancer patients. *Ann Intern Med*, 1980;92:832.
19. Vertinsky IB, Thompson WA, Uyeno D. Measuring consumer desire for participation in clinical decision-making. *Health Serv Res*, 1974;15:121.
20. Haug MR, Lavin B. Public challenge of physician authority. *Med Care*, 1979;17:844.
21. Bales RF. *Interaction process analysis*. Cambridge, MA: Addison Wesley, 1950.
22. Davies AR, Ware JE Jr, Brook RH, et al. Consumer acceptance of pre-paid and fee-for-service medical care: results from a randomized controlled trial. *Health Serv Res*, 1986;21:429.
23. Kasteler J, Kane R, Olsen D, et al. Issues underlying the prevalence of 'doctor-shopping' behavior. *J Health Soc Behav*, 1976;17:328.
24. Ware JE Jr, Davies AR, Kane RL, et al. *Effects of differences in quality of care on patient satisfaction and behavioral intentions: an experimental simulation*. Presented at Research in Medical Education Annual Meeting, New Orleans, 1978.
25. Roter D. Patient participation in patient-provider interactions: the effects of patient question-asking on the quality of interactions, satisfaction and compliance. *Health Educ Monographs* 1977;5:281.
26. Francis V, Korsch BM, Morris MJ. Gaps in doctor-patient communication: patients' response to medical advice. *N Engl J Med*, 1969;280:535.
27. Korsch B, Gozzi EK, Francis V. Gaps in doctor-patient communication: I. doctor-patient interaction and patient satisfaction. *Pediatrics*, 1968;42:855.
28. Woolley FR, Kane RL, Hughes CC, et al. The effects of doctor-patient communication on satisfaction and outcome of care. *Soc Sci Med*, 1978;12:123.
29. Patrick DL, Scrivens E. Charlton JRH. Disability and patient satisfaction with medical care. *Med Care*, 1983;21:1062.
30. Linn LS, Greenfield S. Patient suffering and patient satisfaction among the chronically ill. *Med Care*, 1982;20:425.
31. Stiles WB, Putnam SM, Wolf MH, et al. Interaction exchange structure and patient satisfaction with medical care. *Med Care*, 1979;17:667.
32. DiMatteo R, Hays R. The significance of patients' perceptions of physician conduct: a study of patient satisfaction in a family practice center. *Community Health*, 1980;6:18.
33. Bertakis K. The communication of information from physician to patient: a method for increasing patients' retention and satisfaction. *Fam Prac*, 1977;5:217.
34. DiMatteo MR, Taranta A, Friedman S, et al. Predicting patient satisfaction from physicians nonverbal communication skills. *Med Care*, 1980;18:376.
35. Doyle BJ, Ware JE, Jr. Physician conduct and other factors that affect consumer satisfaction with medical care. *J Med Educ*, 1977;52:793.
36. Feletti GI, Carney SL. Evaluating patients' satisfaction with medical students interviewing skills. *Med Educ*, 1984;18:15.

37. Weinberger M, Greene Jy, Mamlin JJ. The impact of clinical encounter events on patient and physician satisfaction. *Soc Sci Med*, 1981;15:239.
38. Anderson LA, DeVellis BM, DeVellis RF. Effects of modeling on patient communication, satisfaction and knowledge. *Med Care*, 1987;25:1044.
39. Hall JA, Roter DL. Rand CS. Communication of affect between patient and physician. *J Health Soc Behav*, 1981;22:18.
40. Stewart M. What is a successful doctor-patient interview? A study of interactions and outcomes. *Soc Sci Med*, 1984;19:167.
41. Buller MK. Buller DB. Physicians' communication style and patient satisfaction. *J Health Soc Behav*, 1987;28:375.
42. Janis IL. Effectiveness of social support for stressful decisions. In: Deutsch M, Homstein H, eds. *Applying social psychology: implications for research practice and training*. Hillsdale, NJ: Lawrence Erlbaum, 1975.
43. Orth JE, Stiles WB, Scherwitz L, et al. Patient exposition and provider explanation in routine interviews and hypertensive patients' blood pressure control. *Health Psych*, 4 1987;6:29.
44. Starfield B. Wray C, Hess K, et al. The influence of patient-practitioner agreement on outcome of care. *Am J Public Health*, 1981;71:127.
45. Stewart MA, McWhinney IR, Buck CW, et al. The doctor-patient relationship and its effect upon outcome. *J R Coll Gen Pract*, 1979;29:77.
46. Bass MJ,. Buck C. Turner L, et al. The physician's actions and the outcome of illness in family practice. *J Fam Pract*, 1986;23:43.
47. The Headache Study Group of the University of Western Ontario. The predictors of outcome in headache patients presenting to family physicians: a one year prospective study. *Headache Journal*, 1986;26:285.
48. Hulka BS, Kupper LL, Cassel JC, et al. Doctor-patient communication and outcomes among diabetic patients. *J Community Health*, 1975;1:15.
49. Greenfield S, Kaplan SH, Ware JE, Jr. Patient participation in medical care: effects on blood sugar and quality of life in diabetes. *J Gen Intern Med*, 1988;3:448.
50. Kaplan SH, Greenfield S, Ware JE, Jr. *Expanded patient involvement in medical care: effects on blood pressure*. Presented at National Conference on High Blood Pressure Control, April 1985.
51. Stewart AL, Ware JE, Jr, Brook RH. *Construction and scoring of aggregate functional status measures*. Santa Monica, CA: The RAND Corporation, R-2551-1-HHS, 1982.
52. Bergner M, Bobbitt RA, Carter WB, et al. The Sickness Impact Profile: development and final revision of a health status measure. *Med Care*, 1981;19:787.
53. Greenfield S, Kaplan SH, Ware JE Jr. Expanding patient involvement in care: effects on patient outcomes. *Ann Intern Med*, 1985;102:520.
54. Adler IM, Enelow AJ. Instrument to measure skill in diagnostic interviewing: a teaching and evaluation tool. *J Med Educ*, 1966;41:281.
55. Adler IM, Ware JE Jr., Enelow AJ. Changes in medical interviewing style after instruction with two closed-circuit television techniques. *J Med Educ*, 1970;45:21.
56. Klenk DC, Hermanson GT, Krohn RI, et al. Determination of glycosolated hemoglobin by affinity chromatography: comparison with calorimetric anion-exchange methods and effects of common interferences. *Clin Chem*, 1982;28:2088.
57. Cronbach LJ. Coefficient alpha and the internal structure of tests. *Psychometrika*, 1951;16:297.

58. Rodin J. Health, control and aging. In: Baltes M, Baltes PB, eds. *The psychology of control and aging*. Hillsdale, NJ: Lawrence Erlbaum, 1986.
59. Hall JA, Roter DL, Rand CS. Communication of affect between patient and physician. *J Health Soc Behav*, 1981;15:18.
60. Stewart MA. What is a successful doctor-patient interview? a study of interactions and outcomes. *Soc Sci Med*, 1984;19:167.
61. Schulz R. Effects of control and predictability on the physical and psychological well-being of the institutionalized aged. *J Person Soc Psychol*, 1976;33:563.
62. Langer E, Rodin J. The effects of choice and enhanced personal responsibilitics for the aged: a field experiment in an institutional setting. *J Person Soc Psychol*, 1976;34:191.
63. Rodin J. Behavioral medicine: beneficial effects of self-control training in aging. *Int Rev Appl Psychol*, 1983;32:153.
64. Pennebaker JW, Burnam MA, Schaffer MA, et al. Lack of control as a determinant of perceived physical symptoms. *J Person Soc Psychol*, 1977;35:167.
65. Matthews K, Scheier MF, Brunson BI, et al. Attention, unpredictability, and reports of physical symptoms. *J Person Soc Psychol*, 1980;38:525.
66. Pettingale KW, Philathis A, Tee DEH, et al. The biological correlates of psychological responses to cancer. *J Psychsom Res*, 1981;25:433.
67. Janis I, Mann L. *Decision making: a psychological analysis of conflict, choice, and commitment*. New York. Free Press, 1977.
68. Hippocrates. The Physician's Oath.
69. DiMatteo MR, Hays R. Social support and serious illness. In: Gottlieb BH, ed. *Social networks and social support*. Beverly Hills, CA: Sage Publications, 1981.

Information Exchange in Medical Encounters: Problems and Promises

Nurit Guttman

Much of recent research in the area of patient adherence to medical treatment suggests that information exchange between health care practitioners and their patients is crucial in promoting patient participation in health care decision-making and enhancing patient adherence to recommended medical regimens (Meichenbaum & Turk, 1987). Yet, the medical encounter represents a problematic context for information exchange. The caregiver-patient information exchange is often fraught by a variety of obstacles which inhibit competent information exchange (Bochner, 1983; Meichenbaum & Turk, 1987; Waitzkin, 1984). This chapter explores some of the factors that contribute to such obstacles such as the asymmetrical practitioner-patient interaction which typically characterizes the caregiver-patient relationship. The popular, scholarly literature, as well as the press and private and public discussions indicate that dissatisfaction with health care encounters and the health care system as a whole is growing (e.g. Gibbs, 1989). Patients typically only partially adopt health promoting medical recommendations, and the health care system in general is characterized as "in a crisis" with escalating costs and suspicious clients and caregivers.

In the past several decades the primary focus of medical care has been shifting. Despite the prominence of medical technology in medical training and health care delivery, primary health care is becoming more and more concerned with the treatment and care of chronic, asymptomatic diseases as well as with the prevention of illness. Health promoters, including medical practitioners progressively suggest that medical conditions are currently "managed" rather than "treated", and good management requires that patients become active participants in their health care. Therefore, it can be argued that patients should be provided with accurate and appropriate health care information as well as training in the necessary skills to actively participate in health promoting behavior or management of their medical conditions.

Another factor related to the growing emphasis on providing lay people with health information is the rise of the consumer movement. Proponents have been advocating the notions of consumer rights and demands for accountability of service providers, as well as the provision of more information and the participation of the lay person in decision making (Gartner & Reissman, 1974; Rosengren & Lefton, 1975). In the early 1970's, with the growth of the consumer movement, the practices of different professions have come under close scrutiny, including the profession of medicine. Some authors believe that a fundamental change is occurring in the client-practitioner relationship as the professional authority has been challenged by the consumer perspective (Haug & Lavin, 1983; Inlander et al., 1988). The aura of medicine and the authority of the physician have been seriously questioned as people are continually exposed to medical controversies, contradictions, and reversals (Gibbs, 1989; Meichenbaum & Turk, 1987). The rise of consumerism, has promoted an image of the health care client as a discriminating consumer, often "shopping" for medical services (Gibbs,

1989; Haug & Lavin, 1983), while the health care professionals are cast as vulnerable providers of services in a competitive and litigious market (Altman & Rosenthal, 1990; Gibbs, 1989; Haug & Lavin, 1983).

Changing market conditions have contributed to the rise of the consumer trend in health care services. Health care has become, on one hand progressively more expensive, demanding increasing specialization and sophisticated materials, equipment and procedures, while on the other hand, it is a growing competitive business. Therefore, the concern for fostering consumer (i.e. patient) satisfaction has become a major concern (Pascoe, 1983; Pendelton, 1983; Ruben, 1990 and in this volume; Speedling & Rose, 1985; Ware & Davis, 1983). Consistently, it has been found, that patient satisfaction is linked to communication and information exchange factors (Hall & Dorman, 1988; Hall, Roter & Katz, 1988; Ruben, 1990; Waitzkin, 1985 and in this volume). Also, medical professionals are legally required to obtain the "informed consent" of their patients for major as well as many minor medical procedures.

Since the role of the lay person - the health care client - is currently seen more as that of an active participant than that of a passive recipient of medical care: this active participation requires considerable understanding, acquisition of knowledge or skills, as well as motivation to carry out the recommended health care regimen (Meichenbaum & Turk, 1987). Having patients follow the recommended health care regimen, has become one of the major challenges of modern health care (Pryor & Mengel, 1987; Peck & King, 1986 and in this volume).

The Phenomenon of Non-Compliance

Since in the management of diseases or adopting health promotion activities it is often crucial that patients follow a recommended regimen, the latter can be seen as a major goal of practitioners in medical encounters. Not following particular medical recommendations may result in poor patient health, renewed rounds of diagnostic testing, and increased cost to both the patient and the health system (Peck & King, 1986; Meichenbaum & Turk, 1987; Pryor & Mengel, 1987). However, to the distress of many health care practitioners, most studies confirm that at least one third, and frequently up to ninety percent of patients fail to follow their practitioners' recommendations across various medical conditions (Byham & Vickery, 1988; Meichenbaum & Turk, 1987). The failure to follow a recommended medical regimen or health promoting behavior is referred to by authors and practitioners as patient nonadherence, noncompliance, or lack of cooperation on the part of the patient. Although these different terms connote different perspectives regarding the practitioner-patient (or professional-lay) relationship, the main concern is the same: Why is it that so many patients do not follow "the doctors' orders", and what can be done to improve this situation?

Several studies show that physicians tend to underestimate the rates of noncompliance in the general population as well as in their own patients. When confronted with occurrences of patient noncompliance, researchers found that the physicians in tended to attribute its cause to patients' characteristics or traits. Only a minority of practitioners believed that practitioners themselves might contribute to noncompliance (Gillum & Barskey, 1974). Empirical studies, however, have not found a "typical noncompliant personality", nor have studies located a typical set of patient personality traits or sociodemographic variables consistently associated with noncompliance. As Meichnbaum and Turk (1987) state: "Every patient is a potential defaulter" (p. 42).

A great deal of discussion and research has been devoted to this topic in the literature. Hundreds of articles have been published and reviewed in the literature. One review (Trostle, 1988 and in this volume) suggests that more than 4000 scholarly papers have been published in the past two decades. These publications demonstrate the growing recognition in scholarly literature that behavioral factors play an important role in health care interactions, particularly communication and information exchange processes (Meichenbaum & Turk, 1987). While the quality of information exchange in medical encounters is dependent on the relationship or the communication between the interactants, the relationship between patients and health care practitioners is often characterized as problematic (e.g. Stone, 1979; President Commission, 1983), particularly from an information exchange perspective.

Caregiver-patient Information Exchange

The medical practitioner-client relationship has undergone dramatic changes in the past several decades. Some characterize the health caregiver-client relationship as inherently paternalistic, where medical practitioners perform the role of the experts and authority, while the lay persons come to "consult" them in their "sick role" (Parsons, 1951). Other authors maintain that since patients are consumers, they should have greater control and autonomy over information and decision-making factors involved in the health care process (Childress & Siegler, 1984; President's Commission, 1983).

These different perspectives are reflected in the typology of Szasz and Hollander (1956 and in this volume) who present three basic types of doctor-patient relationships and the conditions of illness with which each type is likely to be associated: (1) The model of activity-passivity: the physician is active - the patient, passive. This model is appropriate for the treatment of emergencies, severe injuries or coma. (2) The model of guidance-cooperation: The patient seeks help and is willing to cooperate. The physician is more powerful and expects to be listened to. (3). The model of mutual participation: This model is predicated on the notions of equality. The assumptions underlying this model are that the participants have approximately equal power, are mutually interdependent, and engage in activity that in some ways satisfies both. This corresponds to the consumer oriented approach which implies increasing input and demands by the health care client (President's Commission, 1983). Alternative approaches view the ideal practitioner-lay person interaction as a process of negotiation (Brody, 1980) or mutual persuasion (Smith & Pettegrew, 1986).

In the first two models, the agreement between the physician and patient is taken for granted. In the third model, the physician does not profess to know exactly what is best for the patient. Rather, the determination of what is the best treatment regimen becomes the essence of the therapeutic interaction. The patients' own experiences furnish indispensable information for eventual agreement, as to what 'health' might be for them. Open information exchange in this type of interaction, therefore, can be seen as an essential factor (Brody, 1980).

If we adopt the latter model, particularly in the context of the management of chronic medical conditions (even Parsons, 1975, contends that patients assume a more active role in these situations), we need to address several issues: Are patients in actual practice equally active partners in the medical encounter? What communication and information exchange processes take place in this encounter? What are their effects on medical and sociopsychological outcomes? What are possible approaches to enhance information exchange and collaborative decision-making between lay persons and professionals in the health care context? Substantial theoretical and empirical work point to factors that contribute to inhibited information exchange in the medical encounter.

Stuctural Factors

Some authors believe that the problematic aspects of the relationship between the health care client and the caregiver are embedded in asymmetric power relations and control in health care encounters (Beisecker, 1990; Hardesty, 1988; Nelson & McGough, 1983; Stone, 1979). They point to structural factors which create an asymmetry in the practitioner-patient relationship, which result in an interaction dominated by the caregiver in which patient initiated exposition of their concerns and ideas are relatively inhibited (Hardesty, 1988; Waitzkin, 1985). Although asymmetry in a relationship is often a characteristic of professional-client relationships in general, the factors which contribute to the inhibition of information exchange in this relationship are particularly problematic in the health context (Antonovsky, 1979; Ruben, 1990), since decisions in this context relate to matters that can dramatically impact the welfare of the patient.

Friedson (1975; 1980) characterizes the medical profession as an occupation which has assumed a dominant position in the division of labor, since it has gained control over the determination of the substances of its own work. Medical professionals have been socialized into their professional role or have been working within a framework that provides them with power and dominance. Unlike most occupations, the medical profession is relatively autonomous or self-directing. It claims, and is legally empowered to be the most reliable authority on the nature of the reality it deals with, it changes the definition of and shapes the problems as they are experienced by the lay person, and it tries to manage the problems of its clients in its own fashion, within the confines of its own discipline, specifically, in the biomedical model (Engel, 1978; Stein, 1990).

Practitioners have more power than lay persons because of their professional knowledge and resources. By entering a medical encounter the lay person acknowledges that the medical professional has a particular technical expertise in dealing with certain kinds of problems, or has access to specific resources that the patient does not have. Thus the medical practitioner assumes a relatively superior position of power (Antonovsky, 1979). Also, the medical encounter usually takes place in an environment alien to the patient, such as clinics or hospitals (Cicourel, 1983; Pritchard, 1983; Ruben, 1990), Also disconcerting to the patient is the medical professionals' use of jargon or medical terminology (Barlund, 1976 and in this volume). Further more, the patient invariably perceives the situation as involving anxiety, uncertainly and ambiguity (Antonovsky, 1979), and patients are often anxious or worried about their medical condition and well-being (Barlund, 1976).

Despite the rise of consumer orientation in health care which has created according to Zola and Miller (1973) an erosion of medicine's license and mandate, medicine is spreading its influence even farther in terms of it becoming a major institution of social control. Thus, although new arrangements of service and relationship between health care providers and patients are emerging, medicine (as an institution) remains relatively in control. More over, practitioners, according to Hardesty (1988), are adopting strategies to overcome some of the tensions brought about by the consumer orientation.

An example of how in a situation where the patients clearly identified with a consumer orientation, the physicians managed to maintain control over the actual decision-making is provided in a study by Nelson and McGough (1983). The authors describe how the physicians managed to implement their own favored treatment option, despite their patients' consumer orientation, and their patients' relatively high level of information. The physicians managed to gain their compliance with procedures they previously adamantly expressed their opposition to. The practitioners managed to accomplish this compliance by presenting the procedure as medically necessary when the actual delivery time arrived. Interestingly, these patients did not view their physicians in a negative way, even though they went against their requests. This is because the physicians, suggest Nelson and McGough (1983), offered them what the authors label the "illusion of autonomy". Nelson and McGough (1983) propose that what occurs in such interactions is a process of negotiation: The client's assertions are legitimated by the physician by maintaining an illusion of autonomy, while actually maintaining the physician's control, and avoiding outright conflict between them. These authors predict that as consumer-oriented medical information becomes more available and more accessible to clients, the nature of the relationship between the client and the physician (or any professional) will change. Negotiations will become more overt, and the illusion of the client's autonomy may not continue to produce conflict-free outcomes.

Medical Encounters as an Intercultural Context

In addition to factors relating to differential power in medical encounters, there is an inevitable built-in difference in perspectives of the different interactants, which can be characterized as intercultural (Antonovsky, 1979; Lazare et al., 1976; Ruben, 1990). Practitioners are socialized into the "world of medicine" which becomes their "home territory", while to patients this world is often alien and anxiety provoking. Further more, the patient is mostly concerned with his or her self-interest, while practitioners, in addition to being concerned with the patient's self interest, have additional professional and societal normative commitments (Parsons, 1970).

Interaction-analysis studies have provided empirical data which support the theoretical frameworks regarding the asymmetry in the medical practitioner-patient relationship. Conversation analysts have noted that rules of discourse give differential rights to doctors and patients to pursue topics (Fisher, 1983; Frankel, 1983; Rost, Carter & Inui, 1989), where patients are less likely to introduce topics in the discussion (Shuy, 1983). Doctors and patients utilize different conversational means. For example, physicians employ serial questioning sequences by which they maintain preeminence over the information exchanged during the visit, and patients rarely volunteer information or append comments on other topics (Rost, Carter & Inui, 1989).

Medical consultation and advice are frequently given in circumstances in which discussion, feedback and learning are inhibited (Ruben, 1990). It has been demonstrated that patients are interrupted disproportionately by physicians (Shuy, 1983; West, 1983), seldom ask questions (Waitzkin, 1985; West, 1983) and do not inform their doctors when they do not understand their instructions or explanations (Purtilo, 1978; Waitzkin, 1985; Putnam et al. 1985.) Thus, patients interpret what they have heard to the best of their understanding (Ley & Spelman, 1976; Matthews & Hingson, 1977). DiMatteo and DiNicola (1982) report that patients are often afraid to ask what specific terms mean for fear that the doctor will think they are uneducated or unintelligent.

A common consequence of asymmetrical communicative power, argues Cicourel (1983), is misunderstanding. The professional-bureaucratic setting creates informational constraints and resources for the doctor, but tends to weaken the patient's communicational capabilities. One result is that when people believe they are unable to express their views, or that their feelings and emotions are constrained by the organizational setting, they are likely to have doubts about what they are told, despite a desire to trust the doctor's communication. Cicourel (1983) also suggests that the professional-bureaucratic context can influence the preference for particular medical treatments by the way the problem is framed by the professional. Thus, patients may not be aware, or may be discouraged to opt for health care alternatives which are presented by the professional as the less desirable options. Yet, the professional's criteria for recommending certain treatments may be influenced by their values or preconceptions, and they use persuasive strategies to convince their patients to follow what they believe is best for them or society (Fisher, 1983). Additional factors related to problems in information exchange in medical encounters are gender (Verbrugge & Steiner, 1981), age (Waitzkin, 1985), physical attractiveness (Hadjistavropoulos, Ross & Bayer, 1990), culture (Ellmer & Olbrisch, 1983), social class (Pendelton & Bochner, 1980), perceptions of personality or attributions (Fisher, 1983).

Structural elements of the practitioner-patient relationship, factors of power, dominance and tension, as well an intercultural differences contribute to the problematic nature of information exchange in the practitioner-patient encounter. Practitioners tend to dominate the encounter implicitly or explicitly, and they typically follow a biomedical model of information seeking (categorizing symptoms), problem solving (reaching a scientific diagnosis), and prescription of treatment. Clients, however, may have various, often contradictory concerns which do not necessarily "fit" the scientifically oriented medical model (Engel, 1978; Stein, 1990). Since patients' major concerns may often not be presented to the practitioner as their "chief complaint" in the information exchange process, these concerns may be ignored or belittled by the medical practitioner (Frankel & Beckman, 1989; Shorter, 1985). In addition, since patients may feel inhibited in presenting their sensations, feelings, ideas or suggestions, they are less likely to be involved in negotiating a true partnership with the practitioner. It could be argued that as long as health practitioners are trained and almost exclusively rely on an information seeking model in the biomedical model (Shorter, 1985; Weston & Brown, 1989), information exchange and partnership building in the medical encounter will continue to be sadly impoverished.

Patients Want More Information

Findings consistently indicate that regardless of their sociodemographic background, health care clients are interested in knowing more about their health condition than is offered by their practitioners, and many are dissatisfied with the information provided to them (Blanchard et al., 1988; Covel et al. 1985; Ewles & Shipster, 1981; Korsch, Gozzi & Francis, 1968; Waitzkin, 1985). Yet, despite their dissatisfaction patients are reticent about asking questions because they believe physicians do not have the time to explain to them (Purtilo, 1978).

An example of research which focused on information exchange in patient-physician interactions is reported by Waitzkin (1985). Waitzkin and his colleagues analyzed 336 encounters recorded from several outpatient settings. The researchers coded measures such as the level of technicality of the doctor's explanations, the numerical count of doctors' explanations and patients' requests for information. Their analysis reveals that doctors spent relatively little time informing their patients, overestimated the time they did spend, and underestimated their patients' desire for information.

Findings from several studies indicate that patients' social class or educational background were related to the information provided by their practitioners (Pendelton, & Bochner, 1980; Waitzkin, 1985). Patients from corporate and upper-middle class backgrounds received more physician time, more explanations, more multilevel explanations than patients from lower-middle or working class backgrounds. Also, reports of patient dissatisfaction with how physicians elicit information and ignore the patient's perspective are common in daily discussions by lay persons (Cicourel, 1983). In conclusion, clients are dissatisfied but nevertheless inhibited in their input in many medical encounters. In spite of the often impoverished information exchange that takes place in medical encounters, patients are increasingly expected by their health care providers to actively participate in the increasingly complex and demanding process of the management of their health care.

Knowledge and Beliefs

There is a growing body of literature that focuses on patient beliefs as an important factor that is related to individuals' and community's health related behaviors. A growing body of literature suggests that patients' personal beliefs play an important part in adherence to medical recommendations. Western culture emphasizes the biomedical model of conceptualizing health conditions. Illness is explained in terms of pathophysiology, with practitioners focusing on the disease rather than the person. Yet the experience of illness is unique to each individual, and lay persons' perspective often dramatically diverges from that of their practitioners' (Cassell, 1985; Cicourel, 1983; Bochner, 1983; Hamoson et al., 1990; Mishler, 1984; Weston & Brown, 1989).

Cicourel (1983) suggests that "we need to understand the extent to which beliefs can resist new or contradictory information" (p. 236). This implies that both parties need to explore the assumptions and beliefs of the other and attempt to reach a mutual or a working definition of the health problem and how to address it (Weston & Brown, 1989). If there is a discrepancy in the beliefs of the interactants, if the interactants do not share the meaning of the terminology employed, and if there are inadequate efforts to bridge the gaps between the assumptions of the professionals and lay person - adherence to the medical advice and partnership building in the relationship is likely to be minimal. In other words, information exchange between the parties which does not involve a negotiation of shared meanings (Barlund, 1976; Brody, 1980; Mishler, 1984) may not result in health promoting behavior.

The Health Belief Model formulated by Rosenstock and developed by Becker and his colleagues (Janz & Becker, 1984; Rosenstock, 1990) is the most frequently studied model of patients' health beliefs (King, 1983). It was Originally developed to explain and predict preventive health actions but has since been employed to explain patient adherence as well. Becker and his colleagues suggest that whether or not individuals will undertake a recommended health action is dependent upon their perceptions of several factors: general health motivations; perceived susceptibility or vulnerability; perceived severity of the consequences of the health condition; perceived benefits and costs or barriers involved in taking the recommended health action; and the occurrence of cues which "trigger" the individual to action.

Although the Health Belief Model focused originally predominantly on the patient, some suggest that the patient- practitioner interaction contributes to the health beliefs of the patient (Leventhal et al. 1983). For example, Inui and his colleagues (1976) developed a tutorial aimed at training practitioners in strategies for increasing hypertensive patients' adherence to the prescribed regimen. The results show that the patients of the tutored physicians were more aware of their own susceptibility and more compliant. Thus, enhanced communication between practitioners and their patients was related to enhanced outcomes.

Patient Knowledge

In order to carry out the medical regimen the patient must be sufficiently informed about how to carry out the recommendations. The conceptual framework of the Health Belief Model (Janz & Becker, 1984: King, 1983) implies that patients need to acquire an understanding of why the recommended regimen is needed, as well as knowledge and skills of how to carry it out. Unless lay persons turn to alternative information sources, they are most likely to depend on the information provided by their health practitioner (Gann, 1986). Thus health practitioners can be viewed as "gatekeepers" regarding important health information, and consequently the practitioner-patient interaction is particularly important as a source for the patients' health knowledge.

Knowledge and information enable lay persons to participate in their own health care (Gann, 1987). Some researchers propose that often the failure of patients to adhere to medical treatment can be attributed to patients' lack of appropriate information (Gann, 1986; Geller & Butler, 1981; Hulka, et al. 1975; Hulka et al., 1976) or a simple failure of comprehension (Ley & Spelman, 1967;

Ley, 1983). Research findings demonstrate that individuals often lack knowledge regarding their medical regimen, the location of major organs, or causes of illness (Kreps et al., 1987; Ley, 1983).

Hulka and her associates (1976) suggest that patients often tend to adhere to the best of their knowledge but act on misinformation regarding their treatment regimen. They found that over half of the patients who made mistakes in their administration of medication assumed they understood their treatment, and only five percent asked their doctor for clarification (Gann, 1987). Stewart, Cluff and Leighton (1972) lament that in our society individuals are provided with better instructions when purchasing a new camera or automobile than when they receive a life saving drug.

Although there seems to be conflicting evidence regarding the relationship of information to adherence, a number of studies indicate that providing clear and accurate information is positively related to adherence as well as being cost effective (Gann, 1987; Slack, 1985). Hulka, Cassel, Kupper and Burdette (1976) found that communication of instructions and information was inversely associated with drug error rates: The better the communication, the lower the errors. Neither characteristics of patients nor the severity of the disease were associated with medication errors. Other studies indicate that better informed patients were found to experience less stress and anxiety in the hospital setting or require fewer painkilling drugs and shorter hospital stays (Gann, 1987; Slack, 1985). Thus, the importance of competent information exchange in the medical encounter is a prominent concern in health care (Pendelton, 1983; Waitzkin, 1985). However, providing patients with information is not sufficient to influence health related behavior. As much of the literature points out: Having individuals attend, comprehend and act upon information may greatly depend on the person's values, attitudes or beliefs.

However, communication of information between practitioner and their patients is limited, as reported in a study by this author (Guttman, 1990) which compared practitioners' assessment of the knowledge and attitudes of their patients with their actual responses. The findings of this research point to a gap between what practitioners think their patients know and what they actually know about their health care, which in turn may be related to the problematic factors associated with information exchange in medical encounters.

Davis, Hall and Boutaugh (1981) argue that it is important for health car practitioners to have a careful and comprehensive assessment of patients' needs and their current knowledge base, limitations and readiness to learn. They point out that practitioners' perceptions about the extent of patients' knowledge and self-management have been found to differ markedly from actual measures of these dimensions. Health professionals, like professionals in other fields, face the problem of transmitting technical information and advice to lay-persons (Cicourel, 1983; Meichenbaum & Turk, 1987; Ruben, 1990) as well as the problem of not knowing what their clients want in this interaction (Davis et al. 1981; Diabetes Forecast, 1987; Innes, 1977; Wertz et al. 1988). If indeed, patient knowledge is increasingly important in the health care process, and if the primary care health practitioner is often the major source of this information (Gann, 1986; Thompson, 1986) - it is important to investigate whether what practitioners assume their patients know, corresponds to what patients actually do know. If practitioners over-estimate what their patients know they may not provide them with the necessary information needed to participate in decision making or in the implementation of the recommended health care regimen.

Findings of this author's study (Guttman, 1990) that explored how well primary care medical practitioners assessed their patients' knowledge and attitudes regarding the care of diabetes, indicate that practitioners overestimated the knowledge of their patients and were not well attuned to their patients' knowledge or particular feelings about their medical care. This gap may directly affect the management of these patients' medical condition since successful management of these patients' medical condition - diabetes - relies on considerable knowledge and skills on the part of the patient and their motivation to carry on with the prescribed regimen (Brown, 1988; Chandalia & Bagrodia, 1979; Etzwiller, 1984; Geller & Butler, 1981; Hulka et al., 1975; Romm & Hulka, 1979).

This study focused on a specific domain of knowledge of diabetes, such as nutrition or food exchanges, hypoglycemia and skin care, and utilized knowledge items which were identified as important for diabetics to know in order to control their medical condition. The practitioners were asked to assess how well their patients possess knowledge of diabetes care. The practitioners' assessments were then compared with the responses of the patients. In addition there were items addressing their feelings or emotions (affect) regarding diabetes and well-being in general. Analyses of the findings indicate that the practitioners overestimated their patients' knowledge and the patients themselves also over-estimated their own level of knowledge of certain topics. However, the analysis of the items regarding affect (their feelings) indicated that the practitioners' assessments of the patients' responses to affect items were mostly in accordance with the actual responses of the patients. Yet, practitioners tended to overestimate the amount of concern their patients have with possible complications.

These findings support the notion that information exchange in the health practitioner-patient encounter is problematic. Patients knew less about the care for their medical condition than their practitioners assumed they did (in contrast to McKinlay, 1975), but this gap was undetected. Whether this was a result of lack of comprehension on the part of the patient, poor instruction on the part of the practitioner, reticence on the part of the patient regarding asking questions, or other causes, should be investigated further.

The results of this study support results of a survey conducted by the American Diabetes Association (Diabetes Forecast, 1987) which indicated that while 89% of the health care professionals said that they trained their patients on how to use self-monitoring of blood glucose, only 54% of the patients responded they were instructed in the method. In that survey, however, the diabetics surveyed were not the patients of the health care professionals surveyed. The gap found in this author's study (Guttman 1990), between what the practitioners thought patients knew, and what patients actually knew, or rather, did not know, might have implications for patients' adherence to following a recommended medical regimen. If patients lack appropriate health related knowledge they are not likely to perform the recommended behaviors appropriately (Meichenbaum & Turk, 1987).

Interestingly, findings also indicate that practitioners were relatively accurate in their assessment of patients' affect responses. It is proposed that practitioners may be more attuned to their patients' concerns or feelings than is often attributed to them (Merkel, 1984). Nevertheless, the analysis indicates that regarding complications of diabetes, the practitioners overestimated the concern their patients had. Thus, practitioners may believe their patients feel more susceptible (following the Health Belief Model) to complications of their medical condition than they actually are. This, according the Health Belief Model, may influence patients' motivation to adhere to the recommended regimen.

The results of this study indicate that although what patients knew or did not know, was not communicated well to their practitioners, the patients managed to communicate effectively some of their general concerns to their doctor or nurse. One possible explanation is that patients feel more comfortable expressing what they are "expert" in - their feelings and attitudes regarding their home, family, occupations and general health. Yet, patients might be more reluctant to ask the practitioner questions which refer to medical knowledge and skills. Similarly, practitioners might be more likely to possess social skills which facilitate their finding out about what people feel. They appear to lack skills that would enable them to assess how well their patients understand or know technical or somatic matters. This view is supported by findings that physicians talked more openly to their patients when discussing psychosocial topics than somatic topics (Verhaak, 1988).

As the scholarly literature and everyday experiences suggest: Patients may not possess the knowledge, skill or motivation to effectively participate in promoting their health. Having interactants explore their health beliefs, knowledge and assumptions are key elements in establishing a "common ground" on the definition of the health care problems as well as optimal ways to address them. This goal however, is dependent on a complex process of negotiation which requires the active involvement of the both the professionals and their clients.

Involvement and Negotiation

Goffman (1963) describes involvement in an interaction as the capacity of individuals to give or withhold their concerted attention to some activity at hand. Involvement then is an admitted closeness between the individual and the object of involvement, in which a "working consensus" or a shared definition of the situation come to prevail. The literature on the health practitioner-patient interaction implies that the involvement in the medical encounter is typically not symmetrical. The "working consensus" that generally is established in the medical encounter is characterized by a passive patient, and the situation is controlled by the practitioner. In light of the discussion above, an important question is whether this definition of the situation can undergo fundamental changes. For example, we may ask if it possible to increase patient control of the information exchange in medical encounters.

The "mutual participation" (Brody, 1980; Stone, 1979; Szass & Hollander, 1956) or "mutual persuasion" models (Smith & Pettegrew, 1986) recognize that an inherent conflict between patients' and their practitioners' perspectives is likely to exist, and therefore the process of negotiation between them is crucial. In the same vein, Rost, Carter and Inui (1989) underscore the importance of reaching a mutual agreement on the definition of the (health) problem. These authors suggest that a necessary step in genuinely defining the patients' problem is the introduction of relevant information about the problem by both doctor and patient. These researchers investigated how doctors and patients negotiated what information is relevant in understanding the patient's problem, as it reflects both the patient's and physician's perspective and how it is was related to patient adherence. Their findings support the idea that the physician's willingness to allow patients to contribute input was related to patient adherence to physician recommendations. This, they suggest, might be due to increased partnership at arriving at treatment decisions that have meaning for both patient and physician. These findings support the notion that enhanced information exchange processes in medical encounters can promote positive health related outcomes (Kaplan, Greenfield & Ware, 1989 and in this volume).

Regardless of whether the changes in the doctor-patient relationship are undergoing fundamental revisions or merely adjusting to the marketplace conditions, there is evidence that the medical profession is undergoing changes in some of the elements of the therapeutic relationship with its clientele. This is manifested in the growing cautiousness of medical professionals in making sure they provide patients with certain information as they have entered the era of increased litigations. The medical literature and health practitioners are showing a growing interest in communication aspects of the medical relationship, particularly in communication skills or communicative competence (Leebov, Vergare & Scoot, 1989; Meichenbaum & Turk, 1987).

The Challenge of Enhancing Communication Competence in the Healthcare Context

More and more health care practitioners and medical educational programs recognize the importance of enhancing the communication skills of caregivers. There is a growing body of literature as well as training programs aimed at health care professionals, urging them to enhance their communication skills (e.g. Burgoon et al., 1987; Campbell, et al., 1990; Cline, 1983; Kreps & Thornton, 1984; Leebov, Vergare & Scott, 1989; Meichenbaum & Turk, 1987; Northouse & Northouse, 1985; Ruben, 1990; Thompson, 1986; Wakeford, 1983), and change their style from paternalistic (Taylor, Pickens & Gedden, 1989) to empathetic (Squier, 1990; Suchman & Matthews, 1988) or partnership building (Ballard-Reisch, 1990). Increasingly, it becomes apparent that health care communication interventions should include also the enhancement of patient communication competencies (Arntson, 1989; Ruben, 1990). Not only health practitioners, but lay persons should be provided with health related negotiation skills (Hardesty, 1988).

Active participation of patients in medical encounters might be enhanced by encouraging patients to ask more questions (Roter, 1977); having them initiate topics or proffer their opinions and suggestions, and teaching them negotiation skills (Arntson, 1989; Argyle, 1983; Brody, 1980; Hardesty, 1988; Thompson, 1986). Patients can be encouraged to actively participate in the decision making process by establishing mutual clarification of expectations each party has regarding their respective roles and responsibilities in the health care process (Ballard-Reisch, 1990; Meichenbaum & Turk, 1987; Weston & Brown, 1989). In fact both the American Hospital Association's Patients' Bill of Rights and the American Civil Liberties Union Rights of Hospital Patients, underscore the role of active patient participation and collaborative negotiation in the treatment regimen (Meichenbaum and Turk, 1987).

Although the literature on enhancing health communication of patients is relatively sparse, there is growing empirical evidence that interventions to enhance patients' health communication are successful in increasing patients' input in medical encounters and may be related to long-term adherence or increased control of the medical condition. For example, Roter (1977), Robinson and Whitfield (1985), and Thompson and Nanni (1990) succeeded in increasing the number of questions asked by patients by aiding them to prepare questions ahead of time. In addition, in Robinson and Whitfield's study (1985), patients in the experimental group which received specific information about their condition and some training in interaction management, had better control of their medical condition. In Thompson and Nanni's (1990) study, it was found that "coached" patients were also more satisfied with the visit.

Greenfield, Kaplan and Ware (1985) designed an intervention where patients in one group were helped to read their medical record and coached to ask questions and negotiate medical decisions with their physicians during a twenty minute session before their scheduled visit. Patients in this group showed more active involvement in the interaction than those in the other group, and subsequently better control of their medical condition. Overall, the results of these studies suggest that increasing patient health communication skills can be beneficial to individual patients' well-being as well as to the health care system (Kaplan, Greenfield & Ware, 1989).

Although the findings of these studies indicate that the "trained" patients managed the information exchange relatively better than those who did not, these "improved" medical encounters are still a far cry from the "mutual participation model" (Szasz and Hollander, 1956), from real partnership building (Brody, 1980) or from the "mutual persuasion" model (Smith & Pettegrew, 1986). More so, the recommendations in the literature for enhancing the health communication competence of both practitioners and patients are often commonsensical (Rowland-Morin & Reuben, 1987 and in this volume; Sneider, 1986; Thompson, 1986). Although these efforts might indeed contribute to more effective communication skills of practitioners and clients, they do not address some of the more problematic aspects of the physician-patient interaction, as reviewed above.

In conclusion, Patient-practitioner information-exchange has been portrayed as problematic. In fact, it can be characterized as a "risk factor" among other recognized health risk factors, since impoverished information exchange in medical encounters might be detrimental to individuals' health. Problematic information exchange in medical encounters has implications for dissatisfaction and frustration experienced by caregivers, patients and the public, the inhibition of partnership building, and minimal patient adherence to medical recommendations. With growing dependence of lay persons on sophisticated health services, combined with escalating economic and social costs - scholars, lay advocates and health care professionals are increasingly concerned with both satisfying the public as well as with maintaining a viable health-care system that provides optimal care. Increasingly it is pointed out that shared responsibility in decision making and participation in the implementation of health care delivery may help address the contradictions, as well as ethical and economic constraints that lay persons, health care professionals, administrators and politicians currently face.

However, presently most efforts which aim to address the problematic aspects of information exchange in medical encounters focus on how to enhance practitioners' communication skills, with some minor efforts also aiming to enhance the communication skills of patients' in specific medical contexts. Yet, as this review suggests, communication skills training of individuals may not be sufficient to overcome the asymmetric nature of the professional-lay person relationship which usually takes place in a bureaucratic setting. Such training tends to ignore the inherent problematic issues that are embedded in structural arrangements of the health care delivery system. Such training also fails to address important factors relating to intercultural differences, which stem from socialization of practitioners into medical professions (Bochner, 1983; Ruben, 1990; Stein, 1990) and the predominance of the biomedical model as the ultimate criteria for definitions of health and illness. These can be seen as factors which will continue to perpetuate asymmetrical control of information exchange in the medical encounter.

The promise of enhancing information exchange in medical encounters lies in recognizing and unveiling to all stakeholders the multitude of potential obstacles which can be characterized as structural, systemic, cultural or interactional. The promise lies in developing interventions that focus not only the enhancement of communication skills of caregivers or those of particular patients, but on enhancing and enabling actual negotiations and shared decision-making between all stakeholders regarding all important healthcare related issues: These might include allocation of healthcare resources, decsions on the use of particular medical procedures, or patients' and healthcare givers' rights.

The promise lies also in increased mobilization of resources and the encouragement of developing new approaches in health care delivery that will comprehensively address structural, cultural and other communication barriers in health care partnership building. Consequently, more symmetrical information exchange in medical encounters will be encouraged, and perhaps this will contribute to a more satisfying and effective health care system.

References

Altman, L., & Rosenthal, E. (1990). Changes in medicine bring pain to healing profession. *The New York Times*, February 18, 1.

Antonovsky, A. (1979). *Health, Stress and Coping*. San Francisco:Jossey-Bass.

Argyle, M. (1983). Doctor-patient skills. In D. Pendelton, & J. Hasler (Eds.), *Doctor-Patient Communication*, (pp.57-74). London:Academic Press.

Arntson, P. (1989). Improving citizens' health competencies. *Health Communication*, 1(1), 29-34.

Ballard-Reisch, S.S. (1990). A model of participative decision making for physician-patient interaction. *Health Communication, 2*(2), 91-104.

Barnlund, D.C.(1976). The mystification of meaning: Doctor- patient encounters. *Journal of medical Education*, 51,716-725.

Beisecker, A.E. (1990). Patient power in doctor-patient communication: What do we know? *Health Communication, 2*(2), 105-122.

Blanchard, C.G., Labrecque, M.S., Ruckdeschel, J.C., & Blanchard, E.B. (1988). Information and decision-making preferences of hospitalized adult cancer patients. *Social Science and Medicine*, 27(11), 1139-1145.

Bochner, S. (1983). Doctors, patients and their cultures. In D. Pendelton, & J. Hasler (Eds.), *Doctor-Patient Communication*, (pp. 127-138). London:Academic Press.

Brody, D.S. (1980). The patient's role in clinical decision- making. *Annals of Internal Medicine, 93*(5), 718-722.

Brown, S. (1988). Effects of Educational Interventions in Diabetes care: A meta-analysis of findings. *Nursing Research*, 37(4), 223-229.

Burgoon, J.K., Pfau, M., Parrott, R., Birk, T., Cocker, R., & Burgoon, M. (1987). Relational communication, satisfaction, compliance-gaining strategies, and compliance in communication between physicians and patients. *Communication Monographs, 54*(3), 307-324.

Byham, L. D., & Vickery, C.E. (1988). Compliance and health promotion. *Health Values, 12*(4), 5-12.

Campbell, J.D., Mauksch, H.O., Neikirik, H.J., & Hosokawa, M.C. (1990). Collaborative practice and provider styles of delivering health care. *Social Science and Medicine, 30*(12), 1359-1356.

Chandalia, H. B., & Bagrodia, J. (1979). Effects of Nutritional counseling on the blood glucose and nutritional knowledge of diabetic subjects. *Diabetes Care, 2*(4), 353-356.

Cassel, E.J. (1985). *Talking with Patients: Volume 2* Clinical Technique. Cambridge, MA:MIT Press.

Childness, J. & Siegler, M. (1984). Metaphors and models of doctor-patient relationships: Their implications for autonomy. *Theoretical Medicine, 5*, 17-30.

Cicourel, A.V. (1983). Hearing is not believing: Language and the structure of belief in medical communication. In S. Fisher, & A.D. Todd, (Eds.). *The Social Organization of Doctor-Patient Communication*, (pp. 221-239). Washington, DC:Center for Applied Linguistics.

Cline, R.J. (1983). Interpersonal communication skills for enhancing physician-patient relationships. *Maryland State Medical Journal*, April, 272-278.

Covel, D.G., Uman, G.C., & Manning, P.R. (1985). Information needs in office practice: Are they being met? *Annals of Internal Medicine, 103*, 596-599.

Davis, W.K., Hull,A.L., & Boutaugh, M.L. (1981). Factors affecting the educational diagnosis of diabetic patients. *Diabetes Care, 4*(2), 275-278.

Diabetes Forecast. (1987). What you said about monitoring. February, 25-26.

DiMatteo, M.R. & DiNicola, D.D. (1982). *Achieving Patient Compliance: The Psychology of the Medical Practitioner's Role*. New York: Pergamon Press.

Ellmer, R., & Olbrisch, M.E. (1983). The contribution of a cultural perspective in understanding and evaluating client satisfaction. *Evaluation and Program Planning, 6*, 275-281.

Engel, G.L. (1978). The Biophychosocial model and the education of health professionals. *Annals of the New York Academy of Sciences*, 310, 169-181.

Etzwiller, D.D. (1984). Diabetes education: The reason for its existence. *Diabetes Care, 7*(1), 15-18.

Ewles, L. & Shipster, P. (1981). *One to one: A handbook for the health educator*. Lewes, GB:East Sussex Area Health Authority.

Fisher, S. (1983). Doctor talk/paticnt talk: How treatment decisions are negotiated in doctor-patient communication. In S. Fisher, & A.D. Todd, (Eds.). *The Social Organization of Doctor-Patient Communication*, (pp. 135-157). Washington, DC:Center for Applied Linguistics.

Frankel, R.M., Beckman, H.B. (1989). Conversation and compliance with treatment recommendations: An application of micro-interactional analysis in medicine. In B. Dervin, L. Grossberg, B.J. O'Keefe, & E. Waartella, (Eds.), *Rethinking Communication, Volume 2: Paradigm Examplars*, (pp.60-74). Newbury Park,CA:Sage.

Freidson, E. (1975). *Profession of Medicine: A Study in the Sociology of Applied Knowledge*. New York:Dodd, Mead & Company.

Freidson, E. (1980). Dominant professions, bureaucracy, and client services. In W.R. Rosengren & M. Lefton (Eds.), *Organizations and Clients: Essays in the Sociology of Service*, (pp. 71-92). Columbus, Ohio:Charles E. Merrill.

Gann, R. (1986). *The Health Information Handbook: Resources for self care*. Hants, England: Gower Publishing.

Gartner, & Reissman. (1974). *The service society and the consumer vanguard*. New York: Harper & Row.

Geller, J., & Butler, K. (1981). Study of educational deficits as the cause of hospital admission for diabetes mellitus in a community hospital. *Diabetes Care, 4*(4), 487- 489.

Gibbs, N. (1989). Sick and Tired. *Time*, July 31, 48-53.

Gillum , R.F. & Barskey, A.J. (1974). Diagnosis and management of patient noncompliance. *Journal of the American Medical Association*, 228, 1563-1567.

Goffman, E. (1963). *Behavior in Public Places. Notes on the Social Organization of Gatherings*. Glencoe:The Free Press.

Green L.W. (1978). Health information and health education: There's a big difference between them. *Bulletin of the American Society of Information Science, 4*(40), 15-16.

Greenfield S, Kaplan S, Ware Jr. (1985). Expanding patient involvement in care: effects on patient outcomes. *Annals of Internal Medicine, 102*, 520-528.

Guttman, N. (1990). Practitioner' assumed versus patients' actual knowledge and attitudes regarding diabetes care: Implications fro practitioner-patient communication. Paper presented at the 40th International Communication Association Annual Conference, June 1990, Dublin.

Hadjistavropoulos, H.D., Ross, M.A., Von Bayer, C.L. (1990). Are physicians' rating of pain affected by patients' physical attractiveness? *Social Science and Medicine, 31*(1), 69-72.

Hall, J., & Dorman, M. (1988). What patients like about their medical care and how often they are asked: A meta-analysis of the satisfaction literature. *Social Science and Medicine, 27*(9), 935-939.

Hall, J.A., Roter, D.L., & Katz, N.R. (1988). Meta-analysis of correlates of provider behavior in medical encounters. *Medical Care, 26*, 657-665.

Hamoson, S.E., Glasgow, R.E., & Toobert, D.J. (1990). Personal models of Diabetes and their relations to self-care activities. *Health Psychology, 9*(5), 632-646.

Hardesty, M.J. (1988). Information tactics and the maintenance of asymmetry in physician-patient relationship. In D. R. Maines, & C. J. Couch (Eds.), *Communication and Social Structure*, (pp. 39-58). Springfield, IL:Charles C. Thomas.

Haug, M., & Lavin, B. (1983). *Consumarism in medicine: Challenging physician authority*. Beverly Hills:Sage.

Hulka, B.S., John C. Cassel, Lawrence L. Kupper & James A. Burdette. (1976) Communication, Compliance, and concordance between physicians and patients with prescribed medications. *American Journal of Public Health, 66*(9), 847-853.

Hulka, B.S., Kupper, L.L., Cassel, J.C., & Mayo, F. (1975). Doctor-patient communication and outcomes among diabetic patients. *Journal of Community Health, 1*(1), 15-27.

Inlander, C.B., Levin, L.S., & Weiner, E. (1988). *Medicine on Trial*. Prentice Hall, NY.

Innes, J.M. (1977). Does the professional know what the client wants? *Social Science and Medicine, 11*, 635-638.

Inui, T.S., Yourtee, E.L. & Williamson, J.W. (1976). Improved outcomes in hypertension after physician tutorials. *Annals of Internal Medicine, 84*, 646-651.

Janz, N.K., & Becker, M.H. (1984). The Health Belief Model: A decade later. *Health Education Quarterly, 11*(1), 1-47.

Jaspars, J., King, J., & Pendelton, D. (1983). The consultation: A social psychological analysis. In. D. Pendelton, & J. Hasler (Eds.), *Doctor-Patient Communication* (pp.139-157). London:Academic Press.

Joos, S. K., & Hickam, D.H. (1990). How health professionals influence health behavior: Patient provider interaction and health care outcomes. In K. Glans, F.M. Lewis, & B.K. Rimer, *Health Behavior and Health Education: Theory, Research and Practice*, (pp. 216-241). San Francisco:Jossey-Bass.

Kaplan, S.H., Greenfield, S., & Ware, J.E. (1989). Assessing the effects of physician-patient interactions on the outcomes of chronic disease. *Medical Care, 27*(3), S110-S127.

King, J. (1983). Health beliefs in consultation. In D. Pendelton, Hasler J. (Eds.), *Doctor-Patient Communication*, (pp. 109-125). London: Academic Press.

Korsch B.M., Gozzi E.K., & Francis V. (1968). Gaps in doctor- patient communication: I. Doctor-patient interaction and patient satisfaction. *Pediatrics, 42*, 855-871.

Kreps, G.L. (1987). The pervasive role of information in health and health care: Implications for health communication policy. *Communication Yearbook 11*, 238-276.

Kreps, G.L. & Thornton, B.C. (1984). *Health communication: Theory and practice*. New York:Longman.

Kreps G.L., Ruben, B.D., Baker, M.W., Rosenthal, S. (1987). Survey of public knowledge about digestive health and diseases: Implications for health education. *Public Health Reports, 102*(3), 270-277.

Lazare, A., Eisenthal, S., Frank, A. Stoeckle, J.D. (1976). Studies on the negotiated approach to patienthood. In E.B. Gallangher (Ed.), *The doctor-patient relationship in the changing health scene* (DHEW Publication No. (NIH) 78-183) (pp. 119-139). Washington D.C.:U.S. Government Printing Office.

Ley, P. (1983) Patients' understanding and recall in clinical communication failure. In. D. Pendelton, & J. Hasler (Eds.), *Doctor-Patient Communication* (pp. 89-107). London:Academic Press.

Ley, P. & Spelman, M. S.(1967). *Communicating with the patient*. London:Staples Press.

Leventhal, H., Safer, M.A., & Panagis, D.M. (1983). The impact of communications on the self-regulation of health beliefs, decisions, and behavior. *Health Education Quarterly, 10*(1), 3-29).

Matthews, D., & Higson, R. (1977). Improving patient compliance: A guide for physicians. *Medical Clinics of North America, 61*(4), 879-889.

McKinlay, J. (1975) Who is really ignorant - physician or patient? Journal of health and social behavior, 16, 3-11.

Meichenbaum D, Turk DC. (1987). *Facilitating treatment adherence: A practitioner's guidebook.* New York:Plenum Press.

Merkel, W. (1984). Physician perception of patient satisfaction: Do doctors know which patients are satisfied? *Medical Care, 22*(5), 453-459.

Mirowsky, J., & Ross, C. (1983). Patient satisfaction and visiting the doctor: A self-regulating system. *Social Science and Medicine, 17*(18), 1353-1361.

Mishler, E. G. (1984). *The Discourse of Medicine: Dialectics of Medical Interviews.* Norwood, NJ:Ablex.

Nelson, M.K. & McGough, E. (1983). The informed client: A case study in the illusion of autonomy. *Symbolic Interaction, 6*(1), 35-50.

Northouse P.G. & Northouse, L.L. (1985). *Health Communication: A Handbook for health professionals.* Englewoods Cliffs, NJ:Prentice Hall.

O'Hair, D. (1989). Dimensions of relational communication and control during physician-patient interaction. *Health Communication, 1,* 6(2), 97-115.

Parsons, T. (1951). *The social system.* New York:Free Press.

Parsons, T. (1970). How are clients integrated in service organizations? In W.R. Rosengren & M. Lefton (Eds.), *Organizations and Clients: Essays in the Sociology of Service,* (pp. 1-16). Columbus, Ohio:Charles E. Merrill.

Pascoe, G.C. (1983). Patient satisfaction in primary health care: A literature review and analysis. *Evaluation and Program Planning, 6,* 185-210.

Peck, C., & King, N.J., (1986). Medical compliance. In J.N. King, & A. Remeny. (Eds.), *Health care: A behavioral approach.* Orlando, FL:Harcourt & Brace, Jonavich Publishers.

Pendelton, D.A., & Bochner, S. (1980). The communication of medical information in general practice consultation as a function of patient's social class. *Social Science and Medicine, 14A,* 669-673.

Pendelton D. (1983). Doctor-patient communication: a review. In Pendelton D., Hasler J. (Eds.), *Doctor-patient communication,* (pp. 5-53). London: Academic Press.

President's Commission for the Study of Ethical Problems in Medicine and Biomedical and Behavioral Research (1982). *Making health Care Decisions Vol.1.* Washington DC:U.S. Government Printing Office.

Pritchard, P. (1983). Patient participation. In Pendelton D, Hasler J, (Eds.), *Doctor-patient communication,* (pp. 206- 223). London: Academic Press.

Pryor, B. & M. Mengel. (1987). Communication strategies for improving Diabetics' self-care. *Journal of Communication, 37*(4), 24-35.

Purtilo, R. (1978). *Health Professional/Patient Interaction, Second edition.* Phila. PA:W.B. Saunders.

Putnam, S.M., Stiles, W.B., Jacob, M.C. (1985). Patient exposition and physician explanation in initial medical interviews and outcomes of clinic visits. *Medical Care, 23,* 74-83.

Robinson, E.J. & Whitfield, M.J. (1985). Improving the efficiency of patients' comprehension monitoring: a way of increasing patients' participation in general practice consultation. *Social Science and Medicine, 21,* 915-919.

Romm, F. J. & Hulka, B.S. (1979). Care process and patient outcome in Diabetes Mellitus. *Medical Care, 17*(7), 748-756.

Rosengren, W.R. & Lefton M. (Eds.). (1970). *Organizations and Clients: Essays in the Sociology of Service.* Columbus, Ohio:Charles E. Merrill.

Rosenstock, I.M. (1990). The health belief model: Explaining health behavior through expectancies. In K. Glans, F.M. Lewis, & B.K. Rimer, *Health Behavior and Health Education: Theory, Research and Practice* (pp. 39-62). San Francisco:Jossey-Bass.

Rost, K., Carter, W. & Inui, T. (1989). Introduction of information during the initial medical visit: consequences for patient follow-through with physician recommendations for medication. *Social Science and Medicine, 28*(4), 315-321.

Roter, D. (1977) Patient participation in the patient-provider interaction: the effects of patient question asking on the quality of interaction, satisfaction and compliance. *Health Education Monographs, 5*, 281-315.

Rowland-Morin, P. A. & Reuben, D.B. (1987) Getting the Most from Your Visit to the Doctor: Make your office visit work for you. *Diabetes Forecast, 40*(10), 27-28.

Ruben, B.R., & Bowman, J.C. (1986). Patient satisfaction (Part I): Critical issues in the theory and design of patient relations training. *Journal of Healthcare Education and Training, 1*(1), 1-5.

Ruben, B. D. (1990). The health caregiver-patient relationship: pathology, etiology, treatment. In E.B. Ray & L. Donohew (Eds.), *Communication in Health Care Contexts: A Systems Perspective.* Hillsdale, NJ: Lawrence Erlbaum Associates.

Shorter, E. (1985). *Bedside Manners: The Troubled History of Doctors and patients.* New York:Simon & Schuster.

Shuy, R.W. (1983). Three types of interference to an effective exchange of information in the medical interview. In S. Fisher, & A.D. Todd, (Eds.), *The Social Organization of Doctor-Patient Communication* (pp. 189-202). Washington, DC:Center for Applied Linguistics.

Slack, P. (1988). Cost effective advice. Nursing Times, 81(14) p. 26.

Smith, D.H., & Pettegrew, L.S. (1986). Mutual persuasion as a model for doctor-patient communication. *Theoretical Medicine 7,* 127-146.

Sneider, I. (1986). Patient power: How to have a say during your hospital stay. White Hall, VA:Betterway Publications.

Stein, H.F. (1990). *American Medicine as Culture.* Boulder:Westview Press.

Stewart, R.B., Cuff, L.E. & Leighton, E.D. (1972). Commentary: A review of medication errors and compliance in ambulatory patients. *Clinical Pharmacology Therapy, 13*, 463-486.

Stone, G.C. (1979). Patient compliance and the role of the expert. *Journal of Social Issues, 35*(1), 34-59.

Suchman, A., & Matthews, D.A. (1988). What makes the patient- doctor relationship therapeutic? Exploring the connexional dimension of medical care. *Annals of Internal Medicine, 108*, 125-130.

Squier, R.W. (1990). A model of empathic understanding and adherence to treatment regiments in practitioner-patient relationships. *Social Science and Medicine, 30*(3), 325-339.

Szasz, T.S. & Hollender, M.C. (1956). The basic models of the doctor-patient relationship. *Archives in Internal Medicine, 97*, 585-592.

Taylor, S.G., Pickens, J.M., & Geden, E.A. (1989). Interactional styles of nurse practitioner and physicians regarding patient decision making. *Nursing Research, 38*(1),50-55.

Thompson, S.C., Nanni, C., & Schwankovsky, L. (1990). Patient-oriented interventions to improve communication in a medical office visit. *Health Psychology, 9*(4), 390-404.

Thompson, T. L. (1986). *Communication for Health Professionals*. Lanham, MD:University Press of America.

Trostle, J.A. (1988). Medical compliance as an ideology. *Social Science and Medicine, 22*(12), 1299-1308.

Verbrugge, L.M. and Steiner, R.P. (1981). Physician treatment of men and women patients: sex bias or appropriate care? *Medical Care, 19*(6), 609-632.

Verhaak, P. (1988). Detection of psychologic complaints by general practitioners. Medical Care, 26(10), 1009-1020.

Waitzkin H. (1985). Information giving in medical care. *Journal of Health and Social Behavior, 26*, 81-101.

Wakeford, P. (1983). Communication skills training in United Kingdom Medical Schools. In D. Pendelton, & J. Hasler (Eds.), *Doctor-Patient Communication* (pp. 233-247). London:Academic Press.

Wertz, D.C., J.R. Sorenson and T.C. Heeren. (1988). Communication in health professional-lay encounters: How often does each party know what the other wants to discuss? in B. Ruben, (ed.) *Information and Behavior. Vol.2.* (pp. 329- 342). New Brunswick, NJ:Transaction.

West, C. (1983). "Ask me no questions..": An analysis of queries and replies in physician-patient dialogues. In S. Fisher, & A.D. Todd (Eds.), *The Social Organization of Doctor-Patient Communication* (pp. 75-106). Washington, DC:Center for Applied Linguistics.

West, C. (1984). When the doctor is a "lady": Power, status and gender in physician-patient encounters. *Symbolic Interaction, 7*(1), 87-106.

Weston, W.W., & Brown, J.B. (1989). Importance of patients' beliefs. In M. Stewart, & D. Roter, (Eds.). *Communicating with Medical Patients*, (pp. 77-85). Newbury Park, CA:Sage.

Zola, I.K. & Miller, S. (1973). The erosion of medicine from within. In E. Freidson (Ed.) *The professions and their prospects*, (pp. 153-172). Beverly Hills, CA:Sage.

The Issue of "Patient Compliance"

Compliance and Health Promotion

by Laura D. Byham and Connie E. Vickery

Compliance has long been an area of concern in medical therapies. As efforts toward health promotion and wellness grow, compliance also must be addressed in the context of health promotional lifestyle changes. Research has focused on direct and indirect methods useful in measuring compliance. Results, however, are inconclusive as to which method offers the most useful data. Studies have found related factors of compliance that may help the health-care provider to determine or predict compliance: lack of knowledge, sociodemographic variables, and practitioner-client relationship. Through research on measurement and determinants of compliance, a number of successful strategies for enhancing compliance have surfaced.

The growing number of studies related to enhancement of health through changes in lifestyle is a reflection of the burgeoning interest in health promotion and wellness. This has become known as the "second revolution in public health."[1] Although not synonymous in definition, the terms health promotion, disease prevention, and wellness all imply a means to achieve improved health status. Research in the area of health promotion and wellness seeks to explore the determinants and consequences of health behaviors, so that health-care providers might design effective programs aimed at promoting health-conducive lifestyles.

One aspect of research related to health promotion and wellness is compliance. Typically, compliance is associated with therapeutic regimens for an existing health problem, such as coronary artery disease or diabetes mellitus. Impetus for lifestyle change is based on a disease-prevention or risk-avoidance orientation.[2, 3] Haynes and colleagues defined compliance as, "the extent to which a person's behavior (in terms of taking medication, following diets, or executing lifestyle changes) coincides with medical or health advice."[4]

In concert with a healthy lifestyle, compliance or "adherence behavior" must also be viewed as a positive ingredient in a benefitseeking orientation.[5] In a recent review of adherence issues in health behavior change, Cameron and Best differentiated between "participation compliance," defined as how well prescribed regimens are followed, and "adherence."[6] The latter term, which

Byham, L. D. and Vickery, C. E. COMPLIANCE and HEALTH PROMOTION, Health Values, 12 (4) p. 5-12 (1988).

1 Michael JM: The second revolution in health: Health promotion and its environmental base. *Am Psychol* 1982; 37:936-941.

2 Key JC: Health factors in food choices: Risk avoidance or health seeking? *Clin Nutr* 1987; 6:163-167.

3 Heimbach JT: Risk avoidance in consumer approaches to diet and health. *Clin Nutr* 1987; 6:159-162.

4 Haynes RB, Taylor DW, Sackett DL, (eds): *Compliance in Health Care*. Baltimore: Johns Hopkins University Press, 1979.

5 Hindi-Alexander MC, Throm J: Compliance or noncompliance: That is the question! *Am J Health Promo* 1987; 5-11.

may include the concept of participation compliance, encompasses the extent to which behavior patterns are changed in response to curriculum exposure.

Compliance should not be viewed as coercive obedience to orders, but as a negotiated agreement.[7] Inherent in this definition is an open, candid, helping relationship between client and health professional. Compliance is the outcome of provider-client communication and interaction; while the practitioner demonstrates interest and concern, the client assumes the role of an active participant.

Conversely, the noncompliant individual is one who desires the "benefits of modern medicine," but experiences difficulty making a commitment to the prescribed treatment.[8] Hindi-Alexander and Throm state that compliance/noncompliance is not a have/have not situation.[9] Rather, compliance is on a continuum which spans from blind adherence to total nonadherence with intermediate points covering educated adherence and intelligent noncompliance.

On the average, only one out of three individuals will comply to all components of a treatment plan.[10] Podell and Gray purport that of those individuals for whom medications have been prescribed, one third will follow instructions consistently, one third will take the medications on occasion; the remaining third, with limited frequency.[11] Nevertheless, compliance rates can be variable. The highest rate of noncompliance occurs among those therapies which require lifestyle changes, such as diet or exercise regimens.[12]

The intent of this article is to broaden the concept of compliance as it relates to health promotion and wellness. The review will address three components of compliance: measures of compliance; determining factors of compliance; and strategies for improving compliance.

Measuring Compliance

Measuring compliance is simply an evaluation of behaviors.[13] Essentially, compliance measurements can be categorized into direct and indirect methods. Whether one or a combination of both approaches is applied, the health-care practitioner desires a method that produces accurate, relevant, objective information about the desired behavior. Expenses of the procedure as well as ease of application and acceptability deserve attention as well.

Direct measures of compliance include biochemical assessments such as blood and urinary samples for the presence or amount of constituents. Analysis of lipids, glucose, protein, and electrolytes are examples. Sloan used urinary sodium values to assess compliance of patients to dietary sodium restriction.[14] Body weight is another direct measure of compliance as well as such parameters as blood pressure and body organ function tests. Reliability of results is considered highly acceptable because when defined

---

6 Cameron R, Best JA: Promoting adherence to health behavior change interventions: Recent findings from behavioral research. *Patient Education and Counseling* 1987; 10:139-154.

7 Hindi-Alexander MC, Throm J: Compliance or noncompliance: That is the question! *Am J Health Promo* 1987; 5-11

8 Haynes RB, Taylor DW, Sackett DL, (eds): *Compliance in Health Care.* Baltimore: Johns Hopkins University Press, 1979.

9 Hindi-Alexander MC, Throm J: Compliance or noncompliance: That is the question! *Am J Health Promo* 1987; 5-11.

10 Becker MH: Patient adherence to prescribed therapies. *Med Care* 1985; 23:539-555.

11 Podell R, Gray L: Compliance: A problem in medical management. *Am Fam Phys* 1976; 13:74.

12 Haynes RB, Taylor DW, Sackett DL, (eds): *Compliance in Health Care.* Baltimore, MD: Johns Hopkins University Press, 1979.

13 Westfall UE: Methods for assessing compliance. *Topics Clin Nurs* 1986; 7:23-30.

14 Sloan RS: Achieving compliance to a reduced sodium diet. *Nurse Practitioner* 1985; 10:24-26.

procedures are used data are reproducible with only minor variations.

Physiological assessments as a means of measuring compliance are not without drawbacks; practitioners must be aware of these flaws. All tests must be valid—a true determiner of the parameter desired. For example, evaluating serum calcium to assess dietary intake of the mineral is inappropriate; one is not necessarily reflective of the other. Values must be carefully interpreted. Does an individual's weight loss represent the adoption of health-enhancing behaviors such as increased physical activity and decreased caloric intake, or, has the individual been crash-dieting recently? Individual biological variations can also influence results and ultimate assessment of compliance, if not offered due consideration. Certain laboratory determinations lend themselves to false confirmation of compliance by those whose behaviors are temporarily altered when testing is anticipated.

Pill counts represent another direct measure of compliance.[15] Determining the number of pills allotted and comparing that number with the expected count at a given point in the regimen allows an ultimate estimation of adherence. Although the procedure is simple and cost effective, it is fraught with obvious potential problems. The patient may take the correct number but not in the correct time period; although the expected number of pills remain, they may have spilled and been discarded.

In a report on compliance measurement, Roth noted greater reliability associated with bottle counts than mere pill counts.[16] Emptied bottles of antacid were compared with levels of a blood marker concluding in a positive correlation. Patients received bottles at their homes, a courier later visited to ascertain the number of empty and missing bottles. Bottle count did result in overestimation of intake. Despite less reliability, pill counts are simpler to perform.

Indirect measurements of compliance include clinical assessment, direct observation, self-reporting, interviewing, and therapeutic outcome.[17, 18, 19] Again, individual biological variation resulting in individual differences in response to treatment limits the usefulness of clinical assessments.[20] Direct observation requires defining desired outcome behaviors and training individuals to record those behaviors. In a 1986 study, Westfall highlighted some of the associated difficulties.[21] An observer is not always available, accentuating the fact that "much health care occurs outside the direct observation of the provider." The potential of the Hawthorne effect, purporting that individuals comply when they believe they are receiving special attention, is present. Subjectivity of the observer is also possible.

Direct observations have proven to be no more valid than self-reporting.[22] In the latter method, data are elicited directly from the participant. The mode of eliciting this information may be as informal as asking the individual to maintain a simple diary. More formal and structured methods may require to participant to answer detailed questionnaires. Obvious to the health-care pro-

15 Westfall UE: Methods for assessing compliance. *Topics Clin Nurs* 1986; 7:23-30.

16 Roth HP: Current perspective: Ten year update on patient compliance research, *Patient Education and Counseling* 1987; 10:107-116.

17 Hindi-Alexander MC, Throm J: Compliance or noncompliance: That is the question! *Am J Health Promo* 1987; 5-11.

18 Becker MH: Patient adherence to prescribed therapies. *Med Care* 1985; 23:539-555.

19 Westfall UE: Methods for assessing compliance. *Topics Clin Nurs* 1986; 7:23-30.

20 Gordis L. Conceptual and methodologic problems measuring patient compliance, in Haynes RB, Taylor DW, Sackett DL, (eds): *Compliance in Health Care*. Baltimore, MD: Johns Hopkins University Press, 1979.

21 Westfall UE: Methods for assessing compliance. *Topics Clin Nurs* 1986; 7:23-30.

22 Dunbar JM, Stunkard AJ: Adherence to diet and drug regimen, in Levy R, Rifkind B, Dennis B, Enrnst N (eds.): *Nutrition, Lipids, and Coronary Heart Disease*. New York: Raven Press, 1979.

fessional is the realization that the accuracy is suspect as is the possibility of intentional misrepresentation.

Hilbert used a home interview format to investigate the validity of data obtained in measuring compliance.[23] She concluded that a personal interview based on established rapport yielded more accurate results. Gentle probing is suggested when discrepancies in answers are noted, however, the importance of open communication and trust between both parties is stressed. Of course, the patient needs to be comfortable with the confidentiality of the information secured. However, for the dangerously noncompliant individual, such information must be shared with an appropriate health-care professional, but only after receiving consent from the patient. The face-to-face interview affords the immediate opportunity for this to take place.

Therapeutic outcome is seemingly an ideal manner by which compliance can be assessed. What better way to assess compliance with a weight reduction program than to monitor loss of weight? The answer to this question should serve to highlight problems in using desired therapeutic outcome to evaluate compliance. Other factors unrelated to compliance may impinge on the desired result. Perhaps the individual is experiencing fluid retention; this may not be reflected in scale weight. Perhaps the individual fasts prior to being weighed thus yielding a false impression. Outcome criteria must be clearly defined and attention must be devoted to such unrelated factors which may exert influence on interpretation of compliance. Following, criteria must be tested to determine accuracy, validity, and reliability.

Monitoring appointment records has been proposed as another simple, indirect method of assessing compliance.[24] One would expect that if appointments are kept, the subject is more than likely attempting to comply with the regimen; failing to return could be interpreted as noncompliance. The drawback to this method: it could also mean that the individual feels capable of complying and does not feel the need to continue participation.

Related Factors of Compliance

Underlying causes of noncompliance are many in number and contradictory, in much of the literature. Yet, there are many variables which may help the clinician determine or predict compliance, including lack of patient knowledge, locus of control, sociodemographic factors, types of illness, and practitioner-client relationship.

House and associates categorized compliance difficulties with diets into various constructs. The first, motivation, was defined simply as lack of incentive or desire. Physicians identified this as the major reason for noncompliance with diet. Conversely, patients identified environmental or life factors such as family, employment, or economic conditions as the primary obstacle to dietary adherence. Somatic/physiologic factors, the third category, included physical limitations, i.e., visual or ambulatory restrictions that interfere with food preparation. Of the subjects responding to the survey, none of the 50 physicians and only 16 of the 90 clients perceived this as a problem. Lack of information, knowledge, or education was considered a major factor in noncompliance by physicians but not by patients. House concluded from responses of subjects and physicians that the former group perceived noncompliance as principally out of their control, however, physicians did not concur.

It is widely considered that whenever a knowledge deficit exists, noncompliance is certain. Swain and Steckel reported a study which supports the opposite. They compared patients with hypertension who were part of a patient education

---

23 Hilbert GA: Accuracy of self-reported measures of compliance. *Nurs Res* 1985; 34:319-320.

24 Westfall UE: Methods for assessing compliance. *Topics Clin Nurs* 1986; 7:23-30.

program with those receiving routine care.[25] The educational program included information booklets and access to a nurse to whom they could address questions. Noncompliance, identified by dropout rate, was lowest for those patients receiving routine care. Patients in the education group knew from the education program that they were not complying. They reported a feeling of guilt and therefore did not return to the clinic.

In another investigation of patient education for clients with hypertension, a mastery learning process was studied.[26] Periodic testing of knowledge and understanding followed an initial presentation and further instruction was available. While the program was very effective in increasing knowledge, the authors inferred a lack of relationship between compliance rates and increased knowledge. They concluded that the, "acquisition of health knowledge is insufficient by itself to alter behavior."[27]

In their investigation of reducing health risk behaviors in college-age students, Edwards and Dziuban studied the effectiveness of a post-secondary health education course.[28] Parameters included health risk scores, life change units, locus of control, health ranking, weight, and blood pressure determinations. Pre-, post- and 3-month delayed post-treatment measures revealed a lack of significant differences among an experimental group receiving 45 hours of personal health instruction, a group receiving a computerized lifestyle assessment with no formal health instruction, and a control group.

Results of these and other studies concluding a lack of relationship between knowledge and compliance are challenged in the literature. Powers and Woolridge demonstrated better compliance, defined by adherence to medication regimens, in hypertension patients who demonstrated an increased knowledge of medication and personal responsibility for health care.[29] Similarly, Edwards and Pathy noted improved compliance among clients who received drug counseling.[30] The researchers attributed the improvement to a greater understanding of the therapeutic regimen.

Sennott-Miller and Miller investigated the factor of difficulty as a variable in effecting long-term lifestyle changes.[31] Likelihood of adoption of risk-reducing activities was high at low levels of difficulty. As levels of difficulty increased, likelihood rapidly declined. Convincing the client of the effectiveness of health promotion behavior changes, a hallmark of many intervention programs, may not be sufficient according to these data.

One area which has received much attention is that of the health belief model which postulates that one's beliefs about health are determinants of medical regimen compliance.[32, 33, 34, 35, 36] The

25 Swain MA, Steckel SB: Influencing adherence among hypertensives. *Res Nurs Health* 1981; 4:213-222.

26 Sackett DL, Haynes RB, Gibson ES: Randomized clinical trial of strategies for improving medication compliance in primary hypertension. *The Lancet* 1975; 1:1205-1207.

27 Sackett DL, Haynes RB, Gibson ES: Randomized clinical trial of strategies for improving medication compliance in primary hypertension. *The Lancet* 1975; 1:1205-1207.

28 Edwards MJ, Dziuban CD: Reducing health risk behaviors in college population. *Health Values* 1986; 10:30-36.

29 Powers M, Woolridge P: Factors influencing knowledge, attitudes, and compliance of hypertensive patients. *Res Nurs* 1982; 5:171-182.

30 Edwards M, Pathy J: Drug counselling in the elderly and predicting compliance. *The Practitioner* 1984; 228:291-300.

31 Sennott-Miller L, Miller JL: Difficulty: A neglected factor in health promotion. *Nurs Res* 1987; 36:268-272.

32 Eckerling L, Kohrs MB: Research on compliance with diabetic regimens: Application to practice. *J Am Diet Assoc* 1984; 84:805-809.

33 Rosenstock I: Patients' compliance with health regimens. *JAMA* 1985; 234:402-403.

34 Becker M, Radius S, Rossinstock I, et al: Compliance with medical regimen for asthma: A test of the health belief model. *Public Health Reports* 1978; 39:268-277.

35 Dai Y, Catanzaro M: Health beliefs and compliance with a skin care regimen. *Rehab Nurs* 1987; 12:13-16.

health belief model theorizes that prior to acceptance of a therapeutic regimen, four factors must be "exemplified" in the client: 1) perception of susceptibility to the disease or medical condition; 2) prediction of the impact of the severity of the illness on his/her life; 3) faith in the prescribed treatment regimens; and 4) willingness and ability to surmount barriers to the prescribed therapies.

Merely telling someone what to do and expecting passive obedience is futile; evaluating understanding and reemphasizing unlearned material is also without merit. Health-care providers are beginning to recognize that people possess certain information (beliefs) and develop values (attitudes) about their disease or medical condition and the proposed medical regimen.[37] The individual internalizes beliefs and values which evolve to a set of intentions related to specific behavior or performance. Hence, it is the responsibility of the counselor to educate the client toward health beliefs and attitudes to enable enhanced compliance.

Closely aligned to the association between beliefs in health care and compliance is the theory of locus of control. Those who perceive personal control of actions have an internal locus of control.[38] Conversely, the person denoted as having an external locus of control views behavioral control by outside pressures such as family, friends, chance, luck, or even fate, thus the tendency to comply to prescribed regimens is "out of his/her hands." The individual internally controlled will seek and use information to make decisions, accept responsibility for health behavior, and alter behavior accordingly. Results investigating relationships between locus of control and compliance support the positive relationship between internal locus of control and compliance.

Davis has extensively researched the effect of physical, psychosocial, and demographic variables on compliance.[39] He found no significant correlation between any of these factors and the tendency to adhere to therapeutic regimens. Although his findings have been replicated and substantiated, a closer review is warranted.[40, 41, 42, 43]

Bille investigated the relationship of perceived body image and compliance.[44] His data support a positive correlation between compliance in the individual and a positive body image. Similarly, positive support systems, including family and friends, are also associated with improved compliance.[45] Leventhal[46] and Peck and King [47] compared compliance rates of patients

---

36 Leventhal H, Cameron L: Behavioral theories and the problem of compliance. *Patient Education and Counseling* 1987; 10:117-138.

37 Miller SP, Johnson NL, Garrett MJ, et al: Health beliefs of and adherence to the medical regimen by patients with ischemic heart disease. *Heart & Lung* 1982; 11:332-339.

38 Eckerling L, Kohrs MB: Research on compliance with diabetic regimens: Application to practice. *J Am Diet Assoc* 1984; 84:805-809.

39 Davis MS: Physiologic, psychological, and demographic factors in patient compliance with doctors' orders. *Med Care* 1968; 6:115.

40 Haynes RB, Taylor DW, Sackett DL, (eds): *Compliance in Health Care*. Baltimore, MD: Johns Hopkins University Press, 1979.

41 Litt IF, Luskey WR: Compliance with medical regimens during adolescence. *Pediatrics Clinic of North America* 1986; 27:3-15.

42 Eden I, Kamath SK, Kohrs MB, et al: Perceived control of nutrition behavior: A study of the locus of control theory among health subjects. *J Am Diet Assoc* 1984; 84:1334-1339.

43 Morse W, Sims LS, Guthrie HA: Mothers' compliance with physicians' recommendations on infant feeding. *J AM Diet Assoc* 1979; 75:140-148.

44 Bille D: The role of body image in patient compliance and evaluation. *Heart & Lung* 1977; 6:143-148.

45 DiNicola D, DiMatteo M: Practitioners, patients, and compliance with the medical regimens: A social psychological

living with others and by themselves. A lack of difference in compliance between the two groups is interpreted. The quality of the social support may exert greater influence than access to that social support.

The impact of practitioner-client interaction on therapeutic outcome indices has been significantly covered in the literature. According to Julien, noncompliance is inevitable when rapport is lacking between practitioner and client.[48] Davis' results agree, stating that, "noncompliance (is) related to deviant and difficult physician-patient communication."[49]

The communication pattern impacts positively on client satisfaction which in turn is related to increased compliance. Mazzuca and Weinberger analyzed videotaped encounters between diabetic patients and various health professionals.[50] The researchers noted that acknowledgment of patients' statements, instruction, and clinicians' eliciting comprehension appear to be valued by the patients. The study also reported the relationship of dissatisfaction to clinicians' offering advice without rationale or justification. Although they cautioned against generalizing the data they concluded that active participation of clients is always a preferred goal. The theme of the client's perception of the clinician being interested, caring, and genuinely concerned, resulting in increased compliance, has been noted by other investigations.[51, 52, 53]

Improving Compliance

The foremost step by the health-care provider toward enhancing compliance is the knowledge of compliance strategies and the opportunity to practice these skills. Building rapport between the clinician and client is an important step in promoting compliance. Practitioner warmth and concern and sensitivity to non-verbal behavior are positive factors influencing client satisfaction and thus influencing compliance.[54] Stimulating the individual to participate in the planning of the regimen also is advisable.[55] The client feels a satisfaction of belonging and esteem when included as "a member of the health-care team."[56]

Educating the individual according to learning level is essential.[57] If the clinician does not communicate clearly, the client cannot be expected to adhere to the health advice given. The process must begin by determining what is already known, believed, and what the client thinks is important to learn. This requires active listening on the part of the clinician. In this way, the client is free to express any underlying concerns which

perspective, in: Taylor S, Jirger J (eds): *Hand Tools of Psychology and Health*. Hillside, NJ: Erlbaum, 1984.

46 Leventhal H: Fear appeals and persuasion: The differentiation of a motivational contract. *Am J Public Health* 1971; 61:1208-1224.

47 Peck CL, King NJ: Increasing patient compliance with prescriptions. *JAMA* 1982; 248:2874-2890.

48 Julien JK: Dietary compliance—A partnership between patient and dietitian. *Topics in Clinical Nutrition* 1986; 1:51-57.

49 Davis MS: Physiologic, psychological, and demographic factors in patient compliance with doctors' orders. *Med Care* 1968; 6:115.

50 Mazzuca SA, Weinberger M: How clinician communication patterns affect patients' comprehension and satisfaction. *The Diabetes Educator* 1986; 12:370-373.

51 Feldman R: A guide for enhancing health care compliance in ambulatory care settings. *Journal of Ambulatory Care Management* 1982; 5:1-12.

52 Yoos L: Factors influencing maternal compliance to antibiotic regimens. *Pediatric Nurse* 1984; 10:141-147.

53 Given B, Given C: Creating a climate for compliance. *Cancer Nurse* 1984; 7:139-147.

54 Green CA: What can patient health education coordinators learn from ten years of compliance research? *Patient Education and Counseling* 1987; 10:167-174.

55 Glanz K: Dieticians' effectiveness and patient compliance with dietary regimens. *J Am Diet Assoc* 1979; 75:631-636.

56 Etzwiler DD: The patient is a member of the medical team. *J AM Diet Assoc* 1972; 61:421-423.

57 Ressler MM: Teaching strategies that promote adherence. *Nurs Clin North Am* 1983; 18:799-811.

may ultimately contribute to or detract from client compliance.

To determine the client's learning abilities, the clinician should use the conceptual step-care process: assessment, plan, implementation, and evaluation. To promote acceptance of beneficial "health beliefs," the clinician's educational approach should include explicit objectives, focused instruction, learner demonstration, and feedback evaluation.[58]

Focused instruction will depend on client interest and abilities. Approaches may include one-on-one counseling or group interaction. The clinician may utilize demonstrations, slide-tape or videotape presentation, programmed mastery learning, written client education materials, or a combination of these and others.

Haynes and colleagues cite six general education principles useful in guiding the presentation of information:[59] specificity, organization, repetition, brevity, primacy and readability. That is, both the clinician and the client need to agree on specific goals to be realized. The presentation should reflect organization—clear, careful planning of every aspect of the interaction which affords the opportunity of repeating important information. Because most individuals remember only what was presented in the first third of the presentation and forget half of that presented within the first five minutes, the presentation should be as short as possible without sacrificing vital information and important points should be introduced early. Written materials should be readable by the average individual, targeted for the fourth grade reading level.

Following the educational session, the client's understanding should be ascertained. Merely asking the client is inappropriate, the opportunity should be given to practice or demonstrate that which was taught, asked to recite important aspects, and clarify any information. This affords the clinician the opportunity to evaluate the client's understanding.

As demonstrated earlier and in other studies, education alone will not create satisfactory compliance.[60, 61] In view of the impact of the difficulty factor on the likelihood of adopting health promotional behaviors, assisting the individual to reduce the difficulty of desirable activities is warranted.[62] Although this represents a reversal of the conventional focus of intervention, greater benefits are likely.

Learned behaviors, including undesirable ones, take time to develop; therefore, effecting changes in this behavior will also take time. The emergence of behavioral science principles abound and many behavioral techniques such as contracting, modeling, self-monitoring, and group therapy have been used with varying success.[63] Contracting involves an agreement which specifies rules and rewards for a specific behavior between client and clinician. Acceptable terms are negotiated and specifically stated. Positive reinforcement for reaching desired goals as opposed to punishment for undesirable behavior is characteristic. Contract terms may be changed only by mutual consent of both parties. Modeling is based on the premise that an individual will imitate the behaviors of others and thus can be used to assist the client learn new behaviors and strengthen or weaken existing behaviors. Self-

---

58 Shortridge RC: Learner success or failure? *Journal of Nutrition Education* 1976; 8:18-20.

59 Haynes RB, Taylor DW, Sackett DL, (eds): *Compliance in Health Care*. Baltimore, MD: Johns Hopkins University Press, 1979.

60 Hindi-Alexander MC, Throm J: Compliance or noncompliance: That is the question! *Am J Health Promo* 1987; 5-11.

61 Morse W, Sims LS, Guthrie HA: Mothers' compliance with physicians' recommendations on infant feeding. *J Am Diet Assoc* 1979; 75:140-148.

62 Sennot-Miller L, Miller JL: Difficulty: A neglected factor in health promotion. *Nurs Res* 1987; 36:268-272.

63 Barlow DH, Tillotson JL: Behavioral science and nutrition: A new perspective. *J Am Diet Assoc* 1978; 72:368-371.

monitoring necessitates observing and recording results of therapeutic behaviors. Involvement by the client is highlighted as he observes personal behaviors, evaluates, and alters them accordingly. To have an impact on behavior change, self-monitoring must be associated with goal-setting. Through group therapy, clients find that other people can be a source of safety and strength. The skilled leader uses the group experience to promote change.

Conclusion

Success of a health promotion program can be achieved when the participant is able to make appropriate decisions and adopt those health-enhancing behaviors which are both comfortable and satisfied. To accomplish this, the health-care provider must be cognizant of the uniqueness of participants and prepared with strategies and techniques to help them adopt necessary activities and move closer to the more positive end of the compliance continuum.

The complexity and enormity of the topic of compliance and health promotion and wellness is illustrated by the numerous reports noted in the literature and the number of investigations currently under study. This review is limited by comparison and the reader is encouraged to complement the emphasis of compliance through review of the current literature.

Medical Compliance as an Ideology

James A. Trostle

Introduction

Medical compliance has been defined as "the extent to which the patient's behavior (in terms of taking medications, following diets, or executing other lifestyle changes) coincides with medical or health advice" [1]. Virtually any North American medical journal published since the mid-1970s contains numerous advertisements proclaiming that a particular product's simple dosage or low level of side effects will increase patient compliance. These proclamations are frequently used to advertise treatments for common chronic conditions such as arthritis, diabetes, and hypertension. Studies estimate that about half of the people who have chronic conditions like these are non-compliant with their medication regimens [2].

This paper discusses why therapeutic compliance is an important topic today. I contend that the topic is better approached as an ideology supporting the authority of medical professionals. The basic problem with research on medical compliance is that it is dominated by a series of ideological conceptions of the proper roles of patients and physicians. Though presented as a literature about improving medical services, the research literature about compliance is preeminently, although covertly, a literature about power and control. It is written largely by medical professionals about themselves and their clientele, and it reveals the medical profession's worldview: the problem lies in patients' behavior or in doctor/patient interaction; the solution lies in patient education, behavioral reinforcements, and better doctor/patient communication. By reviewing historical materials of the twentieth century I show that what clinicians now call 'compliance' used to be presented overtly as a matter of physician 'control'.

The clinical, economic, and academic importance of therapeutic compliance

While compliance is an ideology, there are clinical, economic, and academic reasons to study the use of medications. In the clinical realm, the irregular, diminished, or excessive consumption of medicine can reduce health or extend illness. Some medications must be taken long after symptoms disappear, others are dangerous if taken in excess, many are ineffective unless a certain critical minimum level of medication is taken. Consumption that varies from professional expectations, or prescription that varies from accepted standards, can cause a medication's therapeutic effectiveness to be misjudged either in individuals or in large-scale clinical trials.

Compliance is also important today because it affects a large and profitable portion of the economy. The total retail value of drugs and health aids sold in the United States encompassed 1.5% of the nation's gross national product in 1982,

Trostle, J.A. Medical Compliance as an Ideology. SOCIAL SCIENCE AND MEDICINE, 22 (12), (1988), p. 1299-1308.

and more than a third of this portion consisted of pharmaceutical sales over 16 billion dollars [3]. Pharmaceutical companies use compliance today as a promotional strategy to increase market share and product sales. But compliance also serves other latent functions: increased compliance is one of a set of positive attributes (low cost, few side effects, therapeutic efficacy) advertisers use to increase the visibility of their products and to enhance their company's positive image among physicians and the lay public.

Compliance has excited a great deal of contemporary attention both in clinical and social science journals: more than 4000 English-language research and review articles on the topic have been listed in the *Index Medicus* and other bibliographic collections. A cumulative bibliography on the subject [4] listed only 22 articles in English published before 1960, and 850 published by 1978. More than 3200 compliance articles in English were listed in the *Index Medicus* between 1979 and 1985, with more than 1100 appearing in 1984 and 1985. This indicates a dramatic increase in research interest in this aspect of patient-doctor relationships.

Compliance as ideology

My purpose here is not to survey the compliance literature—that has been done often and well [4-6]. Rather I want to argue that therapeutic 'compliance' itself is a problematic concept with its own social history. Most of the many research articles on compliance have evaluated a range of possible determinants and measures, but few have asked why compliance itself has prompted such research enthusiasm, or how it came to be so important. The present popularity of compliance can be better understood if it is analyzed as an *ideology*, that is, a system of shared beliefs that legitimize particular behavioral norms and values at the same time that they claim and appear to be based in empirical truths. Ideologies help to transform power (potential influence) into authority (legitimate control). Compliance is an ideology that transforms physicians' theories about the proper behavior of patients into a series of research strategies, research results, and potentially coercive interventions that *appear* appropriate, and that reinforce physician's authority over health care. (Physicians are certainly not the only professionals involved in patient care, but they still largely determine the direction and intensity of medical interventions.) Looking at compliance as an ideology helps explain why research into the determinants of compliance has been inconclusive: this research has defined patient behavior in terms of professional expectations, and has ignored health-related behavior that contradicts the profession's view of its own centrality to health care.

Social scientists might be expected to adopt an outsider' perspective to facilitate investigating the differences between expert recommendations and lay responses. Unfortunately, those who write about compliance commonly adopt the worldview of the medical profession, a phenomenon once labeled "management bias" by Julius Roth [7]. When differences between expected and adopted behavior arise despite the best intentions and efforts of physicians and patients, research on the day-today use of medications certainly can contribute to improved health care. But the future success of research under the rubric of compliance depends on recognizing that the present definition of the concept poses barriers.

The History of Compliance as an Ideology

To date there has been no historical work done on the topic of compliance, except for a few cursory paragraphs relying on a standard set of anecdotes. R. Brian Haynes, an editor of the first major compliance bibliography, stated facetiously that the "first recorded incident of human non-compliance in Judeo-Christian tradition" occurred when Eve ate the apple in the Garden of Eden [1, p. 3]. Compliance researchers commonly cite Hippocrates as their progenitor because he is reported to have said that [The physician] should keep aware of the fact that patients often lie when they state that they have taken certain medicines" [8]. They also cite the renowned nineteenth century clinician Sir William Osler, who wrote that "The desire to take medicine is perhaps the greatest feature which distinguishes man from animals" [9]. These few anecdotes are inadequate, for the ideology of compliance does have a history.

The origins of compliance research: conventional explanations

Compliance researchers have explained the growth of their literature by linking it to the development of antibiotics in the 1950s, and the subsequent wide availability of these effective treatments. Authors like Robbins [10], Bissonette and Seller [11], and Haynes, [1, p. 4] write that while non-compliance may have been occurring since the time of Hippocrates, only the 1950s did physicians obtain many truly effective medications for the first time, and only then did It become as important for physicians to make sure that these medications were *consumed* by patients as it was to make sure they were properly chosen and prescribed.

This explanation mistakenly assumes that scientific measures of efficacy are the foundation of professional beliefs about clinical efficacy. The explanation is incomplete because it fails to acknowledge that most healers in any historical period (be they physicians, bone-setters, barbers, surgeons, or shamans) believe in and help to reinforce the curative powers of their treatments. Physicians in the eighteenth and nineteenth centuries relied on their so-called "heroic" treatment" which consisted of bleeding, purging, mercurials, and blistering. Dissenting voices were raised, such as a remark by Oliver Wendell Holmes in 1860 that "I firmly believe that if the whole *materia medicus* as now used could be sunk to the bottom of the sea, it would be all the better for mankind—and all the worse for the fishes" [12]. But by and large eighteenth and nineteenth century physicians and healers also believed in the therapeutic effects of their actions, and they probably were just as concerned about compliance as any contemporary physician is. The efficacious treatments of one era become the outmoded therapies of the next.

Belief in therapeutic efficacy fueled a concern for compliance in the treatment of epilepsy in the mid-nineteenth century. W. R. Gowers, a respected physician of the day, explained that non-compliance sometimes caused a patient's epileptic seizures to become more severe after treatment had begun:

> A very frequent occurrence is, that a patient, after a few months' freedom from fits, discontinues the medicine and relapses. He comes again, the fits are again stopped, but less readily than before, again he quits the treatment and the attacks recur, and are not completely arrested [13].

Gowers plainly believed in 1881 that his treatments were effective, and that seizure recurrences were caused by non-compliance. He blamed patient behavior, not ineffective medication, although the first effective anticonvulsant medication, phenobarbital, was not introduced until 1912.

A history of medical compliance must therefore explain the popularity of the concept by referring to cultural beliefs in curative substances and the history of the profession of medicine, as much as the efficacy of pharmaceuticals. The history of compliance as an ideology can be uncovered by looking at legislation, medical journals, and advertisements that address and reveal the self-image of the medical profession. Such a history portrays the origins and growth of concerns about compliance: rather than resulting solely from medical advances in the past three decades, contemporary concern for compliance is also a product of the growing monopoly of the medical profession over the past century.

The origin of compliance research: an alternative explanation

The modern chronicles of compliance have missed a point made by Owsei Temkin, a historian of medicine, who pointed out that patients have had faith in drugs for longer than they have had faith in physicians [14]. The compliance literature suggests that the relationship between physician and patient is—and by inference, should be—the most important factor determining the course of a person's health-related activities (exceptions have been noted by [15-19] among others). Yet Temkin says that obtaining the medical *products* now available (primarily if not solely from physicians) may be more important to patients than their relationships with physicians. Physicians are an historically and geographically bounded profession organized to provide health care, but the consumption of substances to cure illness has no such temporal or spatial boundaries Labeling patients 'non-compliant' because they follow their own ideas about their own care misses the point that this is what people have done since medicines were first used. Those who use the label mistakenly equate health care dominated by physicians—a specific outcome of a contemporary power distribution—with health management in general.

Compliance research makes a crucial historical error. It places undue emphasis on one particular historical relationship between healers and the afflicted, the physician-patient relationship, and neglects the existence of more universal forms of obtaining care: self-management, and relying on family, friends, neighbors, and others. The very notion of compliance requires a dependent layperson and a dominant professional—someone to give advice, suggestions, or orders, and someone to carry them out. Yet even within North American and European societies the structural dominance of the medical profession is not a timeless or universal phenomenon. United States physicians owe their dominance to nineteenth and twentieth century legislative acts that helped to establish the 'monopolizing' and 'gate-keeping' functions of medicine: controlling who may practice the profession and where (licensing of practitioners and educational establishments, malpractice review); who can obtain and prescribe scarce valuable items like pharmaceuticals (controlled substance laws); what reasonable levels of payment are (Medicaid, Medicare); how much is known about costs and charges (restrictive advertising covenants); and a host of other structural constraints [20-28].

Rather than pointing to the efficacy of antibiotics to explain the growth of a concern for compliance with therapeutic regimens in the United States, one might point instead to this developing consolidation of the profession of medicine, and the growth and sales strategies of the pharmaceutical and proprietary drug industries. One example of this comes from advertising in medical journals in the early 1900s, for example, which proclaimed that companies were directing information to physicians rather than to patients. This reinforced physicians' beliefs that they were not just the most skilled but also the only proper source of health care for their patients. A selection of advertisements from campaigns for infant feeding materials shows the development of a new professional and industrial concern for controlling the behavior of the weak and the sick. These advertisements document that a concern for market control combined with a concern for therapeutic power and evolved into a concern for patient compliance.

Nutritional supplements and infant formula: transforming information control into patient compliance

For much of the nineteenth century physicians in the United States had little power: they were poorly trained, disorganized, and had little social prestige. During this time patent medicine companies advertised their products directly to the general public. ('Patent' is a misnomer: their ingredients were copyrighted and thus private rather than patented and public.) Up to the late nineteenth century many miracle cures were touted as cheap alternatives to medical care. At the beginning of the twentieth century, however, both organized medicine and the United States government began to legislate changes in the extent and kind of drug advertising directed at the public. The federal government began with the Pure Food and Drugs Act of 1906, setting initial standards for labeling drug ingredients and claims of efficacy, and in 1938 passed the Food, Drug, and Cosmetic Act with further restrictions and additional enforcement provisions. The American Medical Association (AMA) stopped accepting patent medicine advertisements in its Journal in 1905, and also began to rule on whether various products were acceptable for medical use. In 1924 it reserved the right to reject advertising for approved drugs from companies that derived earnings from other unapproved drugs. Though physicians and politicians both campaigned against misrepresentation of health products they did so with somewhat different goals: the government meant to make consumer information more accurate, while the AMA wanted to make information accurate as well as to control the amount of product information consumers received, and thereby increase physician control over medicines and other health-related products[27, pp. 130-134, 29, 30].

Physicians in the early twentieth century thus began to consolidate their control over the business of healing in the United States and to increase their influence over the health-related activities of their patients. [This was paralleled by the growing public health movement in the United States, which argued for improving (and controlling) the collective health of the country by means of population interventions like putting iodine into salt or, more recently, fluoridating water.] One early strategy in doctors' attempts to control patient behavior was to sell food products containing nutritional additives, thereby, at least ostensibly, circumventing patients' problems in taking nutritional supplements as suggested. This strategy was a means to resolve the problem now called non-compliance.

Some attempts to increase patient compliance were couched in terms of improving patient forgetfulnes. This strategy was used in the 1934 *Journal of the American Medical Association* in an advertisement promoting evaporated milk with cod-liver oil extract, the text of which follows:

> YOU FORGOT again MOTHER. Yes. . . . mothers do forget!
>
> How many mothers forget to give regularly the cod-liver oil you prescribe? Many doctors are now recommending DEAN'S so that the children under their care are assured a regular and definite supply of Vitamin 'D'. DEAN has put Vitamin 'D', extracted from cod-liver oil (by the Zuckerman process), into evaporated milk. And you can't even taste it. Furthermore, DEAN'S is pure, selected, cow's milk from tuberculin-tested herds, unsweetened and evaporated to double richness. Developed especially for infant feeding, DEAN'S is also important in child and adult nutrition. We should like to send you Vitamin 'D' Evaporated Milk Literature and a Standard Feeding Formula. May we [31].

Adding nutritional supplements to food products is a problematic strategy: on the positive side the dietary supplement is consumed whenever the food product is consumed; no extra pills or syrups need to be taken. On the negative side, doctors can rely on a fixed proportion of the additive being consumed only *if the food product is consumed according to directions*. Moreover the product provides the additive but does not require the continuing supervision of the physician. This was an economic hazard to the physician because it did not require return visits [29]. Physicians gained control over return visits by emphasizing that these products could be misused by patients unless they were monitored. They emphasized the potential medical hazards to the patient, and thereby avoided focusing on the economic hazard to their livelihood.

The potential problem was solved for infant formula preparations in a way that increased physician control over patient behavior and increased formula company revenues. It was simple and elegant: formula companies took preparation directions and feeding schedules off containers of infant formulas, and directed advertising at physicians rather than the lay public. Potential consumers could obtain the product only if they were under the care of a physician.

This change took place in a time of increasing government regulation, when infant formula companies decided to entrust physicians with control over their products. (This is called the 'ethical push' route for advertising, while the 'consumer pull' strategy is to advertise in the mass media directly to the public.) Physicians would be more respectable and profitable salesmen than the company sales force; as time passed physician control over the distribution of certain health-related products began to appear natural and even necessary. (For a recounting of the history of the formula-marketing decision see [29, 30]. The sales strategy was expanded to vitamin supplements, and became the model for subsequent marketing of prescription pharmaceuticals. The strategy was forthrightly articulated in the advertising section of the *Journal of the American Medical Association,* where one full-page advertisement concluded with the following paragraphs:

> When the physician reads this class of exploiting advertisement of which patronizingly refers to his endorse the most ridiculous claims, and later hears his patients knowingly repeating these to him, he cannot help asking himself these questions:
>
> (1) Should the layman receive his medical education including his vitamin-mindedness, from the commercial house, or from his doctor?
>
> (2) Should the commercial house exploit vita modern patent medicine style, or should the physician control their intelligent application?
>
> Mead Johnson & Company, for one, continue to feel that vitamin therapy, like infant feeding, should be in the hands of the medical profession, and consequently refuse to lend their aid to exploiting these valuable agents to the public. This house, for one, advertises its vitamin products exclusively to the medical profession and furnishes no directions to the public [32].

This deliberate company decision to advertise their marketing strategy was effective because it reflected and magnified a sentiment already common among U.S. physicians, namely, that the medical profession should maintain control over the distribution of infant formula. That sentiment was formalized in 1932 when the American Medical Association passed a resolution requiring infant food companies that wanted AMA approval of their products to advertise those products only to physicians. This particular advertisement clearly goes beyond infant feeding, addressing vitamin therapy as well. But what is most interesting is that an ideology of physician control itself is being created and promoted here; an explicit announcement of support for physician control over patient behavior is used to sell products.

We see another of the ideology of physician control in another 1931 advertisement by Mead Johnson & Company. This advertisement also promotes a company's products by associating them with a policy of advertising only to the profession. It also points out that professional benefits accrue from having physicians control health-related information. But rather than employing the stark unadorned text of the last advertisement, this advertisement presents an idealized image: the doctor is drawn as the active provider of care, the patient as passive (and grateful) recipient. In this ad the mother cannot read what is written on the page in the doctor's hand, and she has a trusting expression. This is a telling portrayal of the marketing strategy of the producer, but it is also a snapshot of an image-making process. By controlling information doctors gain power. By withholding information they promote passivity and dependence.

Mead Johnson had the most visible "No Laity Advertising" strategy, used in its campaigns up until the mid-1940s for products ranging from infant formula to fish liver oil. But it was not the only company to extol this strategy. Similar claims were also made, for example, by the Corn Products Sales Company for its Karo syrup for infant feeding [33], and by the Nestle Corporation for its Lactogen infant formula [34]. These advertisements demonstrate that: (1) a concern for controlling patient behavior antedated the development of antibiotics; (2) the U.S. medical profession's interest in maintaining control over patients' behavior and access to information was recognized and reinforced throughout the 1920s to 1940s, before many effective medications became available; (3) professional self-interest was a significant factor in the movement to limit popular advertising of infant feeding products and of vitamins; and (4) the contemporary concern for 'compliance' was openly articulated earlier in this century as a concern for patient cooperation' and physician 'control'.

Physician authority and the status of compliance

The concern for compliance is a cultural phenomenon intimately connected with the self-image of physicians. and with their organized (and often successful) attempts to define the limits of their own discipline. Yet the present respect and authority accorded physicians in the United States is of recent origin, and may be diminishing [35, 36]. Physicians have exercised their control over medical technology and pharmaceuticals only in the past century. Now for-profit hospitals and medical groups are employing physicians as salaried workers; their growth is causing reductions in physicians' monopolistic power [27, 37, 38]. Physician control over the technology of medical care is starting to decrease as pharmaceutical companies lobby for the right to advertise directly to consumers, the Food and Drug Administration moves drugs (such as cortisone) from prescription to non-prescription categories, and Health Maintenance Medical Organizations develop limited lists of approved medications. This may eventually reduce physicians' control over the technology of health care. Some would even argue that the last decade's preoccupation with compliance is a consequence of the declining authority of the profession.

Unpacking the contemporary ideology of compliance

Contemporary research on medical compliance is burdened by the multiple meanings of the word 'compliance'. To pursue Haynes' witticism that noncompliance began in the Garden of Eden, if the term 'non-compliance' can apply equally to a patient's non-conformity with medical advice, and to a Biblical figure's non-conformity with God's commandment, then what values does the term express? While Haynes was joking, the biblical example is not serendipitous: Haynes states that his definition of compliance was intended to be non-judgmental. Some researchers urge that terms like 'non-adherence' or 'defaulting' be substituted for 'non-compliance' in an effort to escape the word's connotations of dominance and subservience [18, 39, 40, 41]. Others suggest that we consider cases of 'intelligent non-compliance' or 'capricious compliance', better to conceptualize those instances where non-compliance makes sense, or where compliance does not [42]. Some have proposed to replace 'non-compliance' with labels like patient 'self-regulation' [43], or 'self-management' [44]. This is done to emphasize that patients are ultimately responsible for their behavior, and to counter the prevailing research emphasis that the physician needs to foster compliance. If unmodified, however, these terms overemphasize the patient's contribution to therapy, and they thus mirror the errors of relying on a physician-centered approach to compliance. An editor of the first compliance bibliography explicitly recognized that the term complaint "is troublesome to many people because it conjures up images of patient or client sin and serfdom" ([1, p. 2], but he stated that the editors knew of no acceptable alternative. Another editor called the various alternatives 'technical argon terms', thus implying that compliance is immune from such jargon.

Compliance is an ideology based in theories about the proper relationship between physicians and their clients. Yet its assumptions, definitions, and manifestations have been studied and reified as quantifiable categories of human behavior. Though compliance can be called a non-judgmental concept, it rarely is used or studied in this way. Much contemporary compliance research has manifested the theories about proper patient behavior seen in the following examples:

> Through instruction in health magazines, the Reader's Digest, and radio and television programmes, patients acquire that superficial knowledge which often emboldens them to question their doctor more closely than hitherto about their own complaints. Of course it is unlikely that a patient can have any real understanding about his illness, but the greater risk that he will obtain misguided information from less reliable sources has to be reckoned with. Greater profit, therefore, will be earned if the doctor affords time to talk to each patient with cardiac pain [45].

> Communication between doctor and patient ideally necessitates a certain degree of reciprocity. Each person has certain rights and obligations. When the doctor performs a service, the patient is obligated to reciprocate: first, by cooperating with the doctor in their interaction; and second, by complying with the medical recommendations once he leaves the doctor's office [46].

> In some instances, the patient, because his condition is not improving or is getting worse (due to his failure to follow the prescribed regimen) may start a malpractice action. On a less critical level, the patient, and his or her family and friends may decide to go elsewhere for their health care. In addition, a discontented patient is patient is not likely to help a physician's reputation in the community. That's why it's important for the physician to understand the motivations for the patient's noncompliance [47]. (From an article entitled "Why don't patients do what you tell them?"

> Whether your patient needs to be reassured or warned, he needs to be made aware of his responsibility for taking medication as directed. Just as he decided to seek treatment, so he must decide to take his drug correctly and follow other particulars of his therapeutic regimen. Most patients appreciate the idea of being active partners in their treatment [48].

These examples chart some of the changing rationales for physician concerns with compliance. Writing in the late 1950s, Evans [45] portrayed patients as ignorant and prone to act on misguided information. He championed patient education as a strategy to prevent 'improper' consults rather than to prevent illness. This reflects the paternal role the profession adopted at the time. By the late 1960s many physicians had replaced their role as stewards with a role 'therapeutic partners', but this partnership was a limited one. Davis [46] articulated the doctor-patient relationship as a contract, but whereas most professional contracts stipulate that fees are to be exchanged for services, Davis suggested that patients reciprocate their doctor's services by cooperating with the doctor's agenda during the clinical interaction. and complying with the doctor's recommendations afterward. Writing in the late 1970s, in the era of defensive medicine, Van Camerik [47] was more blunt. Physicians' self-interest should cause them to give effective treatments, try to understand non-compliers, and avoid malpractice suits or a damaged public image. In the 1980s Weibert and Dee [48] portrayed a more subtle variant of the contractual model of doctor-patient relationships: having freely and of his own volition sought treatment, the patient is thus responsible for internalizing the doctor's orders and following the regimen.

All these excerpts assume that the professional consultation signals an end to the patient's decision-making about caring for the complaint. Evans was motivated to protect the patient from other nonprofessional influences, while Van Camerik wanted to protect the physician from legal action. Davis and Weibert and Dee presented more egalitarian models of how physicians and patients should interact, yet they both left no conceptual room for patients to disagree with or reject doctors' advice.

These assumptions about patient-doctor relationships can be summarized as follows: the physician is the proper ultimate authority over the actions of his or her patients; in exchange for a physician's services a patient owes fees, cooperation, and compliance; non-compliance is usually the patient's fault; and physicians offer therapeutic partnerships to patients. not vice versa.

The implications of the compliance ideology for patient care

Health care providers with these assumptions use non-compliance like an epithet, obscuring the variability and denying the legitimacy of behaviors that differ from the clinical prescription. When physicians label their patients 'non-compliant' they often distance themselves from their patients' actions, judging and labeling rather than analyzing and understanding. Compliance is successful as a descriptive term in clinical practice precisely because it assumes that physicians legitimately control patient behavior. Yet thinking about patient behavior in terms of compliance' constrains communication by substituting a simple epithet for a complex act or series of acts over time. We know that a non-compliant patient has not followed a clinical prescription, but we do not know what that patient has done instead. Most compliance research focuses only on the results of doctor-patient interactions, and it therefore misses this important larger context. As Zola [19, 49] has pointed out, people often have many illnesses and attempts to alleviate symptoms before they see a doctor—these prior experiences are likely to influence compliance, but they often are excluded from the examining room. Thinking about drug-taking behavior in terms of non-compliance impedes communication: it marks a patient's 'misbehavior' as being outside the boundaries of a physician's responsibility. The term rationalizes physician withdrawal and blames the patient rather than promoting a reexamination of clinical priorities. It further justifies the dominance of the physician in controlling the type and direction of information given during clinical interactions [50, 51].

If one takes an omniscient position outside the physician-patient relationship one can see that noncompliance can be the behavioral result of many motivations. It can express someone's disagreement or dissatisfaction with clinical advice, a rational response to a series of social realities competing with the clinical agenda (e.g. financial constraints, being labeled a patient, inability to function adequately under a medication's side effects, familial opposition to therapy), a conscious preference of illness to health, an immature response to adult responsibilities, a manipulation of one's physical condition for other goals, or even a rejection of medical intervention altogether [15, 52-54]. Thus non-compliance is an unavoidable byproduct of collisions between the clinical world and other competing worlds of work, play, friendship, and family life.

The compliance literature at its most coercive teaches physicians how to manipulate their patients' behavior without questioning their own beliefs or increasing their patients' understanding (for examples of this, see Refs [5, 55, 56]. One extreme variant of this approach outlines how physicians can build up their own 'motivating power', that is, their ability to make patients internalize their recommendations, by using positive feedback and encouraging self-disclosure in their patients. The authors conclude with what is essentially a recommendation to study how physicians can manipulate patients without being found out:

> Clients are just as aware of the norms of social equity as practitioners, and they, are likely to be suspicious when given overzealous unearned praise or compliments. Practitioners' attempts to use acceptance can have boomerang effects if they give so much praise that they are presumed to be ingratiating with a hidden manipulative intent. *The conditions under which acceptance by, health-care practitioners will and will not be perceived as ingratiating by*

their patients need to be systematically investigated [56, p. 76] (My emphasis.)

This is a call to seek the limits of medical deception, for it never acknowledges that 'motivating power' is being increased precisely *to facilitate a* 'hidden manipulative intent'. Physicians and other health care providers can teach patients techniques for self-assessment, behavioral change, and behavioral reinforcement-this provides patients with the tools to follow through with their professed desire to comply. Physicians can also give positive feedback with a coercive intent-this has been labeled unethical by some compliance researchers [57, 58].

These excerpts highlight some of the basic assumptions of compliance research. They show that a concern for compliance serves professional purposes and that the justifications for this concern change over time. These changes can even be seen in the ways the medical literature on patients' behavior is categorized. *Patient compliance* first appeared as a medical subject heading in the *Index Medicus* in 1975, but was cross-referenced under the heading *Patient dropouts* until 1981. In 1981 *Patient dropouts* was replaced by the heading *Patient non-compliance*. This refined a relatively crude category, but both the old and the new categories still use professional norms from inside the clinic to define and pass judgment on health-related behavior outside the clinic.

Conclusions

The topic of compliance is popular among physicians because it gives a focus to their interactions with 'problem' patients, reflects their ideas about how patients should behave, and addresses their notions about the determinants of proper patient behavior. There was little research literature on patient compliance before the 1960s, but we have no reason to believe that patients before that time had obeyed doctor's orders, or that practitioners before that time had no concerns about compliance. A number of factors must have combined to bring non-compliance to clinical attention: increasing numbers of prescription drugs made non-compliance more possible and thus more visible; drug companies often mentioned compliance in their advertising; social scientists and clinicians convinced the growing biomedical research industry to examine the behavioral correlates of the problem; and health educators designed interventions. None of these should be singled out as the most important influence, but all have combined to create and sustain a long period of research on the topic.

Analyzing compliance as an ideology, is useful because it helps explain why the literature is so large and yet so contradictory and incomplete. Looking at patient behavior in terms of medical compliance perpetuates the notion that health care is (and ought to be) centered around proper use of physicians. The causes of problems in the patient-physician relationship are sought in patient behavior and beliefs. Researchers could hypothesize that all patients are potential non-compliers and that particular kinds of situations cause non-compliance. Instead most of the research hypothesizes that there are non-compliant types of people, and that with sufficient ingenuity their traits can be identified.

Descriptions of patient behavior and interventions designed to influence it have come full circle. Early in this century companies manufacturing infant foods attempted to take product information and responsibility for care away from mothers. They gave doctors frank descriptions of how they might attempt to control their patients, and they loudly proclaimed their efforts to consolidate physician control over infant feeding practices. Patient education became accepted practice somewhat later, accompanied by attempts to increase patient responsibility and self-control, as well as attempts to bring patients subtly around to adopting physician desires as their own. Most recently we can see medical technology used to reduce the need for patient initiative. For example, long-acting medications are recommended over short, injections recommended over pills, and office-centered interventions valued over those in the home. These interventions may be effective, but they risk turning patients from responsible subjects into responsive objects.

If research on people's use of medications continues to be analyzed in terms of their compliance then this research will continue to give a distorted picture of behavior. The word 'compliant' has unfortunate connotations, but the underlying concept also needs reworking. It is valid to investigate what patients do with their medications, and how they respond in daily life to the requests of medical professionals. However, these can be investigated far more comprehensively under rubrics like 'drug-taking behavior', 'clinic attendance', or 'medication consumption' than they can under the rubric of compliance. A behavioral definition can address the complexities introduced by self-care, care by nonmedical specialists, and care by non-specialists. It must be flexible enough, however, to describe what strategies, if any, are adopted in place of those recommended by a healer.

Most of these issues can be distilled into a series of empirical questions. For example, if medication use were better divided into component categories (e.g., taking medication as directed, taking it sporadically), regularly taking less, regularly taking more, discontinuing completely), would these component categories have stronger associations with predictor variables than the broader category of non-compliance? Are these categories associated with recourse to multiple sources of biomedical care, recourse to non-biomedical care, or neither? What situations affect people's use of medications? Do people who modify or reject one medical regimen also modify or reject other medical regimens? Do they modify of reject other non-medical regimens? Do rates or strategies of medication use vary across cultures? If variation exists is it associated with different cultural rules about response to authority, different types of health systems, different expectations by medical professionals, or other factors?

These questions cannot be framed within the present definitions of compliance research. They still need to be asked and answered, however, to better portray the complexity and determinants of health-related behavior outside the examining room.

Acknowledgements—Support during the writing of this paper was provided by the Epilepsy Foundation of America, the Wenner-Gren Foundation for Anthropological Research, the U. C. Berkeley Rennie Endowment, and the National Institute of Mental Health (MHO9039-01 to -03). Lynn Morgan, Laura Nader, Fred Dunn, and two reviewers helped me to clarify prior versions. A shortened version was presented in 1984 before the *American Anthropological Association Annual Meeting*.

References

1. Haynes R. B. Introduction. In *Compliance in Health Care* (Edited by Haynes R. B., Sackett D. L. and Taylor, D. W.), p. 2. Johns Hopkins University Press, Baltimore, Md, 1979.
2. Sackett D. L. and Snow J. C. The magnitude of compliance and non-compliance. In *Compliance in Health Care* (Edited by Haynes R. B., Sackett D. L. and Taylor D. W.), pp. 11-22. Johns Hopkins University Press, Baltimore, Md, 1979.
3. United States Department of Commerce. *Statistical Abstract of the United States*. U.S. Government Printing Office, Washington, D.C., 1985.
4. Haynes R. B., Sackett D. L. and Taylor D. W. (Eds). *Compliance in Health Care*. Johns Hopkins University Press. Baltimore, Md, 1979.
5. DiMatteo M. R. and DiNicola D. D. *Achieving Patient Compliance: The Psychology of the Medical Practitioner's Role*. Pergamon. New York, 1982.

6. Eraker S. A., Kirscht J. P. and Becker M. H. Understanding and improving patient compliance. *Ann. intern. Med.* 100, 258-268, 1984.
7. Roth J. S. "Management bias" in social science study of medical treatment. *Hum. Org.* 21, 47-50, 1962.
8. Lasagna L. Fault and default. *New Engl. J. Med.* 267-268, 1973; also Ref. [1].
9. Cushing 1925, quoted in Becker M. H. and Maiman L.A. Strategies for enhancing patient compliance. *J. Commun. Hlth* 6, 130, 1980.
10. Robbins J. A. Patient compliance. *Primary Care* 7, 703, 1980.
11. Bissonette R. and Seller R. Medical non-compliance: a cultural perspective. *Man Med.* 5, 41, 1980.
12. Quoted in Crout J. R. Self-medication: the government role, part 11. In *Self-Medication: The New Era. A Symposium*, p. 41. The Proprietary Association, Washington, D.C., 1980.
13. Gowers 1964 (1881):211 quoted in Wannamaker B. B., Morton W. A., Gross A. J. and Saunders S. Improvement in antiepileptic drug levels following reduction of intervals between clinic visits. *Epilepsia* 21, 157, 1980.
14. Temkin 0. Historical aspects of drug therapy. In *Drugs in Our Society* (Edited by Talalay P.), pp. 3-16. Johns Hopkins University Press. Baltimore, Md, 1964.
15. Conrad P. The meaning of medications: another look at compliance. *Soc. Sci. Med.* 20, 29-37, 1985.
16. Garrity T. F. Medical compliance and the clinician-patient relationship: a review. *Soc. Sci. Med.* 15, 215-222, 1981.
17. Hayes-Bautista D. Modifying the treatment: patient compliance, patient control and medical care. *Soc. Sci. Med.* 10, 233-238. 1976.
18. Stimson G. V. Obeying the doctor's orders: a view from the other side. *Soc. Sci. Med.* 8. 97-104, 1974.
19. Zola I. K. Structural constraints in the doctor-patient relationship: the case of non-compliance. In The Relevance of Social Science for Medicine (Edited by Eisenberg L. and Kleinman A.), pp. 241-252. Reidel Press, Dordrecht, 1981.
20. Brown E. R. *Rockefeller Medicine Men: Medicine and Capitalism in America.* University of California Press, Berkeley, Calif., 1979.
21. Conrad P. Types of medical social control. *Sociol. Hlth Illness* 1-11, 1979.
22. Duffy J. The changing image of the American physician. *In Sickness and Health in America* (Edited by Leavitt J. W. and Numbers R. L.), pp. 131-137. University of Wisconsin Press. Madison, Wis., 1978.
23. Freidson E. *Profession of Medicine: A Study of the Sociology of Applied Knowledge.* Dodd, Mead, New York, 1970.
24. Freidson E. *Doctoring Together: A Study of Professional Social Control.* Elsevier-North Holland, New York, 1975.
25. Klein R. *Complaints against Doctors: A Study in Professional Accountability.* Knight, London, 1973.
26. Morrow C. K. Sick doctors: the social construction of professional deviance. *Soc. Probl.* 30, 92-108, 1982.
27. Starr P. *The Social Transformation of American Medicine.* Basic Books, New York, 1982.
28. Stevens R. *American Medicine and the Public Interest.* Yale University Press, New Haven, Conn., 1971.
29. Apple R. D. To be used only under the direction of a physician: commercial infant feeding and medical practice, 1870-1940. *Bull. Hist. Med.* 54, 402-417, 1982.
30. Apple R. D. *Mothers and Medicine: A Social History of Infant Feeding,* 1890-1950. Wisconsin Publications in the History of

Science and Medicine, No. 7. University of Wisconsin Press, Madison. Wis., 1987.

31. *J. Am. Med. Ass.* 102, (4), 33, 1934.
32. *J. Am. Med. Ass.* 97, (8), 46, 1931.
33. *New Engl. J. Med.* 220, (2), x, 1939.
34. *New Engl. J. Med.* 220, (5), ix, 1939.
35. Betz M. and O'Connell L. Changing doctor-patient relationships and the rise in concern for accountability. *Soc. Probl.* 31, 84-95, 1983.
36. Haug M. and Lavin B. *Consumerism in Medicine: Challenging Physician Authority,*. Sage, Beverly Hills, Calif., 1983.
37. McKinlay J. B. The changing political and economic context of the patient-physician encounter. In *The Doctor-Patient Relationship in the Changing Health Scene* (Edited by Gallagher E. B.), pp. 155-188. US-DHEW Publication No. (NIH)78-183, Fogarty Center, Washington, D.C., 1978.
38. McKinlay J. B. and Arches J. Towards the proletarianization of physicians. *Int. J. Hlth Serv.* 15, 161 -195, 1985.
39. Barofsky I. Compliance, adherence and the therapeutic alliance: steps in the development of self-care. *Soc. Sci. Med.* 12, 369-376, 1978.
40. Kasl S. V. Issues in patient adherence to health care regimens. *J. Human Stress* 1, 5-17, 1975.
41. Stone G. C. Patient compliance and the role of the expert. *J. Soc. Issues* 35, 34-59, 1979.
42. Weintraub M. Intelligent non-compliance and capricious compliance. In *Patient Compliance* (Edited by Lasagna L.), pp. 39-47. Futura, Mt Kisco, N.Y.. 1976.
43. Schneider J. W. and Conrad P. *Having Epilepsy: The Experience and Control of Illness*. Temple University Press, Philadelphia, Penn., 1983.
44. Buchanan N. Treatment of epilepsy: whose right is it anyway? *Br. Med. J.* 284, 173-174, 16 January. 1982.
45. Evans W. Faults in the diagnosis and management of cardiac pain. *Br. Med. J.* 1, 252, 31 January, 1959.
46. Davis M. S, Variations in patients' compliance with doctor's advice: an empirical analysis of patterns of communication. *Am. J. Publ. Hlth* 58, 284, 1968.
47. an Kamerik S. B. Why don't patients do what you tell them? *Legal Aspects Med. Pract.* 6, 30, 1978.
48. Weibert R. T. and Dee D. A. *Improving Patient Medication Compliance*, p. 9. Medical Economics Company, Book Division, Oradell, N. J., 1980.
49. Zola 1. K. Culture and symptoms—an analysis of patients' presenting complaints. *Am. Sociol. Rev.* 31, 615-630, 1966.
50. Waitzkin H. and Stoeckle J. D. Information control and the micropolitics of health care: summary of an ongoing research project. *Soc. Sci. Med.* 10, 263-276, 1976.
51. Waitzkin H. Information giving in medical care. *J. Hlth Soc. Behav.* 26, 81-101, 1985.
52. Taussig M. Reification and the consciousness of the patient. *Soc. Sci. Med.* 14B, 3-13, 1980.
53. Trostle J. A., Hauser W. A. and Susser 1. S. The logic of non-compliance: management of epilepsy from the patient's point of view. *Cult. Med. Psychiat. 7, 35-56, 1983.*
54. Udry J. R. and Morris N. M. A spoonful of sugar helps the medicine go down. *Am. J. Publ. Health* 61, 30-33, 1971.
55. Benfari R. C., Eaker E. and Stoll J. G. Behavioral interventions and compliance to treatment regimens. *A. Rev. Publ. Hlth* 2, 431-471, 1981.
56. Rodin J and Janis I. L. The social power of health care practitioners as agents of change. *J. Soc. Issues* 35, 60-81, 1979.
57. Jonsen A. R. Ethical issues in compliance. In Compliance in Health Care (Edited by Haynes R. B., Sackett D. L. and Taylor D.

W.), pp. 113-120. Johns Hopkins University Press, Baltimore, Md, 1979.

58. Sackett D. L. Introduction. In *Compliance with Therapeutic Regimens* (Edited by Sackett D. L. and Haynes R. B.). pp, 1-6. Johns Hopkins University Press. Baltimore. Md, 1976.

Patient Satisfaction and Quality of Care

Building Effective Client and Colleague Relationships: Insights From Patients, the Factory, the Classroom, and the Pet Shop

Brent D. Ruben

Dimensions Of Quality of Care: Clinical, Administrative, Relationship

A Louis Harris Poll conducted last year determined that 8 of 9 citizens believe the US healthcare system needs a major overhaul (*USA Today*, May 25, 1989). Growing discontent regarding the health care, health care personnel, and our health care systems, in general, is widespread, and detractors are becoming increasingly visible and vocal. Even physicians, traditionally immune to harsh public criticism have fallen victim to the tide of discontent.

It is clear that a number factors have contributed to the present circumstance. Among these

- Cost Pressures
- More Demanding Consumers Capital and labor Shortages
- Increasing Competition
- Rapid Technological Change
- Threat of Litigation
- New Diseases (e.g. AIDS, substance abuse)

In analyzing the challenges facing healthcare providers, primary attention is focused on *clinical/technical* quality of care, and we are seeing increasing efforts to gather, quantify, and analyze information on clinical outcomes. The largest project of this kind is sponsored by the Joint Commission on Accreditation of Healthcare Organizations (JCAHO) and involves about 400 hospitals (McCormick, 190, p. 34). There are many other substantial initiatives in this area. The Humana group, for example, collects and analyzes data from each of its member hospitals relative to claims, readmission rates, infection rates, complication rates, and length of stay, for 14 clinical departments. System-wide profiles are then fed back to the individual institution as a baseline for quality assessment (McCormick, 190, p. 35).

More recently, emphasis is also being directed toward questions of *administrative* quality—matters related to management procedure and policy. Attesting to the growing interest in administrative quality is the emergence of programs such as Phillip Crosby Associates, Inc., Quality Improvement Process (QIP) and 3M's Total Quality Management (TQM) both of which apply quality assurance methodologies from other industries to the healthcare field.

As central as clinical/medical and administrative practices are to the quality of health care, it appears that much of the discontent with the quality of health care has less to do with clinical or administrative quality, than it does what might be termed *relationship* quality. My own research, and the recent writings of others, confirms that much of the widespread dissatisfaction is the result of a lack of quality in caregiver-patient relationships (e.g. Ruben, 1990a, 1990b; Omachonu, 1990; Ben-Sira, 1990).

What is relationship quality.? Why is it important? What are its components? In the article these issues are explored from the perspective patients, the literature, and the pet shop.

INSIGHTS FROM PATIENTS

Much can be teamed about the nature of relationship quality from patients themselves, and not surprisingly a number of researchers have emphasized the patient perspective in their work (e.g. Bertakis, 1977; Ellmer & Olbrisch, 1983; Greenfield, Kaplan & Ware, 1985, 1986; Kaplan, Greenfield & Ware, 1989; Leebov, 1988; Pascoe, 1983; Ruben, 1985; Ware & Davies, 1983; Waitzkin, 1984, 1986)

One focus of my own patient-centered research over the past several years, has been to determine what patients most remember from hospital stays and visits to health centers. The research involved nearly 4,000 patients at six different hospitals and health services.[1] As a part of the project, patients were asked to:

> "Think back to your stay at the hospital (or visit to the health center) and describe, in a sentence or two, your most memorable positive or negative experience. (This can be any experience related to the hospital (or center), its staff or services)."

The open-ended responses were their content analyzed and categorized, and frequencies were calculated. The six categories which emerged are:

"Most memorable experiences related to. . . "

1. Clinical/technical facets of the treatment (abbreviated as: **clinical**);
2. The institutions policies and procedures (abbreviated as: **policies**);
3. The institutions facilities/accommodations (abbreviated as: **facilities**);
4. Aspects of their treatment relating to personal treatment and/or interpersonal communication (abbreviated as: **interpersonal**);
5. The quality and/or quantity of information provided (abbreviated as: **information**;
6. Other (abbreviated as: **other**

As is apparent from Table 1, in each case, patients' most memorable experiences more frequently involved the quality of their relationships with caregivers—and the way they were treated interpersonally—than circumstances related to either a clinical or administrative quality (Ruben, 1990a, 1990b; Ruben & Bowman, 1986; Ruben, Christensen & Guttman, 1990; B. Ruben & J. Ruben, 1987, 1988).

As shown in Table 1, patients do *not* most remember the clinical or technical care they receive, as might be expected. In five of the six populations studied, the "Clinical/Technical" category ranks second; in the case of the ambulatory healthcare center, the rank is third. Overall, "clinical" aspects of care account for only 27.0% (304/1125) of remembered experiences. Health care facilities—which included food in the case of the hospitals—is even less significant to the more lasting memories of health care. "Facilities" ranked fourth overall, accounting for only 7.3% (82/1125) of the experiences reported.

First, by a substantial margin for all for healthcare institutions, is "Personal Treatment/Interpersonal Communication." Across the six populations, "Interpersonal" accounts for 46.7% (525/1125) of all responses. "Policies and Procedures" accounts for 9.4% of the responses overall. "Quality/Quantity of Information Provided" ranked fifth at 5.8%, and "Other"—which included factors like cost and convenience—ranked sixth at 3.9%.

It can be argued that both "Quality/Quantity of Information Provided" and "Personal Treatment/Interpersonal Communication" are facets of communication. If these two categories were combined the primary role of relationship quality is emphasized even more dramatically. Tables 2–7 provide examples of the patient responses in each category.

Table 1

Factors Associated with Patients' Most Memorable Experiences at Six Health Care Institutions

Rank Order	Acute Care Hospital[1] 582 Bed-Community (N = 204)	Acute Care Hospital[2] 206 Bed-Urban (N = 96)	Acute Care Hospitals[3] 248 Bed-Suburban (N = 286)	Acute Care Hospital[4] 354-Bed Community (N = 217)	Rehab Hospital[5] 88 Bed-Regional (N = 94)	Ambulatory Care Center-University[6] 84,867 Visits (N = 228)	Combined Data-Six Institutions (N = 1125)
	Factor *Percent*	**Factor** *Percent*	**Factor** *Percent*	**Factor** *Percent*	**Factor** *Percent*	**Factor** *Percent*	**Factor** *Percent*
First	**Interpersonal** 39.2%	**Interpersonal** 47.9%	**Interpersonal** 46.5%	**Interpersonal** 58.5%	**Interpersonal** 56.4%	**Interpersonal** 37.7%	**Interpersonal** 46.7%
Second	**Clinical** 34.8%	**Clinical** 25.0%	**Clinical** 33.2%	**Clinical** 24.9%	**Clinical** 19.2%	**Policies** 22.4%	**Clinical** 27.0%
Third	**Information** 6.9%	**Facilities** 12.5%	**Information** 10.1%	**Facilities** 6.5%	**Facilities** 18.1	**Clinical** 18.4%	**Policies** 9.4%
Fourth	**Other** 6.9%	**Policies** 9.4%	**Policies** 5.2%	**Policies** 6.0%	**Policies** 5.3%	**Information** 11.8%	**Facilities** 7.3%
Fifth	**Policies** 6.4%	**Other** 4.2%	**Facilities** 3.2%	**Information** 3.7%	**Other** 1.1%	**Other** 7.9%	**Information** 5.8%
Sixth	**Facilities** 5.9%	**Information** 1.0%	**Other** 1.8%	**Other** .5%	**Information** 0%	**Facilities** 1.8%	**Other** 3.9%

[1]Reported in B. Ruben, Zakahi & Kreps, (1985). [2]Reported in B. Ruben & J. Ruben (1988). [3]Reported in Ruben (1990); Ruben & Bowman (1987); Ruben (1986). [4]Reported in B. Ruben, (1987). [5]Reported in B. Ruben & J. Ruben (1987). [6]Reported in Ruben (1990); Ruben, Christensen & Guttman (1990).

Table 2

Patients' Most Memorable Experiences: Representative Responses

Personal Treatment/Interpersonal Communication

Positive Statements:

"Seeing physician. . . I was very nervous but she made me feel calm. Made me feel comfortable."

"The staff gave me the impression that they were interested in me as a person other than just in doing a job of taking care of me."

"All physicians are nice. . . . They seem to care."

"Without exception, every nurse on the floor took care of my father as if he were their father."

"The most pleasant experience was that most of the people treated me very well."

"The friendly attitude makes you feel relaxed when you are tense."

"I have the highest regard for nurses and staff in the maternity ward. They left me with a positive attitude toward birth."

Negative Statements:

"Need more attentive and listening doctors and nurses."

"Many technicians, in my opinion, lacked compassion and concern. They also had no respect for my dignity or modesty. A friendly smile would have helped. They did what they were trained to do and that's all."

"Nurses discuss each patient openly to other nurses, affording anyone in a nearby room an ear-full."

"Being a new mother, I needed instruction, not criticism"

"Please let us feel like we're human."

"Elderly patients are treated like garbage."

"The guards and the receptionists were very impolite with my family and myself."

"Many Black nurses treated Black patients better that Whites."

Table 3

Patients' Most Memorable Experiences: Representative Responses

Clinical/Technical

Positive Statements:

"Got better fast. Identified problem and gave medicine quickly."

"I was very happy with the services rendered in the Emergency Room. I was admitted and treated quickly."

"Blood test didn't hurt at all."

"The help of the nurses in the maternity ward . . . knew when to help me and when to let me do things on my own."

"They really take time. You're not rushed through."

Negative Statements:

"A female doctor was looking to give me an intravenous without checking my name or room number. She had wrong room, wrong sex."

"I was very unhappy because I had to wait three days for a plastic surgeon for a cut on my lip."

"They don't know what they're doing . . . couldn't find vein."

"The RN almost gave my infection medicine to my roommate who was very allergic to it."

"They never x-rayed anything. Just said it was a sprain."

Table 4

Patients' Most Memorable Experiences: Representative Responses

Policies/Procedures

Positive Statements:

"They let you walk in. You don't need an appointment."

"I was impressed by the lack of waiting."

"Attentions given to siblings of newborn is a nice touch."

Negative Statements:

"Too much paperwork . . . too confusing when you first walk in. You don't know where to go or what to do."

"I was told to come back Monday for a blood test, because they don't do blood tests after 12:00. It was very annoying."

"The admissions testing should all be done on one floor."

"Mental patients should not be allowed on floors with other patients."

"Waiting time is too long. Waited two hours for a shot."

Table 5

Patients' Most Memorable Experiences: Representative Responses

Facilities/Accommodations

Positive Statements:

"The birthing room facilities were peaceful and beautiful."

"I have gone to college previously in New York State. The health service building here is much better that what I am used to."

"I loved having my own shower in my room."

Negative Statements:

"The ER is very dirty."

"Get a nicer waiting area. Chairs are uncomfortable."

"Noisy children unattended and drunken adults bother the patients."

"Smoke from the nurses lounges was *very* unpleasant."

Table 6

Patients' Most Memorable Experiences: Representative Responses

Quality/Quantity of Information Provided

Positive Statements:

"The night before my operation the doctor explained the operation to me. This relaxed me."

"The physician explained everything in detail."

"A staff member told me how she reduces stress . . . was friendly."

"When you need to buy a product at the pharmacy, they are never too busy to give you recommendations."

Negative Statements:

"Doctors should tell patients results of tests, and give more information about patient's illness."

"The emergency room should keep you informed as to why you are lying there for so long."

"The doctor didn't tell me he was going on vacation, so no one knew who was suppose to take out my stitches."

"Wish they could better explain about blood test results."

Table 7

Patients' Most Memorable Experiences: Representative Responses

Other (General Statements, Convenience, Cost)

Positive Statements:

"Everything very nice."

"Came away with positive impression."

"Convenient."

Negative Statements:

"Would go (to another facility) if I could wait."

What do these findings mean? To be sure, these results tell us nothing definitive about how patients were *actually* cared for. They do, however, tell us a great deal about how patients *perceive* they were treated, and perhaps more interestingly, about the *criteria they use* in evaluating the quality of care they receive. By implication, the study also tells us about probable sources of satisfaction and dissatisfaction among patients, and helps us understand the basis upon which images of health services are formed.

The findings from these project argue convincingly that patients in a variety of healthcare settings place a very high premium on personal treatment, interpersonal communication, and relationships in forming their impressions of a health care institution and its staff.

As can be discerned from the sampling of patient responses, the research also indicates that all staff play a vital role in creating the experiences which are most critical and memorable to patients. Nurses, nurse practitioners, receptionists, and other staff, as well as physicians, are mentioned in patient's comments. For instance, in the case of the ambulatory care facility (Ruben, 1990; Ruben, Christensen & Guttman, 1990), nurses and nurse practitioners were most often mentioned. They were referred to in 34.3% of the narratives on memorable experiences, and generally in a positive context (60.6% positive vs. 39.4% negative). Physicians were mentioned in 29.2% of the recounted scenarios (64.3% positive vs. 35.7% negative). Receptionists and other non-technical staff were recalled in 26% of the noted experiences, with a majority (56.0% vs. 44.0%) positive.

Again, it is important to remember that these results refer to patient perceptions. However, it is equally important to remind ourselves of the many reasons why the patient perspective and relationship quality are important. Beyond contributing to a patient's satisfaction or dissatisfaction with health care systems in general, relationship quality impacts upon patient compliance and the course of treatment. It also forms the basis for the reputation and image of individual staff members and health center as an organization, influences the probability of malpractice litigation, and facilitates or impedes the appropriate utilization of health care facilities.

Origins of the Problem: Communication Pathologies

At the heart of the linkage between communication and health care is the interpersonal communication between caregivers and patients, and the nature of the relationship which evolves therefrom. Unfortunately caregiver-patient communication and relationships are as problematic as they are important, embodying all the complexity and challenge—and even greater stress—than is present in other professional-lay encounters.

In the most basic terms, interpersonal communication is a process of sending and receiving messages in an effort to coordinate meaning. Influencing what would seem to be a very simple process are a number of factors, some having to do with the people, some the messages they create and some the channels through which messages are exchanged.

As individuals, we each bring our own unique needs, values, attitudes, styles, cultures, and perspectives to interpersonal communication encounters. Hopefully, each of us has a number of relationships in our lives where communication works well, and the outcomes are very satisfying to the parties involved. In such circumstances, communication works as efficiently and effectively as it does because of the compatibility between sender and receiver in terms of needs, priorities, styles, culture, and perspective.

When incompatibilities of various kinds exist, interpersonal communication and the development of relationships is a much greater challenge. Caregiver-patient communication is perhaps the prototypical example of this circumstance. One reason has to do with differences in needs the individuals bring to the situation. Caregivers bring particular needs to their encounters with patients, including the desire for accurate medical history, information pertinent to diagnosis of the presenting problem, efficient information exchange and patient compliance and cooperation. For their part, patients enter the situation with needs that only partially correspond to those of the physician, including not only clinical care, but also information, explanation, attention, reassurance and empathy

Additional Barriers to Relationship Quality

As with the teacher and student, the attorney and client, or the librarian and the information seeker, the relationship between the caregiver and the patient is characteristically asymmetrical, in that expertise and power are unevenly distributed. And while both parties to such relationships can be said to have a common purpose, they seldom share common perspectives.

For their part, physicians, nurses, lab techs, receptionists, administrators, and other staff come to encounters as knowledgeable professionals, "at home" in the environment in which the interactions are occurring, seeing patients on a schedule which they set. Factors such as time pressures, job stress, the burden of paperwork, threat of malpractice, difficult patients, interpersonal stress and problems of coordination and repetition present barriers for the caregiver. Nonetheless, caregivers are familiar with terminology and protocols, comfortable with the tasks at hand (medical histories, physical exams and diagnostic procedures), and generally equipped with substantial experience regarding the range of medical problems and circumstances which present themselves.

Healthcare providers make their judgments of the quality of care using clinical and technical criteria—Have correct diagnostic procedures been followed? Were appropriate treatment protocols adhered to? Was testing conducted in a technically correct manner? (Droste, 1988; Siegel, 1986; 1990; Steiber, 1988)

In contrast, patients come to the relationship "looking for help" in some form. They do so in an environment that is unfamiliar— one which they often perceive as intimidating. Patients must schedule the encounter at the convenience of the caregivers, and often have to wait to be seen. Frequently they enter the interaction anxious about their health, and lacking medical knowledge or relevant professional expertise. For the patient, even "routine" history-taking, physical exams, and tests are often uncomfortable, because they call for levels of verbal disclosure and physical contact normally reserved for intimate relationships. And, depending upon the outcome of these encounters, patients may be faced with the need to comply with recommendations for behavioral change, undergo additional testing, or accept continuing uncertainty about their health status.

Caregivers make assessments of quality of care based on *clinical and technical criteria, clinical and technical skills or competencies* of providers, and the manner in which patients are treated *medically*. Since most patients and family members lack the knowledge necessary to assess the clinical quality of the care they receive, their evaluations emphasize *relationship quality,* the *interpersonal communication skills and competencies* of caregiver, and the manner in which they are treated *personally.* (Korsch, et al., 1972; Ruben, 1990; 1986; Ruben & Ruben, 1988; Ruben, Christensen & Guttman, 1990, Steiber, 1988).

Over the course of a hospital stay or a visit to a physician's office, a patient is likely to have any number of encounters— each of which in subtle and not so subtle ways shapes the impressions which are formed of the quality of the health care givers, the organization, and by extension, the health care itself. If those encounters include a receptionist who seems to lack compassion, a physician who doesn't seem to be paying attention, or a nurse who seems is impolite, the seeds of dissatisfaction are easily planted.

Critical Incidents in Physician-Patient Communication

Given the potential range of incompatibilities in needs, goals, and perspectives is it any wonder that despite the best intentions by all parties, caregiver-patient encounters are plagued by incomplete communication, mistrust, and misunderstanding? When we listen to the stories patients have to tell, examples are, unfortunately, all too plentiful:

- After weeks of pain and visits to several physicians, a patient has been referred to a "highly-regarded neurologist." The patient introduces herself and begins to describe the problem. The neurologist explains that it isn't necessary to hear her symptoms, that the examination and test results will tell her everything she will need to know.
- A patient considering a vasectomy has a number of questions and concerns, and schedules a consultation visit with a urologist. When the patient asks about possible side effects or complications, the physician responds "There's really no evidence to suggest that there are negative side effects, but who knows. We thought Thalidomide was safe, too." The patient says that he has some concerns about the procedure. The physician hands him a pamphlet "which will answer all the questions," and tells him to call the receptionist to schedule the procedure if he decides to go ahead.
- A patient is waiting to be seen. He overhears a physician speaking angrily to a resident and a nurse about an "echo" that was conducted on the wrong patient.
- A patient who was previously operated on for breast cancer discovers several new lumps and a cough which her physician describes as "suspicious." She is sent to a nearby X-ray group for chest x-rays. The tests completed, the woman is asked to return to the crowded waiting room while the pictures are developed. In ten minutes, the radiologist walks into the waiting room and announces loudly across the still-full waiting room that he has developed the X-rays and has just spoken to the woman's physician. . . . The patient is to take the X-rays and go immediately to the Emergency room of the hospital to meet with physician.

From the patient point of view, each of these instances is a critical incident from the perspective of relationship quality. In each, there is a loss . . . of confidence, trust, information, of the potential for quality health care. This occurs not for the lack of good intention, nor of first-rate clinical skill, but rather for the lack of interpersonal communication skill.

INSIGHTS FROM THE FACTORY

This section of the chapter provides brief summary of three studies from the literature of the behavioral sciences, which may at first seem unrelated to health care relationships or even to one another. Hopefully, their relevance and implications for bettering our understanding of quality relationships with clients and colleagues will become apparent.

"The Western Electric Studies"

What has come to be called "The Hawthorne Effect" was first discovered by F. J. Roethlisberger and William J. Dickson in a two-year study of workers at the Western Electric Company Hawthorne Works in Chicago. Their study was described in detail in the book *Management and the Worker* (1941).

The research focused on working conditions, morale, and productivity. Roethlisberger and Dickson set up experimental work rooms and groups to study the impact of such factors as the length of the work day, length of work week, and the introduction of breaks during the day. Who would have guessed that what began as a rather routine study would produce results the researchers came to refer to as "astonishing" (Roethlisberger & Dickson, p. 87).

Much to their surprise, the researchers found that regardless of what specific changes they introduced into the experimental environment—whether they shortened working hours, days and weeks, for instance—worker productivity improved. Every change they made in the subject's environment seemed to increase productivity. They assumed the finding must somehow be the result of some unrecognized factors in the experimental environment, so they systematically examined the relationship between environmental factors and variations in productivity. Still they found no explanation. By the end of the two-year study, efforts to explain the increased productivity had led to an examination of every imaginable explanation including environmental factors, worker fatigue and monotony, wage incentives, and method of supervision. They went to such levels of detail as to test for the possible impact of temperature, humidity, even seasonal variation.

After all was said and done, their conclusion was this: Differences in productivity were not due to specific changes in the experimental design. Rather, *greater product resulted from the positive interpersonal relationships and unusual level of supervisor attention that was present in the experimental group at every phase of the research.* The experiment had fostered closer working relations, and established greater confidence and trust by workers in supervisors, than was present in the normal working group situation. Supervisor-worker relations in the experimental room were discovered to have more the flavor of an office than a shop, creating an atmosphere in which workers had become the focus of considerable amount of attention from top management. And, indeed it has been the increased attention, along with productive relationships between workers, that heightened productivity.

INSIGHTS FROM THE CLASSROOM

Pygmalion in the Classroom

In their book, *Pygmalion in the Classroom*, Robert Rosenthal and Lenore Jacobson (1968), reported on their research on the impact of teacher expectations on student's intellectual development. They argued persuasively that when teachers expect high or low performance from particular students, their own behavior toward these students is sufficiently different to produce these outcomes through a "self-fulfilling prophecy." That is, if I as a teacher believe John to be a talented child, I'll treat him as if he were, and he will be influenced to become talented by my expectations.

Further studies examined this contention in some depth. Not all studies produced the so-called "pygmalion effect," and controversies swirled as to whether these inconsistencies were the result of inappropriate research methods, or whether there were underlying problems with the theory.

Despite occasionally inconsistent findings, the weight of evidence supports the original theory: *Teachers' beliefs that particular students are of superior or inferior in ability, tend to lead to student achievement levels consistent with the expectations.* When teachers expectations are high, student performance matches these expectations; conversely, when teachers have low expectations, lower levels of performance result (Seaver, 1973).

A Study of Adaptation to Junior College

In 1986, John Herrling, a doctoral candidate in the Rutgers Graduate School of Education undertook a thesis study designed to gain a better understanding of dynamics of student adaptation to junior colleges. It is well documented in the literature, that attrition rates are very high during the first semester of enrollment, and a chief goal of this study was to try to identify the factors leading to this outcome. Herrling designed a qualitative, ethnographic study in which he met with students at several points during the semester for open-ended, taped conversations about the process of adapting to college, with the goal of gaining an in-depth understanding of the dynamics of adaptation and attrition processes from a student point of view.

In designing the study, Herrling felt it very important to select an appropriately large enough initial sample of students. Otherwise, if too many students dropped out during the semester, he would be unable to make comparisons between "drop out" and "adapter" groups at the conclusion of the study. Herrling determined that the average first semester attribution rate for the institution where the study was taking place was 30–40%. He wanted the final sample size to be in the range of 20, so he began, with random sample of thirty-two students. He reasoned that even with a 40% drop-out rate, he would be left with a study population of 19 or 20 students who would complete the first semester.

But, Herrling was to be very surprised by his results in this regard. At the end of the first semester, only 3 of the 32 students had left the college—an attrition rate of 9%—rather than the usual 30 to 40%.

What are we to make of this finding. Initially, Herrling feared that somehow his initial sample had been a biased one. He carefully considered a variety of possibilities. However, in reexamining the demographics of his sample, he confirmed that the group was a very representative one in terms of high school grades, SAT scores, curriculum being studied, and so on and so on. After much deliberation and careful analysis of the tapes and transcripts from the interviews he concluded that rather than being an unfortunate circumstance of an unrepresentative sample, the low attrition rate in the study group was instead a truly significant finding in its own right. *Unlike the typical group of college students this group of 32 in effect, had their own personal counselor meeting with them regularly throughout the semester, talking with them, and taking a genuine interest in their concerns and in their experiences.*

The Moral?

What lessons do these studies hold? In some respects these three studies were quite different. The Western Electric study focused on the workplace; Pygmalion, the classroom; and the Herrling study, adaptation to college. Yet, at the same time each of these is a study of relationships. Collectively, the "Hawthorne effect," "the Pygmalion effect" and the "Herrling effect" demonstrate the incredible power of quality relationships. Moreover, they provide a persuasive lesson about the remarkable significance of being noticed, paid attention to, listened to, believed in and cared about.

INSIGHTS FROM THE PET SHOP

It's now time to end the suspense for those wondering about the portion of the subtitle dealing with lessons from the pet store. Hopefully, by the conclusion of this portion of the article it will become apparent that the pet store is a neglected, but nonetheless a valuable source of have lessons regarding relationship quality.

Pet stores sell pets and pet supplies. Nearly every major mall has such stores, and they are generally crowded with shoppers cooing and smiling at creatures through the glass and screens. A moment ago it was suggested that pet stores sell *pets*. Actually, it may be more accurate to say, they sell potential *companionship*. (No wonder they're nearly as crowded as Baskin Robbins). There are the cute little bunnies, cuddly kittens, exotic fish, high and low verbal birds, and perky puppies. And for the less "warm and fuzzy" types there are snakes, rats and gerbils and cousins of all colors, shapes and sizes.

It seems to me there is a lot to be learned about quality human relationships from pets. You may be as surprised as I was to learn that there has been a fair amount of research done on pets and the impact of the relationships we have with them.

For instance, one study found that introducing pets into the lives of terminal cancer patients (Muschel, 1984) or geriatric patients (Brickel, 1986) has significant positive consequence psychologically and socially. Other studies (Friedmann, Ketcher, Lynch & Thomas, 1980) have suggested that pet ownership is a strong predictor of one-year survival among post-coronary patients. Research also shows that older people (65 and over) who are closely attached to a pet are less likely to exhibit symptoms of depression (Garrity, Stallones, Marx, & Johnson, 1989). Studies (Garity et al. 1989; Ory & Goldberg, 1983) have also indicated that individuals with greater attachment to pets have better mental health. In essence, these studies suggest that attachment to—having a significant relationship with—a pet may serve the same beneficial role as significant human attachments in times of stress, providing not only a source of companionship, but an aid to health and relaxation.

A particularly striking piece of research takes this perspective a bit further to examine whether pet ownership has an effect upon the extent of use of physician services (Siegel, 1990). And, remarkably, the study finds that elderly individuals with pets had fewer contacts with doctors (total doctor contacts and respondent-initiated contacts) than those without pets. Even more remarkably, the study found that individuals with stressful lives, who did not own pets, had significantly more doctor contacts than did non-pet owners (10.37 contacts per year vs. 8.38 p.005).

Are all pet relationships equally effective in this regard? Apparently not. Dogs seem to make better relationship partners than cats or birds. For individuals who did not own a dog, doctor contacts increased as levels of stress increased (10.39 contacts for high stress individuals compared to 8.37 for low stress, p.0 1). However, for dog owners with high and low levels of stress, there was not a significant difference between their total annual number of doctor contacts. (Siegel, 1990). This result did not occur for the owners of both cats and birds.

Thus, this study tells us that older people who don't have pets can expect more doctor contacts than individuals with pets. Furthermore, individuals with pets—particularly dogs—are helped by these relationships in times of stress (Siegel, 1990).

There are other lessons to be learned from our relationships with pets, dogs in particular—lessons about relationships and what makes them work. What is it, exactly, that dogs do for their part in relationships that apparently makes them such ideal relationship partners? Some dogs provide protection. But this is certainly not the case with the majority of pet dogs. Even if they lack the ability to protect their owner, they may still be wonderful companions. Actually, the reason dogs are capable of being such great pals is that they exhibit a number of the qualities that are highly valued in human companions. Think about it: Dogs are attentive, interested, trusting, loyal and tolerant. They are nonargumentative, and seem able at times to demonstrate compassion and empathy. Some are even masters of good eye contact. Collectively, these behaviors provide a sense of security and reassurance and confirm our sense of worth as human beings.

Walking on boardwalk last week, I couldn't but help but overhear an interesting conversation. The topic: What else, dogs: "To your dog, it doesn't matter what you look like, whether you've had a good day or bad, whether you have performed brilliantly or ineptly that day, how you feel or what you say, you walk in the door and your dog comes running up to you and wags its tail like you're the most important, wonderful person in the world . . . and loves you."

Whether we take our lessons from patients, the literature, the pet store—even the boardwalk—a common theme emerges. Quality relationships are a valued, valuable and all-too-scarce resource in medical encounters, and contemporary life, in general. But this is not an inevitable circumstance. We each have the power to build and maintain more meaningful, satisfying relationships, through a very fundamental communication process that begins with the genuine expression of interest, empathy, concern and caring for those around us.

Notes

1. "Building Effective Client and Colleague Relationships: Lessons from Patients, the Literature, and the Pet Shop," was first presented at the Annual Conference of the Mid-Atlantic College Health Association, October 1990. The version published here is a revision of that manuscript.

2. The research consisted of surveys of a total of 3,868 patients at six institutions in the Northeast:

1. Acute Care Hospital (Community): Random sample–1,000; returns–253; response rate–25.3%.
2. Acute Care Hospital (Urban): Random sample–381; returns–96; response rate–25.2%
3. Acute Care Hospital (Community): Random sample–1,000; returns–226; response rate–22.6%
4. Acute Care Hospital (Suburban): Random sample–927; returns –338; response rate–36.5%
5. Rehab Hospital (Regional): Total patient population was surveyed–360; returns–130; response rate–36.1.
6. Ambulatory Care Center (University)–random point of departure interviewer-aided surveys at three sites–200; returns–200; response rate–100%.

REFERENCES

Argyle, M. (1983). Doctor-patient skills. In D. Pendleton & J. Hasler (Ed.), *Doctor-patient communication* (pp. 57-74). New York: Academic Press.

Ben-Sim, Z. (1990). Primary care practitioners' likelihood to engage in a bio-psychosocial approach: An additional perspective on the doctor-patient relationship. *Social Science and Medicine,* 31(5), 565-576.

Bertakis, K. D. (1977). The communication of information from physician to patient: A method for increasing patient retention and satisfaction. *Journal of Family Practice, 5*(2), 217-222.

Bowman, J. C., & Ruben, B. D. (1986). Patient satisfaction: Critical issues in the implementation and evaluation of patient relations training. *Journal of Healthcare Education and Training 1*(2), 24-27.

Cline, R. J. (I 983). Interpersonal communication skills for enhancing physician-patient relationships. *Maryland State Medical Journal, April,* 272-278.

DiMatteo, M. R., & DiNicola, D. D. (1982). *Achieving patient compliance: The psychology of the medical practitioner's role.* New York: Pergamon.

Droste, T. (1988). Quality care: Elusive concept deserves defining. *Hospitals, April 15,* 58-59.

Ellmer, R & Olbrisch, M. E. (1983) The contribution of a cultural perspective in understanding and evaluating client satisfaction. *Evaluation and Program Planning, 6,* 275-281.

Ernstene, A. C. (1957). Explaining to the patient: A therapeutic tool and professional obligation. *Journal of the American Medical Association,* (November 2), 1110-1113.

Fine, V. F., & Therrien, M. E. (1977). Empathy in the doctor-patient relationship: Skill training for medical studies. *Journal of Medical Education, 52*(752),

Friedman, E., Katcher, A. H., Lynch, J. J., & Thomas, S. A. (1980). Animal Companions and One-year Survival of Patients After Discharge from a Coronary Care Unit. *Public Health Reports, 95,* 307-312.

Garrity, T. F., Stallones, L., Marx, M. B., & Johnson, T. P. (1989). Pet Ownership and Attachment as Supportive Factors in the Health of the Elderly. *Anthrozoos*, 3, 35-44.

Gilman, S. L. (1988). *Disease and representation: Images of illness from madness to AIDS*. Ithaca, NY: Cornell University Press.

Greenfield, S., Kaplan, S., & Ware, J. E. (1985). Expanding patient involvement in care: Effects on patient outcomes. *Annals of Internal Medicine, 102*, 520-528.

Greenfield, S., Kaplan, S., & Ware, J. E. (1986). Expanding patient involvement in care: Effects on Blood Sugar. *Annals of Internal Medicine, 34*(2), 819A.

Herrling, J. L. (1986). *Student adaptation to a community college*. Rutgers University, New Brunswick, NJ: Doctoral Dissertation.

Hulka, B. S., Kupper, L. L., Cassel, J. C., & Mayo, F. (1975). Doctor-patient communication and outcomes among diabetic patients. *Journal of Community Health, l*(l), 15-27.

Inui, T. S., Yourtee, E. L., & Williamson, J. W. (1976). Improved outcomes in hypertension after physician tutorials. *Annals of Internal Medicine, 84*, 646-65 1.

Kaplan, S. H., Greenfield, S., & Ware, J. E. (1989). Assessing the effects of physician-patient interactions on the outcomes of chronic disease. *Medical Care, 27*(3, Supplement), S110-S127.

Kelly, E. W. J. (1979). *Effective interpersonal communication: A manual for skill development*. Washington, DC: University Press of America.

Kleinman, A. (1980). *Patients and healers in the context of culture: An exploration of the borderland between anthropology, medicine, and psychiatry*. Berkeley, CA: University of California Press.

Klinzing, D., & Klinzing, D. (1985). *Communication for allied health professionals*. Dubuque, IA: Wm. C. Brown.

Korsch, B. M., & Gozzi, E. K. (1968). Gaps in doctor-patient communication: I. Doctor-patient interaction and patient satisfaction. *Pediatrics, 42*, 855-87 1.

Korsch, B. M., & Negrete, V. F. (1972). Doctor-patient communication. *Scientific American, 227*(2), 66-74.

Kreps, G. L., & Thornton, B. C. (1984). *Health communication*. New York: Longman.

Leebov, W. (1988). *Service excellence: The customer relations strategy for healthcare*. Chicago: American Hospital Association.

Ley, P., & Spellman, M. S. (1967). Communication with the Patient. London: Staples Press.

Lynch, J. J. (1977). *The broken heart: The medical consequences of loneliness*. New York: Basic Books.

Northouse, P. G., & Northouse, L. L. (1985). *Health communication: A handbook for health professionals*. Englewood Cliffs, NJ: Prentice-Hall.

Okrent, D. (1987). You and the doctor: Striving for a better relationship. *The New York Times Magazine*, (March 29), 20-21, 92-94.

Omachonu, V. K. (1990). Quality of care and the patient: New criteria for evaluation. *Health Care Management Review, 15*(4), 43-50.

Pascoe, G. C. (1983) Patient satisfaction in primary health care: A literature review and analysis. *Evaluation and Program Planning, 6*, 185-210.

Pendleton, D., & Hasler, J. (1983). *Doctor-patient communication*. London: Academic Press,

Roethlisberger, F. J., & Dickson, W. J. (I 94 1). *Management and the worker*. Cambridge, MA: Harvard University Press.

Rosenthal, R., & Jacobson, L. (1968). *Pygmalion in the classroom*. New York: Holt, Rinehart and Winston.

Rost, K., Carter, W., & Inui, T. (1989). Introduction of information during the initial medical visit: Consequences for patient follow-through with physician recommendations for medication. *Social Science and Medicine, 28*(4), 315-321.

Ruben, B. D. (1985). *The Bottomline: A patient relations training program*. Morristown, NJ: Morristown Memorial Hospital.

Ruben, B. D. (1986). *Patient perceptions of quality of care: Survey Results*. No. 2. Unpublished Report.

Ruben, B. D. (1987). *Patient perceptions of quality of care: Survey Results*. No. 3. Unpublished Report.

Ruben, B. D. (1990a). The health caregiver-patient relationship: Pathology, etiology, treatment. In E. B. Ray & L. Donohew (Ed.), *Communication and health: Systems and applications* (pp. 51-68).

Ruben, B. D. (1990b). Building Effective Client and Colleague Relationships: Lessons from Patients, the Literature and the Pet Shop. Paper presented at the general session of the Annual Conference of the Mid-Atlantic College Health Association, Seven Springs Center Champion, PA, October, 1990.

Ruben, B. D. (1988). *Communication and Human Behavior*. (2nd ed.). New York: Macmillan.

Ruben,B.D and J.C. Bowman (1986). Patient satisfaction: Critical issues in the theory and design of patient relations training. *Journal of Healthcare Education and Training, l*(l), 1-5.

Ruben, B. D., Christensen, D., & Guttman, N. (1990). *College health service: A qualitative analysis of the patient perspective*. Unpublished Report.

Ruben, B. D., & Ruben, J. M. (1988). *Patient perceptions of quality of care: Survey Results*. No. 5. Unpublished Report.

Ruben, B. D., & Ruben, J. M. (1987). *Patient perceptions of quality of care: Survey Results*. No. 4. Unpublished Report.

Ruben, B. D., W. Zakahi, and G. Kreps (1985). *Patient perceptions of quality of care: Survey Results*. No. 1. Unpublished Report.

Seaver, W. B. (1973). Effects of naturally induced teacher expectancies. *Journal of Personality and Social Psychology, 28*(3), 333-342.

Shorter, E. (1985). *Bedside manners: The troubled history of doctors and patients*. New York: Simon and Schuster.

Siegel, B. S. (1986). *Love, medicine and miracles*. New York: Harper & Row.

Siegel, J. M. (1990). Stressful life events and the use of physician services among the elderly: The moderating role of pet ownership. *Journal of Personality and Social Psychology, 58*(6), 1081-1086.

Stewart, M., & Roter, D. (1989). *Communicating with medical patients*. Newbury Park, CA: Sage.

Thompson, T.L. (1986). *Communication for healthy professionals*. Lanham, MD: University Press of America.

Waitzkin, H. (1984). Doctor-patient communication: Clinical implications of social scientific research. *Journal of the American Medical Association, 252*(17), 2441-2446.

Waitzkin, H. B. (1986). Research on doctor-patient communication: Implications for practice. *The Internist*, (August), 7-10.

Ware, John E., Jr. & Allyson R. Davies. (1983). Behavioral consequences of consumer dissatisfaction with medical care. *Evaluation and Program Planning, 6*, 291-297.

Wertz, D. C., Sorenson, J. R., & Heeren, T. C. (1988). Communication in health professional-lay encounters. In B. D. Ruben (Ed.), *Information and Behavior: Volume 2* (pp. 329-342). New Brunswick, NJ: Transaction.

Woolley, F. R., Kane, R. L., & Associates. (1978). The effects of doctor-patient communication on satisfaction and outcomes of care. *Social Science and Medicine, 12*, 123-128.

Patient Relations for Malpractice Claim Prevention

Midwest Medical Insurance Company Risk Management Committee

Patients coming to a clinic are frequently under great stress. They are looking not only for good technical medical care, but also for reassurance, concern, good communication and respect from the physicians and clinic staff. Few patients are equipped to evaluate the clinical skills of physicians and other health care professionals; it is by these more personal aspects of their medical encounters, therefore, that most patients judge the quality of the care they receive.

Plaintiff attorneys estimate that 70-80% of the patients who seek legal assistance to file a malpractice claim do so because they are angry; angry not just because of an adverse outcome, but because of breakdowns in communication, long waits, failures of physicians or clinic staff to provide information, or other nontechnical factors that create a perception of lack of care, concern and respect for the patient. As explained by the U.S. Department of Health, Education and Welfare in its 1973 report on medical malpractice: "The quality of the relationship between the patient on one hand and the doctor ... on the other hand may stimulate the patient either toward or away from filing a malpractice suit. In plain truth, the suit itself is merely tangible proof of the final breakdown of that relationship."[1]

The risk management benefits of good patient relations are twofold. First, open communication with patients can have a direct impact on the quality and outcome of the medical care rendered. Patients who have a good rapport with their health care providers are more likely to be forthcoming with information necessary to provide appropriate treatment; those who are educated about their care by the health care team are likely to be more compliant with the treatment protocols recommended.

Secondly, patients who feel they have a good relationship with, and receive respect from, their physicians and clinic staff are less likely to turn to an attorney and the litigation process when the results of their treatment are less than optimal.

Good patient relations begin the moment a patient has any contact—direct or indirect—with the clinic and are dependent on the efforts of every clinic staff member. Everyone—from the administrative and clerical staff, to the allied health professionals, to the physicians—must take responsibility for ensuring that all patient encounters are handled professionally, efficiently and with respect for the patient.

Many different patient relations issues are cited by patients/plaintiffs as factors that influenced their decision to file a lawsuit against their physician and/or clinic. Areas to which particular attention should be paid include:

Adapted from *Risk Management: Meeting Your Goals*, Midwest Medical Insurance Company, 1991; and *Minnesota Physician*, July 1990. Reprinted by permission.

1 U.S. Department of Health, Education and Welfare, **Report of the Secretary's Commission on Medical Malpractice** p. 671.

Patient Information

Failure to ensure that patients understand what their clinic experience will involve can lead to misunderstanding, anger and frustration. Many clinics have addressed this problem by developing brochures explaining clinic services, appointment procedures, emergency coverage and other pertinent administrative aspects of the treatment to be provided. Each clinic should determine the appropriate content of their own brochure based on the size of the clinic, specialties offered, patient population, etc.

An identified patient representative is another excellent means of facilitating the exchange of information with patients. Patient representatives can serve a wide variety of functions, including disseminating clinic information, answering patients' general questions, informing patients of community services and responding to patient complaints. Clinics that have established patient representative programs report that they have had very positive feedback from their patients and have found the programs to be very good public relations tools for their clinic.

Patient Feedback and Complaints

Because so many malpractice claims evolve out of patient dissatisfaction, finding out about patients' perceptions of the clinic is a positive way to help reduce malpractice liability. Periodic patient surveys can be useful for obtaining this i n format i on. In order for such surveys to be effective, the results should be carefully reviewed and appropriate changes made in response to patient input.

Frequently, the clues that a patient may sue are present long before any legal documents are drawn up. Because many patients are still intimidated by their physician, often it is a staff member who first becomes aware of complaints which may signal an impending malpractice suit. Regardless of how minor they may seem, all complaints deserve a prompt, professional response. A formal complaint policy can help to ensure that appropriate action is taken on all patient complaints.

Many clinics have found it effective to document patient complaints on a complaint form. The complaint can then be easily and accurately reported to the administrator and the patient's physician if one is involved. The follow-up on all complaints may also be documented on the form to enable the clinic administration to monitor the action taken. Documentation by the staff of patient complaints will also enable the clinic to track the number and type of complaints generated and identify recurring problems which need to be addressed on a broader scale.

Generally, complaints related to issues tangential to the patient's medical care (waiting time, etc.) should not be documented in the patient's chart. However, if the physician discusses a treatment-related problem with the patient, the discussion should be documented as part of the medical record.

Waiting Time

In a 1989 poll published by *Medical Economics*, 68% of patients said they consider a wait of more than 15 minutes for an appointment to be unreasonable. Only one patient in five said they are tolerant of a delay of more than 20 minutes. Patients who are already angry when they see their physician may be more likely to vent their frustration through a malpractice lawsuit if an adverse outcome occurs.

Patients in the reception room should be notified if the physician is running late. If the delay will be more than one-half hour, an attempt should be made to contact patients at their home or work place before they leave for their appointments. If the delay will be significant, patients should be given the opportunity to reschedule. The responsibility for notifying patients of delays can be delegated to the receptionist, but he/she must be kept well-informed of schedules by the physician or nurse.

Many clinics help minimize delays by establishing scheduling guidelines, leaving a certain percentage of time slots open each day to accommodate same-day appointments. The clinic should consider the average time for specific types of appointments with each physician and make certain that sufficient time is allotted for patient visits.

Telephone Contact

In most cases, a patient's first contact with a clinic is by telephone; the patient's perception of this initial communication may color his/her perception of the entire clinic experience. It is imperative that this initial encounter portray a professional, efficient, caring attitude toward the patient.

Particular problems frequently found in telephone communication with patients include:

- Insufficient telephone lines resulting in patients being unable to get through to the clinic.
- Patients being placed on "hold" for extended periods of time.
- Patients being placed on "hold" without first ascertaining whether the call may be an emergency.
- Transferring patient calls to other extensions without an explanation of what is being done, often leaving the patient questioning whether they have been disconnected.
- Failure to inform patients of when physicians are likely to return their calls and failure of physicians to respond to calls in a timely manner.
- Staff members being overly aggressive in screening patient calls, thereby creating a barrier between physicians and patients.

Protecting Patient Confidentiality

All clinic staff and physicians must be acutely aware of the importance of maintaining the confidentiality of all patient information. Conversations in the clinic which can be overheard by unauthorized persons are a common problem and may result in complaints of breach of patient confidentiality as well as create the impression that clinic staff are less than professional.

Patients checking in for clinic appointments should not be asked about their reason for seeing the doctor within earshot of other patients in the reception room. Billing matters should be addressed in a private setting. No conversations regarding any patient information should be held in any area where they could be overheard by other patients.

Clinic staff and physicians must use caution never to release confidential information to persons other than the patient without the patient's express written consent. Frequently, schools and employers will call to verify patient appointments. A patient's friends or relatives may request status reports on the patient's health or recent medical treatment. Without the patient's written authorization for the release of information to the particular person inquiring, no patient information should be disclosed.

Confidentiality must be a job requirement for all clinic employees; discussion of the more subtle ways that patient confidentiality can be breached should be part of staff orientation and in-service education.

Billing and Collections

Many malpractice claims are asserted in response to billing and collection efforts, particularly when patients are dissatisfied with their treatment and have not received satisfactory explanations of their medical care before receiving a bill. Honest and candid communication with the patient can resolve many billing complaints before collection measures are begun or a malpractice claim is filed.

The physician should always be notified before any account is turned over to a collection agency. Many disputes over bills are due to misunderstandings about the care rendered which can be resolved if the physician discusses the bill with the patient. The physician may also be aware of problems in treatment that would make postponing aggressive collection actions advisable. If and when an account is turned over to a collection agency, the patient should be notified by letter with the conditions of future treatment clearly stated.

Termination of the Physician/Patient Relationship

While patients may unilaterally sever their relationship with a physician at any time, clinics and physicians have a duty to give the patient sufficient time to find a new physician and effect a transfer of his/her records. Failure to give sufficient notice may result in charges of abandonment.

If a patient is dismissed from the clinic, the patient should be notified in writing; certified or registered letters are recommended by many attorneys. The letter should clearly state that, between the time notice is given and services are terminated. the clinic will continue to provide emergency treatment and necessary care for ongoing chronic conditions. Physicians should always be consulted before services to a patient are terminated to evaluate the medical status and needs of that patient.

Clinics may differ in the length of time they offer emergency care when services to a patient are terminated. Location of the clinic, specialty of the physician, type of treatment being rendered, availability of alternative treatment sites and speed with which the patient's records can be transferred may affect the amount of notice necessary. The clinic should evaluate all of these factors carefully in establishing a policy and granting any necessary exceptions.

Notice of termination should inform the patient that, with appropriate authorization, his/her medical records will be forwarded to the physician of the patient's choice. Including the name and phone number of a physician referral service will ensure that the patient is able to easily locate alternative medical care. A copy of the letter informing the patient of termination of the clinic services should be retained in the patient's medical chart.

Self-Assessment Questionnaire

Critical self-assessment is the first step in any effective risk management program. How does your clinic rate on these issues of patient relations?

First Impressions

1. The clinic presents a professional appearance, both inside and out.
   YES NO
2. The receptionist greets patients promptly, pleasantly and professionally.
   YES NO
3. The reception room is pleasantly decorated with adequate space and comfortable chairs.
   YES NO
4. The reception room is visible to the receptionist so that all waiting patients and activity can be monitored. YES NO
5. The reception room contains current reading material (including health education material) of interest to the clinic's patient population. YES NO
6. All clinic staff present a positive, professional image of the clinic and treat patients with courtesy and concern.
   YES NO
7. Personal conversations among clinic staff are conducted out of the hearing of patients.
   YES NO
8. Clinic staff conduct periodic maintenance and safety inspections of the clinic facilities.
   YES NO

Patient Information

1. The clinic has written material available to patients explaining clinic services, appointment procedures and other pertinent administrative aspects of the clinic.
   YES NO

2. The clinic has a patient representative or other administrative person identified to patients as a source for information, problem solving, etc. YES NO

Patient Feedback and Complaints

1. The clinic conducts periodic patient surveys to determine the level of patient satisfaction with clinic services. YES NO
2. The clinic has a patient complaint procedure which includes mechanisms for documenting, resolving and monitoring all patient complaints. YES NO
3. Physicians are notified of all treatment-related complaints from patients. YES NO
4. The number and type of patient complaints are tracked in order to identify and correct recurring problems in the clinic. YES NO

Waiting Time

1. The wait for patients to obtain an appointment is reasonable. YES NO
2. The clinic has scheduling guidelines to help determine the amount of time necessary to schedule for particular types of appointments, appointments with particular physicians, etc. YES NO
3. Patients are seen by the physician (or other health professional with whom they are scheduled) within 20 minutes of their appointment time. YES NO
4. Patients are informed and given the opportunity to reschedule if their physician is running late. YES NO
5. The clinic conducts periodic time studies to monitor waiting times and takes corrective action when unreasonable waiting times are identified. YES NO

Telephone Contact

1. The clinic has an adequate number of telephone lines to allow patients to contact the clinic without delay. YES NO
2. Clinic staff make a positive, professional impression in answering the telephone. YES NO
3. Clinic staff wait for the caller's permission before placing a call on "hold". YES NO
4. Clinic staff are careful to avoid placing a call on "hold" for an unreasonable length of time. YES NO
5. Callers are told when their calls are being transferred to another extension to avoid any question about whether they have been disconnected. YES NO
6. Callers are told approximately when their calls will be returned by the physician or nurse if they are not handled immediately. YES NO
7. Clinic staff are careful not to build a barrier between patients and physicians by screening calls too aggressively. YES NO

Protecting Patient Confidentiality

1. Clinic staff are careful not to discuss confidential patient information anyplace it could be overheard by other patients (in the reception room, exam rooms, hallways, etc.). YES NO
2. Medical questions, including the patient's reason for seeing the physician, are discussed in private, not where the conversation may be overheard by other patients. YES NO
3. Billing matters are discussed with patients in private, not where the conversation may be overheard *by* other patients. YES NO
4. Clinic staff are careful not to disclose confidential patient information to anyone

other thanthepatient without the patient's written authorization. YES NO

5. Maintaining the confidentiality of patient information is a job requirement and staff members are well-trained on how to uphold this requirement. YES NO

Billing and Collections

1. Clinic billing policies are explained to patients before services are provided. YES NO
2. Before patient accounts are turned over for collection procedures, any conditions for continued treatment (e.g., cash only) are explained to the patients. YES NO
3. The patient's physician is informed and given the opportunity to review the patient's medical record before an account is turned over to a collection agency. YES NO

Termination of Services

1. Before the clinic terminates services to a patient, a determination is made that adequate alternative care is available. YES NO
2. If the clinic terminates services to a patient:
   - The patient is notified by certified or registered letter. YES NO
   - Adequate time is provided before services are terminated to enable the patient to find alternative care and effect a transfer of records. YES NO
   - The clinic offers to transfer the patient's records to a physician of the patient's choice upon receiving appropriate authorization by the patient. YES NO
   - The telephone number of a physician referral service is provided to the patient. YES NO

Enhancing Communication Competencies and Patient Rights

Interpersonal Communication Skills for Enhancing Physician-Patient Relationships

Rebecca J. Cline, PhD.

Far too often, both physician and patient walk away from each other with a vague sense of dissatisfaction, or worse, but often are unable to identify the source of their feelings. Accumulating evidence suggests that ineffective interpersonal interaction occurs with relatively high frequency in physician-patient relationships and may account for the dissatisfaction of both parties. The quality of provider-client interaction is a central issue in health care and promotion. Ironically, a growing dissatisfaction with physician-patient relationships by patients[1, 2] has persisted at the same time that the medical profession's literature has increasingly advocated the use of cooperative, patient-involving models of health care, which imply an increasing valuing of the patient as a responsible participant in health care processes.[1, 3, 4]

Neither physicians nor their patients seem very satisfied with the state of their relationships. Physicians tend to blame patients; a multitude of professional articles have been dedicated to determining what is wrong with patients who do not understand, accept, or follow through on the messages from their physicians (that is, noncompliance). Patients, and a wealth of essays and studies in medical journals, [5-13] tend to blame physicians for dissatisfying and ineffective communication. But in physician-patient relationships, like all other interpersonal relationships, responsibility for the personal satisfaction and quality of communication in the relationship, as well as effective medical outcomes, lies with both parties. Placing blame does little to improve interaction. Neither physicians nor patients can afford the ineffective communication to which they both contribute. Both parties need to take active steps to improve communication and thus to facilitate their mutual health-related goals.

Because medical journals best reach physicians, rather than patients, this essay is directed toward physicians and the role they can play in improving communication with their patients. The essay has two primary purposes: to provide a rationale to physicians for the use of interpersonal communication skills and to identify and describe the specific interpersonal communication skills needed by physicians.

Effective Communication: An Unaffordable Luxury?

Many physicians realize the ineffectiveness of some physician-patient communication but argue that enhancing the quality of communication is an unaffordable luxury. They recount the costs of spending more time with patients. But two compelling sets of evidence argue against this view. First, research suggests that satisfaction with the quality of interaction and the clarity of the diag-

Cline, R.J. INTERPERSONAL COMMUNICATION SKILLS FOR ENHANCING PHYSICIAN-PATIENT RELATIONSHIPS, Maryland State Medical Journal, April 1983; 32(4): 272-78. Reprinted with permission of the author.

nosis provided are not related to the length of the interaction;[14] apparently some other qualitative aspects of the interpersonal communication account for the negative response. There is little reason to assume that changing qualitative aspects of communication requires additional time or that spending more time, in and of itself, will alter patient perceptions. Second, and more compelling, the magnitude of the costs (in terms of medical outcomes) associated with ineffective communication mandates change.

Ineffective, rather than effective, communication is the unaffordable luxury. Research published in a variety of medical journals shows that satisfaction and understanding are not mere "niceties." Rather, the quality and effectiveness of medical care hinges on the establishment of positive relationships (characterized by openness and trust). Several medical outcomes depend on effective communication: the adequacy of diagnosis and treatment processes (which are based on information obtained in the medical interview), compliance with prescribed regimens, satisfaction with health care (also related to compliance), and perceptions of positive medical outcomes by both physicians and patients.

Interview Adequacy Accurate diagnosis and effective treatment are built on information gathered by the practioner. Some information is available through direct observation, other information through tests. However, the practitioner is heavily dependent on patients' words. The patient holds major responsibility for providing information to the physician, but physicians can use interpersonal skills to facilitate a patient's openness. If a patient withholds information about drugs taken, the length of time symptoms have persisted, or the failure to take prescribed drugs, the accuracy of the diagnosis or appropriateness of treatment may be endangered. An effective interviewer can gain the trust of many reluctant patients, elicit focused and full disclosure of information, clarify that information, and assess the role of social and psychological factors in the illness.[14] Thus, the adequacy of the interview is a matter of interpersonal skills.

Compliance Estimates of levels of noncompliance run as high as 72 to 96 percent in some cases,[15, 16] for an average of 33 percent.[15, 16, 17] The problem can be summarized in terms of the "rule of one-thirds." One-third of all patients do not comply at all, one-third comply at a level insufficient to facilitate the outcomes for which the regimen was intended, and one-third comply at a level that, if successful, will facilitate positive outcomes.[18] Rampant noncompliance translates into wasted resources by both physicians and patients, increased future illnesses and medical complications, and is a major source of reduced cost-effectiveness in health care. A commonly found predictor of noncompliance is physician conduct or problems in physician-patient communication.[19, 20] Compliance is increased when physician and patient achieve agreement on which problems require followup.[21, 22] Where physicians have displayed a businesslike rather than friendly style, and where information about cause of illness and diagnosis was expected by the patient but was not forthcoming, higher levels of noncompliance resulted.

Communication skills can be used by the physician to assure agreement and understanding between physician and patient and to communicate friendliness toward the patient. Thus, the physician can have a major impact on patient compliance through the use of interpersonal skills.

The medical establishment has tended to blame the patient; but research seeking to identify the characteristics of compliant versus noncompliant patients has been dishearteningly unfruitful. A more useful approach than assuming that the problem lies with the patient or with the physician (or varies with the illness or prescribed treatment) is to assume that compliance varies with the social context or situation.[15] The question for physicians then becomes, "How can I assist in creating relationships that encourage patients to be responsibly involved with their own treatment?" Such an approach is valid, given evidence linking the communication process to compliance, and is more useful for generating solutions since the communication process can be altered readily, while personal and demographic characteristics of patients, the nature of the illness, and mode of treatment are not open to change. Thus interpersonal communication training for physicians needs to focus on communication skills that encourage patient responsibility.

Satisfaction Quality of physician-patient communication also affects patient satisfaction with outcomes.[14] Satisfaction has been cited as important in several medical journal articles because it is associated with compliance[11, 13] and with patients' perceptions of functional outcomes of treatment.[23] Further, the satisfaction level is associated with keeping appointments and continued use of health services and may predict the probability of initiation of malpractice suits.[9, 14] Each of these translates directly into dollars. Patient dissatisfaction levels run as high as 64 percent,[2] and because physician conduct is a primary determinant of patient satisfaction,[1, 5, 25, 26] researchers have agreed that more training of practitioners in interpersonal communication skills is needed. Yet "few, if any, medical schools routinely teach the range of communication skills necessary to ensure adequate patient care."[14]

Medical Outcomes Agreement by physician and patient about what problems are important, and therefore, require follow-up, is the product of effective interaction. Where patients and their physicians agree, there is greater compliance by patients, and both patients and practitioners report better medical outcomes, regardless of the severity of the problems.[3, 27] Complete agreement is not the rule; research published in *Annals of Internal Medicine* found agreement in only 47 percent of the researched cases.[28]

In summary, in terms of medical outcomes, the costs of engaging in ineffective physician-patient communication are high. These costs can be measured in terms of probability of accurate diagnosis and effective treatment, patient compliance level, patient satisfaction level, and perceptions of outcomes by both practitioner and patient. Further, at least some of the losses due to ineffective communication can be measured in dollars and cents.

The Probability of Failure

Rather than blaming each other for their mutual dissatisfaction, both physicians and patients need to realize that their interaction is inherently problematic. The very nature of the traditional physician-patient relationship is at the source of many of the communication problems. Where parties are dissatisfied, it is probably not because they are doing things unusually "wrong"; rather they are engaging in "typical" or "normal" physician-patient relationships.

Two aspects of physician-patient relationships almost assure dissatisfying communication outcomes. First, the relationship is traditionally structured as a one-up/one-down power relationship in which the physician has control. As a result, patients often do not know how, or are unwilling, to become active participants in the interaction. Second, the practitioner is most often called on when the patient has a problem and thus takes on the role of evaluator. Evaluation is inherently threatening; the physician is forced into a role likely to increase the patient's defensiveness.

The Power Differential Even where physicians have adopted the philosophics of cooperative or participatory models, patients are likely to enter the relationship in the one-down position due to the patient's perception of how the relationship works. Even patients who desire participatory relationships are likely to yield their responsibilities in the face of the medical expertise of the physician. Because of the long-standing history of the physician-patient relationship (as one in which the physician takes control of the interview and takes sole responsibility for medical outcomes), both physician and patient need to take active steps if the structure of the relationship is to change. Patients need to learn how to provide information clearly, how to ask questions, and how to assert themselves without threatening their physicians. Physicians need to learn how to encourage patients' questions, how to invite openness, how to gain information, and how to make nonthreatening medical evaluations.

There are additional negative effects of defining the relationship as one in which one person has control while the other is passive. Social psychologists have shown the consequences can be devastating: (1) the powerful tend to devalue the performance of the less powerful, (2) as power increases, so do the number of attempts to influence the less powerful, (3) those with power view the less powerful as objects of manipulation, and (4) those in power prefer to increase their psychological distance from the less powerful.[29] Think of the implications if these generalizations hold true for the physician-patient relationship: physicians would tend to view their patients as having little value, being open to manipulation, and unworthy of anything other than distant association. The point here is not that physicians are cold and manipulative; rather that, in general, when people have power over others, they may unknowingly begin to change how they treat those others in subtle ways. There is no reason to assume that physicians are immune to these human tendencies. The problem calls for skills that will help define the relationship as a partnership among relative equals. The physician's role in this change is to use interpersonal skills that increase the status of the patient and that communicate a valuing of the patient.

The Threat of Evaluation The second problem inherent in the nature of the interaction is that the relationship exists, most often, for the purposes of evaluation. The patient's health is under evaluation by the physician. While cooperative education-oriented programs encourage the involvement and responsibility of the patient, the patient is still dependent on the physician's expertise and is still subject to evaluation in the interaction. Research in interpersonal communication shows that evaluation is threatening. Where people are threatened, they tend to be come defensive in their communication, they become less willing to change, and the defensiveness on the part of one party is likely to threaten and thus elicit defensiveness on the part of the other party.[30] That is, the more the patient feels threatened and responds with defensiveness, the more the physician is likely to feel threatened and become defensive also. Thus, because physician and patient most often meet to evaluate the patient's health, they meet under conditions that virtually assure communication problems, regardless of the physician's expertise and goodwill. The problem calls for communication skills by both physician and patient that are directed toward creating supportive rather than threatening environments.[30] The physician can help by using communication skills that reinforce the value of the patient and communicate support to the patient.

In summary, communication in the practitioner-provider relationship is inherently problematic due to the status/power differences of participants and the evaluative nature of their encounters. There is little reason to lay blame on either party; the very nature of the relationship causes problems. Instead, both parties need to work at altering the nature of the relationship. Physicians' skills need to be directed toward communicating the enhanced value of the patient and toward creating supportive rather than threatening environments.

Avoiding Common Physician-Patient Communication Problems

"Putting the ill at ease" is the challenge faced by physicians who realize the need for effective physician-patient communication." Many practitioners acknowledge the importance of communicating that the patient is an independent, worthy person held in high esteem.[31] But nearly all the communication problems commonly observed by researchers that are attributable to the physician involve the failure to communicate the worth of the patient. Communication that negates the value of the other person is called "disconfirmation."[32] Disconfirming communication may take many forms. The list is nearly matched, one-for-one, by a list of the communication problems in physician-patient interactions. While patients frequently disconfirm their physicians, the focus here is on physician behavior. A summary of specific forms of disconfirmation follows with the corresponding communication problems typical of physician-patient interaction.

Disconfirming communication is how one responds to another person's attempt to communicate. Five categories of responses are disconfirming, communicating that the other person is of low value.[32] Here, they are translated into possible physician behaviors that need to be avoided if the physician wishes to communicate that the patient is valued.

1. Ignoring the presence of the person and/or ignoring his or her attempts to communicate.

Silence when a reply is expected For example, the patient asks, "Will I be all right?" and no reply is given. Or the physician has just presented a diagnosis that uses a moderately technical term, and the patient has a questioning look on her face—but the physician goes on without acknowledging the patient's possible confusion. In another case, prior to an office visit involving a possibly painful procedure, the physician asks "How are you?" The patient replies in a shaky voice, "Scared." If the physician ignores the patient's response and continues to prepare materials for the procedure, the patient has been blatantly disconfirmed.

Leaving the scene while the other is speaking The physician asks how the patient is progressing following surgery but walks away from the patient, turns his or her back, or leaves the room for any reason while the patient replies, disconfirming the patient.

Engaging in unrelated tasks while the other is speaking Because physicians are so busy, they often try to do several things at once. While this cannot always be avoided, note taking, further examination, or preparation of materials while the patient is discussing deep-seated feelings or important information regarding his or her responses to treatment is disconfirming and is likely to result in the patient being "closed" (unwilling to provide needed information).

Responding by ignoring the topic of the other person's concern, changing the topic abruptly, inappropriately, or without warning This form of disconfirmation is likely to occur when patient and physician disagree about the problem that needs to be addressed or when the patient does not understand the larger picture. For example, a patient may present him- or herself to the physician with particular symptoms. When the physician realizes the symptoms are part of a larger problem, the physician may appear to change the topic or problem of concern. Making clear how the patient's concern is related to the questions the physician is asking or to the diagnosis made may alleviate the perception that the patient's concern has been ignored.

Several documented communication problems common to physician-patient relationships fall into the category of ignoring the other person. For instance, a common complaint among patients is that they are forced to spend large amounts of time waiting to see a physician. While forcing patients to wait is not a personal act ignoring their presence, the waiting patients are not being acknowledged. As a result, they tend to feel ignored and worse, devalued. When patients encounter the practitioner, they may find themselves ignored at other levels. Researchers who observed interactions of pediatricians noted that the physicians frequently ignored the chief concern of the mother about her child, even when the mother made repeated efforts to engage the physician in conversation about those concerns. Further, they sometimes ignored questions, or responded by asking questions on another topic.[5]

2. Using a communication style that prohibits or discourages the participation of the other person.

Interrupting The patient begins to list a series of concerns; the physician begins to see a trend and interrupts the patient to ask several questions. By the time the physician has concluded, the patient has forgotten the other concerns or is too intimidated to ask about them. As a result, the physician is denied information that may be critical to diagnosis and treatment, and the patient is less likely to provide detailed information in the future.

Engaging in monologue The physician makes a hospital visit. He or she rushes in, begins reading several items from the chart aloud, prescribes changes in medication, predicts the patient probably can go home tomorrow, and leaves quickly, discussing the next case with the nurse at his or her side. While responsibility for raising concerns or asking questions lies with the patient, this physician has communicated clearly that this patient should not participate in the process.

Relying on closed questions or other behaviors that limit the range of the other's responses The question, "Tell me how you are responding to the treatment," will gain more information than will "Are you doing O.K.?" The open question gives the patient freedom in how to respond; closed questions tend to limit responses to "yes," "no," or other single-word answers and therefore yield minimal information. In addition, the overuse of closed questions tends to make patients defensive.

Evidence suggests that beyond blatantly ignoring the communication attempts of their patients, physicians can discourage those attempts in many ways. Doctors do most of the talking in interactions.[5] While this may result from patients' reticence, interviewing techniques often used by physicians discourage patient involvement. Physicians studied frequently relied on closed questions and made few attempts to clarify the main complaints presented by patients." Typical history-taking techniques limit rather than encourage disclosure of information.

3. Using behaviors that function to disaffiliate or distance oneself from the other person.

Avoiding eye contact The physician who avoids eye contact with patients (as a means of maintaining professionalism or patient privacy) unknowingly communicates a lack of desire to be involved with patients.

Using impersonal language The classic example of impersonal language occurs when the physician asks, "How are we doing today?" Using the third-person "you" or "we" when the second-person "you" or "I" is meant, is impersonal. Using impersonal formalities, such as titles, also communicates a lack of personal involvement.

Concealing feelings Physicians may mask their feelings as a matter of professionalism; they purposely avoid showing happiness or sadness, surprise, or anger. Patients often believe that physicians have no feelings or misinterpret their physicians because the masking of feelings conceals important information from the patient.

Denying the other person's feelings or meanings ("You don't really feel that way" or "What you really mean is ...") If a patient recovering from surgery winces while being examined, and the physician responds with "It doesn't really hurt that much, does it?" the patient's level of pain has been denied by the physician. The patient is likely to yield to the physician's comment, and the physician now has a less accurate picture of the patient's recovery rate. The physician who says "You will have to learn to live with the pain," may discourage the patient from providing an accurate report.

This third category of disconfirmation, distancing self from patients, often is assumed to be desirable; the distancing is defended as "professional objectivity." But that same behavior functions to disaffiliate and, thus, communicates that the patient is of minimal personal value. Researchers report that the physicians they observed engaged in little affective communication; typical rules of conversation, such as the rules that people introduce themselves or that questions demand responses, were violated.[5, 34] The authors speculated that the distancing functioned to enhance the patient's image of the physician as an authority. Less than 5 percent of the physicians' communication was personal or friendly, and the observed physicians rarely responded to patients' verbal and nonverbal cues about their emotional state.[34]

Distancing is also created by denying feelings and needs of patients. Although research consistently has indicated that the primary concerns of patients include getting a diagnosis, an indication of cause, and a prognosis for treatment,[5, 35, 36] physicians frequently ignore those needs.[5, 38-40] In fact, research with cancer patients showed that physicians tended to deny their patients' desire for information; more than 90 percent of patients wanted full information,[14] yet elaborate means of evasion and misinformation and the issuance of false hopes were used to avoid providing that information.[40]

4. Using messages that are contradictory or ambiguous.

Mystifying (using overly technical jargon that confuses or evades) Physicians' use of jargon is the most common example of an ambiguous message. In their study published in Scientific American, Korsch and Negrete observed physicians using terms such as "SBE" and "Coombs," failing to understand the patient had been mystified.[14]

Using incongruent messages (messages or parts of messages, such as verbal and nonverbal parts that contradict each other) Physicians may be incongruent when they are trying to hide information or their own feelings. Saying "You seem to be doing fine" in a depressed tone of voice suggests that not all is well. Patients are more likely to believe nonverbal behaviors when verbal and nonverbal messages are contradictory.

Confirming selectively (acknowledging part of the other's message for one's own purposes while ignoring other parts) Because physicians are generally pressed for time, they may tend to hear their patients selectively in order to move on to what the physician perceives as important.

As with the previous categories, research indicates that the use of contradictory and ambiguous messages is common in physician-patient interaction. One of the most common complaints among patients (further evidenced in professional literature) is the tendency of physicians to engage in mystification. Doctors observed by researchers tended to denote themselves to a technical discussion of the patient's condition, often using lengthy scientific terms, without checking the patients's understanding, while sometimes ignoring requests for clarification.[5, 22] In more than half the cases, physicians resorted to the use of jargon.[5] Mystification communicates a disregard for the patient, a devaluing of the patient's need and right to information. Even an interested and involved patient can be mystified easily. Careful translation into language appropriate to the specific patient is needed.

5. Rejecting (putdowns, negative evaluations, and other forms of direct disparagement).

This final category probably occurs least frequently in physician-patient interaction. Outright rejection is the exception, not the rule. Research showed little evidence of disapproval, hostility, or criticism of patients by physicians.[6] Where such rejection occurred, dissatisfaction and noncompliance were likely to result. Although the instances of outright rejection are probably infrequent, the costs are high, in terms of medical outcomes and dollars and cents. Research indicated that physicians who were repeatedly the object of malpractice suits tended to be derogatory about patients, dismissed their complaints as trivial, and generally rejected those patients.[20, 24, 41]

In summary, the majority of patients' common complaints about their relationships with physicians, as well as communication problems observed by researchers, involve cases of disconfirmation. When used by physicians, each of the five types communicates that the value of the patient is minimal. In contrast, confirmation is the communication process by which individuals endorse one another. Regardless of the specific content, confirming communication always contains the message "I value you." The evidence and examples presented point to the need for physicians to use confirming communication with their patients.

Interpersonal Communication Skills for Physician-Patient Relationships

Other authors have come to similar conclusions about the need for communication skills but have identified the skills needed in vague or abstract terms. Some say physicians need to elicit open communication or physicians should engage in education only after establishing a good relationship;[42] others point to the need to attend to the emotional component of the relationship[22] or to establish strong rapport.[20] However, few attempts have been made to identify specific behaviors needed to achieve these abstract goals.

The identified goals of communicating the value of the patient and creating a nonthreatening (supportive) climate can be achieved by learning and using the following interpersonal skills: confirming responses, reflective listening, and "I-messages."

Confirming Responses Confirming responses communicate the value of the other person. They consist of behaviors that acknowledge the other person, communicate a willingness to affiliate, and express a value of the person. When translated into appropriate physician behaviors, confirmation includes:

- Looking directly at the patient
- Leaning forward, when seated, to convey interest
- Giving direct responses to the patient's communication, including answers to questions
- Discussing concerns raised by the patient, rather than changing topics
- Giving full attention to the patient's communication (avoiding other activity)
- Allowing the patient to speak without interruption
- Asking the patient if the physician may use his or her first name, then using it
- Asking some open questions, particularly at the beginning of the encounter
- Nodding the head to show that he or she is listening
- Smiling, as appropriate to the situation, to show friendliness
- Asking if the patient has questions
- Suggesting that the patient write down questions before the appointment and bring them along, then asking for the patient's questions
- Asking, at the end of the appointment, if the patient has other concerns Asking the patient to repeat back any instructions given, to check the patient's understanding of the prescribed regimen

Confirmation also includes the use of verbal responses communicating empathy, acceptance, and respect. Both reflective listening and "I-messages" are verbal responses that meet those goals; they also help create a supportive climate.[30]

Reflective Listening Reflective listening is an active response to another person.[43] When engaging in reflective listening, one paraphrases the other person's words and meanings while focusing on the other's feelings. Effective reflective listening "tunes in" to both verbal and nonverbal cues, identifies the other person's feelings, and thus communicates empathy. For example, a physician who notices that a patient is engaging in "nervous" nonverbal behavior while awaiting the results of tests might comment, "You are worried about the results of the tests." Rather than frightening the patient, this physician acknowledges, empathizes with, and accepts the patient's feelings. If the comment happens to be "off-target," the patient is likely to clarify what is really going on. In either case, the reflective response tells the patient that the physician is trying to understand. Reflective listening is conceptualized as an accepting form of communication in which the listener simply accepts and reflects the other's experiences but does not intervene with judgments, evaluations, suggestions, or advice. The listener's verbal and nonverbal cues must be congruent to be effective; saving, "I guess you have been in a lot of pain," is not believable unless a warm tone of voice accompanies the words.

While relying solely on reflective listening would interfere with other goals of physician-patient interaction, the skill is useful for establishing rapport in the initial interview, or in early moments of subsequent meetings. Reflective listening also could be used to respond to patients' verbal and nonverbal communication of emotion for encouraging the patient to discuss sensitive topic; (such as sexuality), for exploring social or psychological factors affecting one's health, for clarifying the physician's understanding of a patient's description of symptoms or responses to tests, or for problem solving when a patient is reluctant to undergo tests or other procedures.

I-Messages "I-messages" can be used to communicate the physician's concerns, feelings, opinions, or ideas in a relatively nonthreatening manner. "I-messages" also tend to communicate empathy, acceptance, and respect. Developed as a skill by Gordon,[44] "I-messages" offer an effective alternative to the threatening messages people generally use. "I-messages" usually (but not always) contain the word "I" and focus on the speaker and his or her feelings, perceptions, or experiences. They tend to communicate a sense of personal responsibility, while conveying that the other person is also responsible for him- or herself. Because "I-messages" focus on feelings and perceptions, they tend to contain an element of tentativeness and are not arguable. For example, a physician might respond to a patient who is not complying with prescribed high-blood pressure medication, "I know how you hate being dependent on medication, but I am worried about you. I am also concerned for your family and if they will be able to handle the eventual results of your illness." Rather than giving an order (Take your medication) or making a threat (You will have a stroke if you don't take the medication), the physician has left the responsibility to the patient, has clearly and strongly communicated his or her professional concerns and fears but in a manner more understanding, accepting, and respectful than the commonly used "You-messages." The use of less threatening forms of communication enhances the possibility of the patient being open to change (and maintaining the change) because the decision was a personal one.

Like reflective listening, physicians probably will find it unuseful to rely solely on "I-messages." Rather, they are useful for particular goals and circumstances. Physicians may find "I-messages" effective for communicating feelings (fears, concerns, empathy for another's feelings); for conveying opinions in a nonauthoritarian but professionally responsible manner in instances where physician and patient disagree about treatment choices, tests, or procedures; to communicate tentativeness where the physician is uncertain; or to present opinions in a conflict situation.

Training in the skills of confirmation, reflective listening, and "I-messages" is proposed as one cost-effective means of achieving positive physician-patient interactions, thereby reducing the costly medical outcomes resulting from ineffective communication. While reading these brief descriptions may be helpful to practitioners, the development and maintenance of a high level of interpersonal communication skills will require at least a brief training program. Medical schools need to institute ongoing interpersonal communication programs, while hospitals and other professional groups may need training programs and refresher workshops.

References

1. Jensen, P.S. "The Doctor-Patient Relationship: Headed for impasse or Improvement?" *Ann Intern Med* 95:769, 1981.
2. Koos, E.L. "Metropolis—What City People Think of Their Medical Services." *Am J Public Health* 45:1551, 1955.
3. Starfield, B. *et al.* "The Influence of Patient-Practitioner Agreement on Outcome of Care." *Am J Public Health* 71:127, 1981.
4. Szasz, T.S. and Hollander, M.H. "The Basic Models of the Doctor-Patient Relationship." *Arch Intern Med* 97:585, 1956.
5. Korsch, B.M. and Negrete, V.F. "Doctor-Patient Communication." *Sci Am* 227:66, 1972.
6. Freidson, E. *Professional Dominance.* Chicago: Aldine, 1970.
7. Kasteler, J. *et al.* "Issues Underlying Prevalence of 'Doctorshopping' Behavior." *J Health Soc Behav* 17:328, 1976.
8. Poole, A.D. and Sanson-Fisher, R.W. "Understanding the Patient: A Neglected Aspect of Medical Education." *Soc Sci Med* 13A:37. 1979.
9. Vaccarino, J.M. "Malpractice: The Problem in Perspective." *JAMA* 238:861.
10. Francis, V.; Korsch, B.M.; and Morris M.J. "Gaps in Doctor-Patient Communication: Patients' Response to Medical Advice." *N Engl J Med* 280:535, 1969.
11. Korsch, B.M.; Gozzi, E.K.; and Francis. V. "Gaps in Doctor- Patient Communication: I. Doctor-Patient Interaction and Satisfaction." *Pediatrics* 42:855, 1968.
12. Becker, M.H. and Maiman. L.A. "Sociobehavioral Determinants of Compliance with Health and Medical Care Recommendations." *Med Care* 13:10, 1975.
13. Freemon, B. *et al.* "Gaps in Doctor-Patient Communication: Doctor-Patient interaction Analysis." *Pediat Res* 5:298, 1971.
14. Sanson-Fisher, R. and Maguire, P. "Should Skills in Communicating with Patients be Taught in Medical Schools?" *Lancer* September 6, 1980:523.
15. Stimson. G.V. "Obeying Doctor's Orders: A View from the Other Side." *Soc Sci Med* 8:97, 1974.
16. Fine, V.F. and Therrien, M.E. "Empathy in the Doctor-Patient Relationship: Skill Training for Medical Students." *J Med Educ* 52:752, 1977.
17. Davis, M.S. "Variations in Patient's Compliance with Doctor's Orders: Analysis of Congruence between Survey Responses and Results of Empirical Investigations." *J Med Educ* 41:1037, 1966.
18. Becker, M. Presentation, Congressional Seminar, Washington, DC, May, 1982.
19. Stone, G.C. "Patient Compliance and the Role of the Expert." *J Soc Issues* 35:34, 1979.
20. DiMatteo, M.R. "A Social-Psychological Analysis of PhysicianPatient Rapport: Toward a Science of the Art of Medicine." *J Soc Issues* 35:12, 1979.
21. Hulka, B.S. *et aL* "Communication, Compliance and Concordance between Physicians and Patients with Prescribed Medications.' *Am J Public Health* 66:847, 1976.
22. Korsch, B.M.; Freemon, B.; and Negrete, V.F. "Practical Implications of Doctor-Patient Interaction Analysis for Pediatric Practice." *Am J Dis Child* 121:110, 1971.
23. Woolley, F.R. *et al.* "The Effects of Doctor-Patient Communication on Satisfaction and Outcome of Care." *Soc Sci Med* 12:123, 1978.
24. Blum, R.H. *The Management of the Doctor-Patient Relationship.* New York: McGraw-Hill, 1960.

25. Caplan, E.K. and Sussman, M.B. "Rank Order of Important Variables for Patient and Staff Satisfaction with Outpatient Service." J *Health Hum Behav* 7:133, 1966.
26. Doyle, B.J. and Ware, Jr., J.E. "Physician Conduct and Other Factors that Affect Consumer Satisfaction with Medical Care." *J Med Educ* 52:793, 1977.
27. Starfield, B.; Steinwachs, D.; and Morris, 1. "Patient-Provider Agreement about Problems: Influence on Outcome of Care." *JAMA* 242:344, 1979.
28. Friedin, R.B., Goldman, L., and Rosellen, R.C. "PatientPhysician Concordance in Problem Identification in the Primary Care Setting." *Ann Intern Med* 93:490, 1980.
29. Kipnis, D. "Does Power Corrupt?" *J Pers Soc Psychol 24:33,* 1972.
30. Gibb, J.R. "Defensive Communication." *J Commun* 3:141, 1961.
31. Bernarde, M.A. and Mayerson, E.W. "Patient-Physician Negotiation." *JAMA* 239:1413, 1978.
32. Cissna, K.N.L. and Sieburg, E. "Patterns of Interactional Confirmation and Disconfirmation." In C. Wilder and J.H. Weakland *(eds.). Rigor and Imagination.* New York: Praeger, p.253, 1981.
33. Wiener, S. and Nathanson. M. "Physical Examination Frequently Observed Errors." *JAMA* 236:852, 1976.
34. Rosenhan, D.L. "On Being Sane in Insane Places." *Science* 179:250, 1973.
35. Wadsworth, M.E.J. "Illness Behavior and Studies of Communications between Doctors and Patients." *J Psychasom Res* 20:317. 1976.
36. Balint, M. *The Doctor, His Patient and the Illness.* London: Pittman Medical Publications, 1957.
37. Ley, P. and Spelman, M.S. "Communications in an Outpatient Setting." *Br J Soc Clin Psychol 4:114,* 1965.
38. Kelly, W.D. and Friesen, S.R. "Do Cancer Patients Want to Be Told?" *Surgery* 27:822, 1950.
39. Gilbertson, V.A. and Wangensteen, O.H. "Should the Doctor Tell the Patient that the Discase is Cancer?" *Cancer* 12:82, 1962.
40. McIntosh, J. "Processes of Communication, Information Seeking and Control Associated with Cancer: A Selective Review of the Literature." *Soc Sci Med* 8:167, 1974.
41. Blum, R.H. *The Psychology of Malpractice Suits.* San Francisco: The California Medical Association, 1957.
42. Finnerly, Jr., F.A. "The Problem of Non-Compliance." *Med Times* 16:71, 1978.
43. Rogers, C.R. *On Becoming a Person.* Boston: Houghton Mifflin, 1961.
44. Gordon, T. *Parent Effectiveness Training.* New York: Peter H. Wyden, 1970.

Getting the Most from Your Visit to the Doctor
Make Your Office Visit Work For You

Pamela A. Rowland-Morin and David B. Reuben

Going to the doctor may seem as simple as arriving on time. But that kind of thinking can lead to poor communication between doctor and patient, unmet expectations, and disappointment. By preparing for your visit and asking the right questions, you can improve the quality of your health care. For people with diabetes, establishing an effective means of exchanging information with your doctor cannot be overemphasized.

Selecting A Physician

Over the past decade, the process of choosing a doctor has become increasingly complex as health maintenance organizations (HMOs) and other health plans have become widely available. Coverage under individual plans varies widely, and you should consult with someone in your company's personnel office to determine which plan is best for you.

Once you select a health insurance plan, you must choose a personal physician. Although endocrinologists have the most extensive diabetes care training, many internists, family physicians, and pediatricians have developed expertise in caring for patients with this disease. Your choice should be guided by the availability of such specialists in your area and an examination of the physician's credentials. These include the doctors medical school, residency, and reputation. Or, you might follow a reference from another doctor.

You may be able to tell a good deal about the staff, the doctor, and the treatment you will receive by observing the waiting room. Is the decor pleasant and comfortable? Or, is the room overcrowded with patients who seem frustrated by delays?

Are you greeted courteously by a staff person as soon as you arrive? Patients who feel expected and appreciated also tend to be more satisfied with their visits.

After checking in, calculate how long before you are taken into the examination room. If you wait longer than 15 minutes, ask the receptionist if there is a reason for the delay. You may decide to reschedule your appointment or select another doctor.

Preparing For Your Visit

You will get the most from your office visit if you're prepared.

Some of this preparation, such as monitoring your blood-sugar levels and forwarding your medical records (if you're seeing a new doctor),

Rowland-Morin, P. A. and Rueben, D. B., "Getting the Most From Your Visit to the Doctor: Make Your Office Visit Work For You", *Diabetes Forecast*, October, 1987, pp. 27-28. Reprinted with permission from *Diabetes Forecast*, October, 1987.

Editorial note: This article was written specifically for diabetics, but the adapted version published here has been edited to be relevant to persons with other medical conditions as well.

should be done well in advance of your visit. Other steps, such as gathering your medications, can be done later.

Here's a simple checklist:

- Be sure your medical records have arrived at your new physician's office.
- List your questions for the doctor.
- Record your blood-sugar levels (or other indicators) if you're doing self-monitoring.
- Compile your families medical history, including cause of death of parents and siblings, and specific illnesses of family members.
- List the types of foods you eat for breakfast, lunch, dinner, and snacks.
- List the kinds of exercise you do.
- Consider bringing a "support person," such as a spouse or friend, to participate in the interview. This person can ask questions you might forget and then help you remember the treatment program.
- Bring all your medication (or a list of them).
- Wear easy-to-remove clothing since you may have to undress for your physical exam.

Interview With The Doctor

After the initial greeting, allow a few minutes for the doctor to look over your chart. Reviewing your history will help your physician better address your current concerns.

Some tips to improve communication with your doctor:

- Share the conversation. The doctor should talk about 60 percent of the talking time, the patient about 40 percent. Remember that you are there to listen to what the doctor says, not to hear yourself.
- Don't be intimidated by technical vocabulary. When you don't understand something, interrupt and ask for an explanation.
- Don't be afraid to bring up sexual or other personal topics.
- Don't be afraid to discuss money. Compassionate doctors realize financial worries can increase patient anxiety and will discuss payment options.

The Physical Exam

Your doctor usually will ask you to undress for the physical examination. Make certain a gown is available and that you know how to put it on. Many doctors also provide a sheet for you to cover up and keep warm.

When you're asked to undress, ask your doctor how much clothing to remove. Some exams can be performed without removing undergarments.

A physical exam for a person with diabetes usually includes the following: weight, blood pressure, heart and lung examination with a stethoscope, foot inspection, and specific examination of problem areas (e.g., a sore shoulder or abdominal pain).

You should also expect to undergo some examinations and tests to determine your overall health. These often include a blood cholesterol level, stool specimen analysis, and an eye exam to detect glaucoma.

For women, recommended tests also include a pap smear, mammogram, and gynecological and rectal exams. Men should receive prostate and rectal examinations.

Unanswered Questions

You've probably come to your doctor with questions regarding your medical condition. And, probably, many of them may have been answered during the course of the interview.

However, check your list to make sure your most important questions have been addressed. If they haven't been, decide whether they could best be answered by the doctor, a nurse, or a health educator.

Here's a general guide for finding answers to commonly asked questions.

Ask the nurse or health educator about:

- problems with self-monitoring (e.g., of blood glucose)
- administering medication
- foods you can eat
- travel on planes or trains across time zones

Ask the doctor about:

- your personal regimen
- kinds of over-the-counter medications you can use.

Last Two Minutes Of The Interview

Before you leave the doctor's office, make sure you have answers to the following questions:

1. When do I need my next medical checkup?
2. Will I be seeing the doctor or nurse then?
3. What type of information (like blood-sugar levels) should I collect between now and the next visit?
4. Where can I find other people with similar health problems?
5. Where can I obtain more information about my condition?

Ask for the doctor's business card with office and emergency phone numbers, and keep it in your wallet or pocketbook.

Finally, don't leave the doctor's office if you're confused about any subject. Ask questions until you understand.

After The Interview

If you were pleased by your doctor, consider sending a note of thanks. Few patients take the time to express satisfaction, even though the effort may encourage continued good treatment.

Also, consider sending a letter to your local chapter (e.g., American Diabetes Association chapter) telling why you were satisfied. This information will help the chapter make appropriate referrals.

If things didn't go right with your visit, consider calling the doctor to discuss why you were disappointed. Sometimes your concern can be resolved.

If confronting the doctor in person is difficult for you, write a letter. If the matter isn't handled in a satisfactory manner, think about filing a complaint with the institution the doctor is affiliated with, members of the group practice, or the doctors employer. Above all, remember you are the person most affected by the quality of medical care you receive. Obtaining the highest quality care requires you to become an active participant in your visit to the doctor.

Asking and Telling

Miriam Shuchman and Michael S. Wilkes[1]

Some years ago, a New York woman was informed by her by her gynecologist that she had an ovarian tumor and needed immediate surgery. Naturally, she was upset, and, as a former cancer researcher with special knowledge of the subject, began to ask the doctor specific questions. He had a timer on his desk. He set it, and told he she had exactly three minutes to ask questions. She got up and left, and never went back. More recently, another patient, who had already had a cancer surgery, asked her physician about future risks. The physician launched into a nonstop treatise on every conceivable danger. The patient's husband, also a doctor, watched as his wife became increasingly alarmed. Finally, he interrupted to ask what the chances were that any of the dangers being described would occur. The chances were less than 1 percent.

The two cases illustrate changes that have taken place in the patient-doctor relationship. Clearly, the days of the all-knowing, intimidating, unchallengeable, imperious physician are gone, or mostly so. But how profound is the change in terms of doctors' real openness and willingness to share medical information with patients? Are most doctors really forthcoming, or just perfunctory? On the other hand, how much, in fact, does a patient really need to know? What should a patient insist on knowing?

Statistics alone don't answer the questions, but clearly there have been significant changes.

In a 1961 study of cancer patients, only 1 in 10 doctors told patients they had cancer; by 1970 1 in 4 doctors said cancer diagnoses were shared with patients; by 1977, 97 percent of 700 doctors surveyed said they preferred to disclose cancer diagnoses.

One impetus for doctors to tell more has been laws on informed consent, which began to develop in the late 1950's, as the courts upheld the principle that patients have a right to know the truth about a diagnosis. Doctors are *required*, at a minimum, to tell patients about conditions and to discuss the risks and benefits of treatments and alternatives.But experts on informed consent content that in practice it is often more a medical rite than a patient's real right. Dr. Paul Appelbaum, a University of Massachusetts Medical School professor, says informed consent often means a doctor comes into a patient's room 15 minutes before a procedure is to take place and hands the patient a form. As the obviously busy doctor stands at the bedside, the patient quickly reads the first word in each paragraph, and the last word in the paragraph. When the doctor asks, "Any questions?" the patient says no, embarrassed in not having read the form, and signs it. In medical jargon, the person has been "consented," a formality that for both doctors and

---

1 Miriam Shuchman is chief resident in psychiatry at the Massachusetts General Hospital; Michael Wilkes is the Robert Wood Johnson Clinical Scholar at the U.C.L.A. Medical Center.

patients has little connection with patients' being involved in decisions about their care.

For a person to know enough about a medical condition to actually consider treatment options involves far more than simply reciting facts or listing them on a piece of paper. It requires time on the part of doctors and patients for explanations and questions. Ideally, this should take place over a period of several meetings, because complex medical information cannot usually be absorbed in a single visit. Research shows that most people—though not all—want to be informed about their medical problems, and need a sufficient time to understand what is happening or going to happen to them.

Of course, it is not always possible to be informed fully or accurately; the process of rehabilitation and the pain involved in some medical procedures may be nearly impossible to describe fully; understandable only by experiencing them. One bone specialist, whose patient had two bone-marrow transplants—an extremely painful and frightening procedure—said it was only with the second one that the patient was truly prepared to give an informed consent. But the patient, in such circumstances, must be told, in general terms at least, that there may be severe pain over a specified period of time.

Some doctors, however, feel that telling a patient the pertinent facts about the pain or side effects of a procedure will, in fact, help lead to pain or side effects through the power of suggestion. Yet one recent study found that people who were adequately informed about the side effects of their medication were better able to discriminate inconsequential effects from more dangerous reactions. And greater knowledge did not lead either to greater side effects or more anxiety about the treatment. Many people, if they know pain is coming, can steel themselves against it. Others, who may be less able to handle pain or don't want to risk the side effects, must be given the option of saying: "Look, forget the procedure. I'd rather suffer the consequences of not having it."

The studies show that people want the medical news about themselves, even when it's bad and even when there is virtually nothing to be done about it. Shielding patients from the truth is usually not in the patient's best interest. It leads to mistrust and a feeling of betrayal just at the time that the doctor needs to be seen as an ally. In the 1988 study, more than 200 people given a description of a 54-year-old patient with Alzheimer's disease were asked if they would want to be told about the diagnosis if they were the patient. The majority said yes. When asked to consider whether they would want to know the diagnosis if they were a different age, respondents over age 65 were more likely than younger persons to say they would want to be told at ages 70 to 90.

In another recent study, investigators in San Francisco found that patients with high blood pressure wanted more information than their doctors realized, but at the same time they wanted to be less involved in decision making than the doctors had thought. Some people simply prefer to leave decisions to the doctor; one man in his early 5O's said that when he was hospitalized for surgery a few months ago, he was feeling very sick and did not want to know the intimate details of his condition. To the anesthesiologist who asked if he preferred spinal or general anesthesia, and the surgical residents describing the risks and benefits of the proposed surgery, he said: "Please, you decide." That man's feelings are shared by others. In one study, a third of the patients asked about preparations for a certain procedure said they would prefer not to hear about details in advance.

The laws on informed consent do not require that information be forced on a person who does not want it, though the individual may be asked to sign a waiver. Doctors are often unaware of that, so people may hear a litany of frightening details that they want no part of because the doctor thinks it is their "right." Still, the more common problem is that people want more information than they get. This sometimes happens when a person goes for a consultation or test. One pregnant woman known to us had a routine ultrasound exam during which the doctor did not speak. At one point, he appeared to concentrate on a small area of her protruding stomach, positioning and repositioning the lubricated probe, as he observed the ultrasonic images on a small screen. The young woman became frightened, convinced that the doctor must have found something abnormal. But when she asked what he had seen, his only reply was, "You'll need to speak with your obstetrician." The woman, believing there was a serious problem, became angry. She insisted on knowing the results, and reminded the radiologist that she was paying his bill. He shrugged, and walked out.

Several days later, she finally reached her obstetrician, who told her everything was normal. She was relieved but still furious, feeling that she had been unnecessarily frightened. Here, perhaps some exaggerated sense of propriety about which doctor ought to do the informing overrode the needs of the patient. This information belongs to the patient. Granted, more complex Information may need special interpretation by the primary physician, but this, too, can be explained to the patient.

It is through answering questions that doctors provide needed reassurance. And medical training gives most doctors experience in responding to all sorts of questions at any time of the day or night. But often a person who may be terribly sick and in a hospital bed, or sitting in a skimpy gown in an examining room on a paper-covered table, is not in the best position to interrogate the doctor. Nor is the patient who has been awakened by a group of doctors making early rounds always able to remember the questions that seemed so pressing the night before. So it may be helpful to have a family member present to do the asking.

It must be pointed out, too, that the patient who asks questions is more likely to get answers than one too shy or nervous to ask.

Regardless of who does the asking or how much spunk is required in getting the answers: all patients need this information: What Is the most likely diagnosis? What treatments are available? Are there alternatives? What are the risks of the proposed treatment? What will be the consequences if the condition Is not treated? In the end, the patient who does not get the answers he needs and wants should seriously consider finding another doctor.

Patients' Rights

Morton Hunt

"My doctor put me on a beta blocker," a friend told me last week. "I hate the side effects but I couldn't argue with him." Many, perhaps most, patients feel that way: they don't really have much say in the matter. Yet, according to the famous New York Court of Appeals decision in 1914, "Every human being of adult years and sound mind has a right to determine what shall be done with his own body." A doctor who does anything to the patient without consent can be sued for having committed battery, malpractice and civil-rights violations (unless the patient is incapable of giving consent).

In other words, you and I have certain rights we should know about—and, when necessary, insist upon. Here, then is a bill of patients' rights.

The Right to Choose Your Treatment

First, you have a right, established in a series of landmark cases, not to have anything done to you without your *informed* consent. Nevertheless, 59 percent of doctors polled by a Presidential commission take that to mean no more than informing patients about their condition and treatment; they ignore the *consent*.

Still, you have an absolute right to reject the recommended treatment and ask for another. Does that mean you can require a treatment the doctor doesn't believe in? Most experts say no. As Daniel Callahan, head of the Hastings Center of bioethical studies, says, that would deny the doctor *his* rights.

Can a doctor simply refuse to take care of you if you reject the recommended treatment? Generally not. A doctor who fails to continue to provide care until you are accepted by another physician can be charged with abandonment and sued for malpractice. (You might have to tell this to the doctor.)

Even in a hospital, you can say no to X-rays, laxatives, excessive probing and puncturing of your body. Few have the courage to do so. A 1983 study found fewer than five patient refusals of any procedure during the course of 100 days of patient treatment. As Professor Vincent Barry of Bakersfield College says, patients "are inclined to act in ways they think will please the doctors and nurses."

The right of refusal extends to hospitalized mental patients: 45 states have laws giving them a qualified right to reject antipsychotic medications, many of which have serious side effects. In most cases, patients must ask a review board to find that they are mentally competent to decide.

The Right to See Your Records

The right of informed consent implies a right to know the truth.

Learning this may mean more than asking the doctor questions; it may necessitate seeing one's medical records—X-rays, lab reports, other data. But doctors and hospitals have traditionally refused to let patients see such records. Not until 1984 did the American Medical Association say that doctors should make them available to patients on request. However, in 15 states patients now have a specified legal right to see doctors' records, and, in 23 states, to see hospital records. Still, a patient may have to fight for that right. Dr. Sidney Wolfe of the Public Citizen Health Research Group, says, "It is much easier to obtain copies of our C.I.A. or F.B.I. files than to get our medical records."

Doctors justify withholding records on the ground that it is often confusing or harmful for patients to know the facts. But four recent studies found that seeing records had *mostly* favorable effects. Even when the news is terrible, a panel of 10 eminent doctors recently declared in *The New England Journal of Medicine*, "The anxiety of dealing with the unknown can be far more upsetting than the grief of dealing with a known, albeit tragic, truth."

The Right to Considerate Care:

This is the very first item in the American Hospital Association's recommended (but not legally binding) Patient's Bill of Rights, published in 1973. But, 16 years later, many patients are subjected to inconsiderate and disrespectful treatment, such as unreasonably long waits in the doctor's office, or being told to undress in an inner office and wait. It is demeaning to be seen by the doctor when clutching only a paper gown around one's nakedness. Some doctors still treat patients like children. My wife described her symptoms to one specialist in medically precise terms, to which he smarmily replied: "Let's not use fancy words. Why don't you just call things by their everyday names?"

Experts agree that there is usually no way to force medical professionals to be considerate and respectful; you can only walk out. But in a few specific areas, the right is enforceable.

In hospitals, says John Robertson of the University of Texas Law School in "The Rights of the Critically Ill," if the patient objects, medical and other hospital personnel not connected with the patient's case may not enter the room to observe. (Teaching hospitals may be an exception.) The patient's right here stems from the basic right to privacy, which also makes the doctor-patient relationship confidential; generally, a doctor can be sued for conveying medical information about a patient without the patient's consent. (An exception is made in many states when conveying the information is necessary to protect others from contagion, crime or other harm.)

The Right to Hospital Treatment:

Congress has recently taken steps to combat "patient dumping"— turning away emergency cases by private hospitals and redirecting them to public ones if patients are uninsured or cannot guarantee bill payment.

New Federal laws governing Medicare and Medicaid provide that any hospital participating in such programs must accept and treat emergency cases, whether or not they have sufficient funds. Nearly all acute-care hospitals do participate in Medicare and Medicaid.

In 1986, Medicare policy was modified to assure hospitalized Medicare recipients of their right to *enough* treatment. If patients receive a notification of discharge from the hospital stating that their Medicare-covered time is up and they no longer need in-patient care, they can appeal by writing or telephoning their state's peer-review organization, panels selected and paid by the Government.

If they appeal, Medicare must pay their bills for two more days; the review panel must reply within three. If the panel approves a continued stay, Medicare continues to pay; if not, the patient pays. And the patient with unpaid bills of $200 or more has a right to appeal an adverse decision to a Social Security administrative law judge.

The Right to Die:

A recent poll conducted for the A.M.A. found that 73 percent of the public approves of withdrawing life-support systems from hopelessly ill or from irreversibly comatose patients if they or their families have requested it.

More leading doctors are writing in medical journals that maintaining the lives of such patients is cruel and that suspending treatment is morally justifiable.

In a number of court cases, patients or their representatives have won the right to stop unwanted treatment. Most important, in recent years legislators in 38 states and the District of Columbia have enacted laws granting patients some control over whether they are to receive life-sustaining treatment. Many of these laws are based on "living wills"—documents signed by patients while they are mentally competent, stating their wishes. Some laws permit a patient to execute a "durable power of attorney," giving power to some trusted person to refuse treatment, on the patient's behalf, if he becomes incompetent.

Even without a living will or power of attorney, family members or other appropriate persons can in some states act for an incompetent patient by stating that, in their judgment, the patient would not have wanted to be kept alive in the present condition; or, if the patient's preference is not known, stating that it is not in the patient's best interest to be maintained on life-support systems. Despite law or precedent, if doctors or hospitals think the case is not clear-cut, they are likely to insist on sustaining life until the patient's family or lawyer gets a court order. Details of your state's laws or court decisions on the right to die can be obtained from most state health departments.

Another crucial step to insure this right: "Tell your doctor once a year if you *really* don't ever want to be on a respirator," says Fenella Rouse, director of legal services at the New York City Society for the Right to Die. "If you do care about your right to die, it's up to you to pursue it."

The Right to Ask Questions.

This is the simplest but probably the most important right, in the sense that it is the one the patient should energetically exercise most often.

It is hard to do so. Asking doctors questions implies that the patient has a right to share in the decision-making, yet a centuries-old tradition holds that "doctor knows best." Many doctors resent having their advice questioned, and many patients are afraid to question it.

Despite all that has been said and written about patients' participation in decision making, both the American Hospital Association's Patient's Bill of Rights and the A.M.A.'s judicial council hold that the doctor may withhold information when he deems it medically advisable. "Sick human beings," asserts Dr. Richard Sherlock, a medical ethicist, in *The American Journal of Medicine*, "want, often desperately, to entrust themselves and their care to the physician."

So the point must be re-emphasized: the law grants patients the right to understand their own cases. How much knowledge, how many questions does that imply? "What the patient has a right to, as established by many court decisions," says Professor Robert Veatch of the Kennedy Institute of Ethics at Georgetown University, "is as much information as a 'reasonable person' would need to feel that he or she is capable of giving informed consent."

You need accept no less.

Medicine, Society and Culture: Alternative Perspectives on the Context of Caregiving

The Medicalization and Demedicalization of American Society

Renée C. Fox

The statement that American society has become "medicalized" is increasingly heard these days. During the past decade or so, the allegation has been made by social scientists, jurists, politicians, social critics, medical scientists, and physicians. In many instances, it has been accompanied by the claim that the society is now "overmedicalized," and that some degree of "demedicalization" would be desirable. There are those who not only espouse "demedicalizing the society," but who also predict that, in fact, it will progressively come to pass.

One of the most extreme statements of this kind is Ivan Illich's monograph, *Medical Nemesis,* which opens with the assertion that "the medical establishment has become a threat to health," and goes on to develop the many damaging ways in which the author considers modern medicine to be responsible for "social" as well as "clinical" and "structural" iatrogenesis:

> The technical and non-technical consequences of institutional medicine coalesce and generate a new kind of suffering: anesthetized, impotent and solitary survival in a world turned into a hospital ward. . . . The need for specialized, professional health care beyond a certain point can be taken as an indication of the unhealthy goals pursued by society. . . . The level of public health corresponds to the degree to which the means and responsibility for coping with illness are distributed amongst the total population. This ability to cope can be enhanced but never replaced by medical intervention in the lives of people or by the hygienic characteristics of the environment. The society which can reduce professional intervention to the minimum will provide the best conditions for health. . . . Healthy people are those who live in healthy homes on a healthy diet; in an environment equally fit for birth, growth, work, healing and dying: sustained by a culture which enhances the conscious acceptance of limits to population, of aging, of incomplete recovery and ever imminent death. . . . Man's consciously lived fragility, individuality and relatedness make the experience of pain, of sickness and of death an integral part of his life. The ability to cope with this trio autonomously is fundamental to his health. As he becomes dependent on the management of his intimacy, he renounces his autonomy and his health *must* decline. The true miracle of modern medicine is diabolical. It consists not only of making individuals but whole populations survive on inhumanly low levels of personal health. That health should decline with increasing health service delivery is unforeseen only by the health managers, precisely because their strategies are the result of their blindness to the inalienability of life.[1]

There are numerous grounds on which Illich's thesis can be criticized. He minimizes the advances in the prevention, diagnosis, and treat-

---

"The Medicalization and Demedicalization of American Society" by Renée C. Fox is reprinted from DOING BETTER AND FEELING WORSE, Health in the United States, Edited by John H. Knowles, M.D., by permission of W. W. Norton & Company, Inc.

1 Ivan Illich, *Medical Nemesis: The Expropriation of Health* (London, 1975), pp. 165-69.

ment of disease that have been made since the advent of the bacteriological era in medicine, and he attributes totally to non-medical agencies all progress in health that has ensued. He implies that modern Western, urban, industrialized, capitalist societies, of which the United States is the prototype, are more preoccupied with pain, sickness, and death, and less able to come to terms with these integral parts of a human life, than other types of society. Although his volume appears to be well documented, a disturbing discrepancy exists between the data presented in many of the works that Illich cites in his copious footnotes and the interpretive liberties that he takes with them. Perhaps most insidious of all is the sophistry that Illich uses in presenting a traditional, orthodox, Christian-Catholic point of view in the guise of a vulgar Marxist argument. For he repeatedly claims that "when dependence on the professional management of pain, sickness and death grows beyond a certain point, the healing power in sickness, patience in suffering, and fortitude in the face of death must decline."[2] In Illich's view, this state is not only morally dubious, but also spiritually dangerous. Because it entails the "hubris" of what he deems arrogant and excessive medical intervention, it invites "nemesis": the retribution of the gods.

But whatever its shortcomings, Illich's essay is a kind of lightning rod, picking up and conducting the twin themes of medicalization and demedicalization which have become prominent in the United States and a number of other modern Western societies. These themes will concern us here. We shall begin by identifying the constellation of factors involved in what has been termed "medicalization," offer an interpretation of these phenomena, and consider and evaluate certain signs of demedicalization. Finally, some speculative predictions about the probable evolution of the medicalization-demedicalization process in American society will be offered.

One indication of the scope that the "health-illness-medicine complex" has acquired in American society is the diffuse definition of health that has increasingly come to be advocated: "a state of complete physical, mental, and social well-being," to borrow the World Health Organization's phrase. This conception of health extends beyond biological and psychological phenomena relevant to the functioning, equilibrium, and fulfillment of individuals, to include social and cultural conditions of communal as well as personal import. Such an inclusive perspective on health is reflected in the range of difficulties that persons now bring to physicians for their consideration and help. As Leon Kass picturesquely phrased it:

> All kinds of problems now roll to the doctor's door, from sagging anatomies to suicides, from unwanted childlessness to unwanted pregnancy, from marital difficulties to learning difficulties, from genetic counseling to drug addiction, from laziness to crime. . . .[3]

A new term has even been coined by medical practitioners to refer to those clients who seem to have some legitimate need of their therapeutic services, but who technically cannot be considered to be ill. With discernible ambivalence, such persons are often called "the worried well."

Accompanying the increasingly comprehensive idea of what constitutes health and what is appropriate for medical professionals to deal with is the growing conviction that health and health care are rights rather than privileges, signs of grace, or lucky, chance happenings. In turn, these developments are connected with higher expectations on the part of the public about what medicine ideally ought to be able to accomplish and to prevent. To some extent, for example, the rise in

2 Illich, *Medical Nemesis, passim.*
3 Leon R. Kass, "Regarding the End of Medicine and the Pursuit of Health," *The Public Interest* 40 (Summer, 1975), p. 11.

the number of malpractice suits in the United States seems not only to be a reaction to the errors and abuses that physicians can commit, but also a reflection of the degree to which the profession is being held personally responsible for the scientific and technical incertainties and limitations of their discipline. The vision of an iatrogenesis-free furthering of health, which social critics such as Illich hold forth, is also an indicator of such rising expectations.

One significant form that the process of medicalization has taken is the increase in he numbers and kinds of attitudes and behaviors that have come to be defined as illnesses and treatment of which is regarded as belonging within the jurisdiction of medicine and its practitioners. In an earlier, more religiously oriented era of a modern Western society like our own, some of these same kinds of attitudes and behaviors were considered sinful rather than sick, and they fell under the aegis of religious authorities for a different kind of diagnosis, treatment, and control. In a more secular, but less scientifically and medically oriented, stage of the society than the current one, certain of these ways of thinking, feeling, and behaving were viewed and dealt with as criminal. Although sin, crime, and sickness are not related in a simple, invariant way, there has been a general tendency in the society to move from sin to crime to sickness in categorizing a number of aberrant or deviant states to the degree that the concept of the "medicalization of deviance" has taken root in social-science writings. The sin-to-crime-to-sickness evolution has been most apparent with respect to the conditions that .are now considered to be mental illnesses, or associated with serious psychological and/or social disturbances.[4] These include, for example, states of hallucination and delusion that once would have been interpreted as signs of possession by the Devil, certain forms of physical violence, such as the type of child abuse that results in what is termed the "battered child syndrome," the set of behaviors in children which are alternatively called hyperactivity, hyperkinesis, or minimal brain dysfunction, and so-called addictive disorders, such as alcoholism, drug addiction, compulsive overeating, and compulsive gambling.

This "continuing process of divestment[5] away from sin and crime as categories for abnormality, dysfunction, and deviance and toward illness as the explanatory concept has entailed what Peter Sedgwick calls "the progressive annexation of not-illness into illness." "The future belongs to illness," he proclaims, predicting that "We . . . are going to get more and more diseases, since our expectations of health are going to become more expansive and sophisticated. If we include into what is going to become more expansive and sophisticated.[6] If we include what is considered to be sickness or, at least, non-health in the United States, disorders manifested by subjective symptoms which are not brought to the medical profession for diagnosis and treatment, but which do not differ significantly from those that are, then almost everyone in the society can be regarded as in some way "sick."

> At least two . . . studies have noted that as much as 90 percent of their apparently healthy sample had some physical aberration or clinical disor-

---

4 In his novel *Erewhon,* written in 1872, Samuel Butler satirized this evolution, and the degree to which what is defined as illness is contingent on social factors. In Erewhon (the fictitious country that Butler created by imagining late nineteenth- and early twentieth-century England stood on its head), persons afflicted with what physicians would call tuberculosis are found guilty in a court of law and sentenced to life imprisonment, whereas persons who forge checks, set houses on fire, steal, and commit acts of violence are diagnosed as suffering from a "severe fit of immorality" and are cared for at public expense in hospitals.

5 Nicholas N. Kittrie, *The Right To Be Different: Deviance and Enforced Therapy* (Baltimore, 1971). See especially chapter 1, "The Divestment of Criminal justice and the Coming of the Therapeutic State," pp. 1-49.

6 Peter Sedgwick, "Illness-Mental and Otherwise," *The Hastings Center Studies,* 1:3 (1973), p. 37.

> der. . . . It seems that the more intensive the investigation, the higher the prevalence of clinically serious but previously undiagnosed and untreated disorders. Such data as these give an unexpected statistical picture of illness. Instead of it being a relatively infrequent or abnormal phenomenon, the empirical reality may be that illness, defined as the presence of clinically serious symptoms, is the statistical *norm.*[7]

Such a global conception of illness acutely raises the question of the extent to which illness is an objective reality, a subjective state, or a societal construct that exists chiefly in the minds of its social "beholders," a question that will be considered in greater detail below.

The great "power" that the American medical profession, particularly the physician, is assumed to possess and jealously and effectively to guard is another component of the society's medicalization. In the many allusions to this medical "power" that are currently made, the organized "autonomy" and "dominance" of the profession are frequently cited, and, in some of the more critical statements about the physician, these attributes are described as constituting a virtual "monopoly" or "expropriation" of health and illness. The "mystique" that surrounds the medical profession is part of what is felt to be its power: a mystique that is not only spontaneously conferred on its practitioners by the public but, as some observers contend, is also cultivated by physicians themselves through their claim that they command knowledge and skills that are too esoteric to be freely and fully shared with lay persons.

However, it is to the biotechnological capacities of modern medicine that its greatest power is usually attributed: both its huge battery of established drugs and procedures and its new and continually increasing medical and surgical techniques. Among the actual or incipient developments that are most frequently mentioned are the implantation of cadaveric, live, or mechanical organs, genetic and other microcellular forms of "engineering," and *in vitro* fertilization, as well as various chemical, surgical, and psychophysiological methods of thought and behavior control. The potentials of medicine not only to prevent and to heal, but also to subjugate, modify, and harm are implicated in such references.

The high and rapidly growing cost of medical and health care is still another measure of increased medicalization. In 1975, Americans spent $547 per person for health care and related activities such as medical education and research. This represented 8.3 per cent of the GNP. In 1950, 4.6 per cent and in 1970, 7.2 per cent of the GNP was spent. From 1963 to the present, health expenditures have risen at a rate exceeding 10 per cent annually while the rest of the economy as reflected in the GNP has been growing at a rate between 6 and 7 per cent.

In addition to allocating an ever increasing proportion of society's economic resources for health care, greater amounts of political and legal energy are also being invested in health, illness, and medical concerns. The pros and cons of national health insurance, which continue to be vigorously debated in various arenas, are as much political, ideological, and legal issues, as they are economic ones. The volume of legislation relevant to health care has grown impressively. In 1974, for example, more than 1,300 health-care bills were introduced in the Congress, and more than 900 such bills in the state legislature in New York alone. The health subcommittees of the Senate and the House of Representatives are particularly active, and they have become prestigious as well. Furthermore, partly as a consequence of various congressional investigations and hearings, the federal government is now significantly involved in bioethical questions (es-

7 Irving Kenneth Zola, "Culture and Symptoms—An Analysis of Patients' Presenting Complaints," *American Sociological Review*, 31:5 (October, 1966), pp. 615-16.

pecially those bearing on human experimentation) in addition to their more traditional interests in medical economic and health-care-delivery problems.

During the past few years, a number of medico-legal decisions have been made that are of far-reaching cultural importance, affecting the society's fundamental conceptions of life, death, the body, individuality, and humanity. These include: the Supreme Court's decisions in favor of the legal right of women to decide upon and undergo abortion; the Court's ruling against the involuntary, purely custodial confinement of untreated, mentally ill persons; the Uniform Anatomical Gift Act, adopted in fifty-one jurisdictions, which permits persons to donate all or parts of their bodies to be used for medical purposes after their death; death statutes passed in various states which add the new, "irreversible coma" criterion of "brain death" to the traditional criteria for pronouncing death, based on the cessation of respiratory and cardiac function; and, in the case of Karen Ann Quinlan, the New jersey Supreme Court's extension of "the individual's right of privacy" to encompass a patient's decision to decline or terminate life-saving treatment, under certain circumstances.

One other, quite different, way in which medical phenomena have acquired central importance in the legal system is through the dramatic escalation of malpractice suits against physicians. An estimated 20,000 or more malpractice claims are brought against doctors each year, and the number seems to be rising steadily. In New York, for example, the number of suits filed against physicians rose from 564 in 1970 to 1,200 in 1974; in the past decade, the average award for a malpractice claim grew from $6,000 to $2 3,400, with far more very large awards being made than in the past.[8]

Increasing preoccupation with bioethical issues seems also to be a concomitant of the medicalization process. Basic societal questions concerning values, beliefs, and meaning are being debated principally in terms of the dilemmas and dangers associated with biomedical advances. Consideration of particular medical developments such as genetic engineering, life-support systems, birth technology, organ implants, and population and behavior control have opened up far-reaching ethical and existential concerns. Problems of life, death, chance, "necessity," scarcity, equity, individuality, community, the "gift relationship," and the "heroic" worldview are being widely discussed in medical, scientific, political, legal, journalistic, philosophical, and religious circles. A bioethics "subculture" with certain characteristics of a social movement has crystallized around such issues.

The unprecedented number of young people who are attempting to embark on "medical careers is also contributing to the medicalization process. In this country, on the average, more than three persons apply for each medical-school place available to entering first-year students, and there is as yet no sign of a leveling off. Paradoxically, this is happening during a period when medicine and the medical profession are being subjected to increased scrutiny and criticism.

Complex, and by no means consistent, the process of medicalization is not an easy one to analyze. Several preliminary *caveats* seem in order. In part, they are prompted by two sorts of assumptions made by critics of medicalization in America: one is that the central and pervasive position of health, illness, and medicine in present-day American society is historically and culturally unique, and the other, that it is primarily a result of the self-interested maneuvers of the medical profession. Neither these assumptions is true without qualification.

To begin with, in all societies, health, illness, and medicine constitute a nexus of great symbolic as well as structural importance, involving and

8 These figures were cited in the June 9, 1976, issue of *Newsweek*, p. 59.

interconnecting social, psychological, and cultural systems of action. In every society, health, illness, and medicine are related to the physical and psychic integrity of individuals, their ability to establish and maintain solidary relations with others, their capacities to perform social roles, their birth, survival, and death, and to the ultimate kinds of "human condition" questions that are associated with these concerns. As such, health, illness, and medicine also involve and affect every major institution of a society, and its basic cultural grounding. The family, for example, is profoundly involved in the health and illness of its members, and, especially in non-moderm societies, the kinship system is as responsible for health and illness as are specialized medical practitioners. The institutions of science, magic, and religion are the major media through which the "hows" and "whys" of health and illness, life and death are addressed in a society, and through which culturally appropriate action for dealing with them is taken. The economy is also involved in several ways: the allocation of resources that health, illness, and medicine entail; the occupational division of labor relevant to diagnosis and therapy; and the bearing of health and illness on the individual's capacity and motivation for work. The deviance and social-control aspects of illness have important implications for the polity which, in turn, is responsible for the organized enforcement of health measures that pertain to the community or public welfare. And in all societies, the influence, power, and prestige that accrue to medical practitioners implicate the magico-religious and stratification systems as well as the polity.[9]

As the foregoing implies, there are certain respects in which health, illness, and medicine are imbued with a more diffuse and sacred kind of significance in nonmodern than in modern societies. For example, in traditional and neo-traditional Central African societies, the meaning of health and illness, the diagnosis and treatment of sickness, And the wisdom, efficacy, and power of medical practitioners are not only more closely linked with the institutions of kinship, religion, and magic than in American society; they are also more closely connected with the overarching cosmic view through which the whole society defines and orients itself. One indication of the larger matrix into which health, illness, and medicine fit in such a society is that in numerous Central African languages the same words can mean medicine, magico-religious charms, and metaphysically important qualities such as strength, fecundity, and invulnerability, which are believed to be supernaturally conferred.

In the light of the multi-institutional and the cultural significance of health, illness, and medicine in all societies it is both illogical and unlikely to believe that the current process of medicalization in American society has been engineered and maintained primarily by one group, namely, the physicians. What the manifestations of medicalization that we have identified do suggest, however, is that the health-illness-medical sector has progressively acquired a more general cultural meaning in American society than it had in the past.[10]

Within this framework, the medicalization process entails the assertion of various individual and collective rights to which members of the society feel entitled and which they express as "health," "quality of life," and "quality of death." The process also involves heightened awareness of a whole, range of imperfections, injustices, dangers, and afflictions that are perceived to exist in the society, a protest against them, and a re-

9 These ideas are presented in more detail in the monograph I am currently writing on "Medical Sociology" which will appear as a volume in the Prentice-Hall *Foundations of Modern Sociology* series.

10 See article by John H. Knowles, "The Responsibility of the Individual," in J.H. Knowles (Ed.), *Doing better and feeling worse: Health in the United States* (pp. 57-80). New York: Norton & Company.

solve to take action that is more therapeutic than punitive. Medicalization represents an exploration and affirmation of values and beliefs that not only pertain to the ultimate grounding of the society, but also to the human condition, more encompassingly and existentially conceived.

Thus, in American society, health and illness have come to symbolize many positively and negatively valued biological, physical, social, cultural, and metaphysical phenomena. Increasingly, health has become a coded way of referring to an individually, socially, or cosmically ideal state of affairs. Conversely, the concept of illness has increasingly been applied to modes of thinking, feeling, and behaving that are considered undesirably variant or deviant, as well as to more forms of suffering and disability. In turn, this medicalization of deviance and suffering has had a network of consequences.

Talcott Parsons's well-known formulation of the "sick role" provides important insights into what these effects have been. According to him,[11] the sick role consists of two interrelated sets of exemptions and obligations. A person who is defined as ill is exonerated from certain kinds of responsibility for his illness. He is not held morally accountable for the fact that he is sick (it is not considered to be his "fault"), and he is not expected to make himself better by "good motivation" or high resolve without the help of others. In addition, he is viewed as someone whose capacity to function formally is impaired, and who is therefore relieved of some of his usual familial, occupational, and civic activities and responsibilities. In exchange for these exemptions which are conditionally granted, the sick individual is expected to define the state of being ill as aberrant and undesirable, and to do everything possible to facilitate his recovery from it. In the case of illness of any moment, the responsibility to try to get well also entalls the obligation to seek professionally competent help. In a modern Western society, such as the United States, this obligation involves a willingness to confer with a medically trained person, usually a physician, and to undergo the modes of diagnosis and treatment that are recommended, including the ministrations of other medical professionals and hospitalization. Upon entering this relationship with institutionalized medicine and its professional practitioners, an individual with a health problem becomes a patient. By cooperating and collaborating with the medical professionals caring for him, the patient is expected to work toward recovery, or, at least, toward the more effective management of his illness.

The fact that the exemptions and the obligations of sickness have been extended to people with a widening arc of attitudes, experiences, and behaviors in American society means primarily that what is regarded as "conditionally legitimate deviance" has increased. Although illness is defined as deviance from the desirable and the normal, it is not viewed as reprehensible in the way that either sin or crime is. The sick person is neither blamed nor punished as those considered sinful or criminal are. So long as he does not abandon himself to illness or eagerly embrace it, but works actively on his own and with medical professionals to improve his condition, he is considered to be responding appropriately, even admirably, to an unfortunate occurrence. Under these conditions, illness is accepted as legitimate deviance. But this also implies that medical professionals have acquired an increasingly important social-control function in the society. They are the principal agents responsible for certifying, diagnosing, treating, and preventing illness. Be-

11 Talcott Parsons's formulation of the sick role is the most important single concept in the field of the sociology of medicine. For his own elaboration of this concept, see, especially, Talcott Parsons, *The Social System* (Glencoe, Illinois), pp. 428-79, and "The Sick Role and the Role of the Physician Reconsidered," *Milbank Memorial Fund Quartery, Health and Society* (Summer, 1975), pp. 257-77.

cause a greater proportion of deviance in American society is now seen as illness, the-medical profession plays a more important role than it once did in defining and regulating deviance and in to forestall and remedy it.

The economic, political, and legal-indicators of a progressive medicalization cited above also have complex origins and implications. For example, the fact that activities connected with health, illness, and medicine represent a rising percentage of the gross national product in the United States is a consequence of the fee-for-service system under which American health-care delivery is organized; the central importance of the modern hospital in medical care; the mounting personnel, equipment, and maintenance costs that the operation of the hospital entalls; and the development of new medical and surgical procedures and of new drugs, most of which are as expensive as they are efficacious. Some of this increase in costs results from the desire for profits that medical professionals, hospital administrators, and members of the pharmaceutical industry share to varying degrees. But how much is difficult to ascertain, though radical ideological criticisms and defensive conservative statements on the point are both rife at present.

In addition to such political and economic factors, the heightened commitment to health as a right and the medicalization of deviance have also contributed to the growth of health expenditures. Because health is both more coveted and more inclusively defined, and because a greater amount of medical therapeutic activity is applied to deviance-defined-as-illness, increasing economic resources are being invested in the health-illness-medicine sector of the society.

The political and legal prominence of questions of health care and medicine in American society at the present time reflects in part a widespread national discontent with the way medical care is organized, financed, and delivered, and with some of the attitudes and behaviors of physicians. The inequities that exist in access to care, and in its technical and interpersonal excellence, are among the primary foci of political and legal activities. Another major area of current political and legal action concerns the internal and external regulation of the medical profession better to insure that it uses its knowledge and skill in a socially as well as medically responsible way, and that it is adequately accountable both to patients and to the public at large. Various new measures, which represent a mixture of controls from within the medical profession and from outside it, have been set into motion. For example, in 1972, the Professional Standards Review Organization was established through the passage of amendments to the Social Security Act which were designed to provide quality assessment and assurance, utilization review, and cost control, primarily for Medicare and Medicaid patients. Over the course of the years 1966 through 1971, a series of government regulations were passed which mandate peer review for all biomedical research involving human subjects, supported by the Department of Health, Education, and Welfare (and its subunits, the National Institutes of Health and the Public Health Service), as well as by the Food and Drug Administration. In 1975, the American College of Surgeons and the American Surgical Association set forth a plan for systematically decreasing the number of newly graduated doctors entering surgical training. In part, this plan represented an organized, intraprofessional attempt to deal with what appears to be an oversupply of surgeons in the United States, and thereby to reduce the possibility that federal health manpower legislation would have to be passed to remedy this maldistribution.

The fact that an extraordinary number of young people are opting for careers in health, particularly as physicians, is the final concomitant of medicalization previously mentioned. Reliable and valid data are not available to explain the mounting wave of young persons who have been attracted to medicine since the nineteen sixties. We do not know as much as we should about how they resemble their predecessors, or differ from them. We are aware that more women, blacks, and members of other minority groups are being admitted to medical school than in the past, partly because of "affirmative action" legislation. But we do not have overall information about the characteristics of those who are accepted as compared with those who are not. Only sketchy materials are available on the impact of those changes in medical-school curricula during the past decade that were designed to make students more aware of the social and ethical dimensions of their commitment to medicine. We do not know whether their attitudes, their professional decisions, or their medical practice actually changed. More data are needed before we can interpret the short- and long-term implications of the rush of college youth toward medicine. As premedical and medical students themselves are first to testify, the prestige, authority, "power," autonomy, and financial rewards of medicine attract them and their peers to medicine, along with scientific interests, clinical impulses, and humanitarian concerns. But there is also evidence to suggest that even among those who readily contend that their reasons for choosing medicine are self-interested, a "new" medical-student orientation has been emerging. In fact, the very candor that medical students exhibit—and in some cases flaunt—when they insist that, regrettably, like their predecessors, their competitiveness, desire for achievenient, and need for security have drawn them into medicine is part of this new orientation. Activist and meditative, as well as critical and self-critical, the "new medical student" not only wants to bring about change in the medical profession, but to do so in a way that affects other aspects of the society as well. The structural and symbolic meaning acquired by health, illness, and medicine has led such students to hope that their influence will be far-reaching as well as meliorative. How many students with this ostensibly "new" orientation will maintain it throughout their medical training and whether their entrance into the profession will significantly alter the future course of medicalization in American society remain to be seen.[12]

Along with progressive medicalization, a process of demedicalization seems also to be taking place in the society. To some extent the signs of demedicalization are actions to what is felt by various individuals and groups to be a state of "*over*- medicalization." One of the most significant manifestations of this counter-trend is the mounting concern over implications that have arisen from the continuously expanding conception of "sickness" in the society. Commentators on this process would not necessarily agree with Peter Sedgwick that it will continue to "the point where everybody has become so luxuriantly ill" that perhaps sickness will no longer be "in" and a "backlash" will be set in motion;[13] they may not envision such an engulfing state of societally defined illness. But many observers from diverse professional backgrounds have published works in which they express concern about the coercive" aspects of the "label" illness and the treatment of illness by medical institutions.[14] The admonitory perspectives on the enlarged domain

12 12. See Renee C. Fox, "The Process of Professional Socialization: Is There a 'New' Medical Student? A Comparative View of Medical Socialization in the 1950's and the 1970's," in Laurence R. Tancredi, ed., *Ethics in Health Care* (Washington, D.C., 1974), pp. 197-227.

13 Sedgwick, "Illness—Mental and Otherwise," p. 37.

14 In addition to Illich, *Medical Nemesis,* and Kittrie, *The Right To Be Different,* see, for example, Rick J. Carlson, *The End of Medicine* (New York, 1975); Michael Foucault, *Madness and Civilization* (New York, 1967); Eliot Freidson, *Professional Dominance* (Chicago, 1970); Erving Goffman, *Asylums* (New York, 1961); R. D. Laing, *The Politics of Experience* (New York, 1967); Thomas J. Scheff, *Being Mentally Ill* (Chicago, 1966); Thomas S. Szasz, *The Myth of Mental Illness* (New York, 196 1); and Howard D. Waitzkin and Barbara Waterman, *The Exploitation of Illness in Capitalist Society* (Indianapolis, 1974).

of illness and medicine that these works of social science and social criticism represent appear to have gained the attention of young physicians- and nurses-in-training interested in change, and various consumer and civil-rights groups interested in health care.

This emerging view emphasizes the degree to which what is defined as health and illness, normality and abnormality, sanity and insanity varies from one society, culture, and historical period to another. Thus, it is contended, medical diagnostic categories such as "sick," "abnormal," and "insane" are not universal, objective, or necessarily reliable. Rather, they are culture-, class-, and time-bound, often ethnocentric and as much artifacts of the preconceptions of socially biased observers as they are valid summaries of the characteristics of the observed. In this view, illness (especially mental illness) is largely a mythical construct, created and enforced by the society. The hospitals to which seriously ill persons are confined are portrayed as "total institutions": segregated, encompassing, depersonalizing organizations, "dominated" by physicians who are disinclined to convey information to patients about their conditions, or to encourage paramedical personnel to do so. These "oppressive" and "counter-therapeutic" attributes of the hospital environment are seen as emanating from the professional ideology of physicians and the kind of hierarchical relationships that they establish with patients and other medical prefessionals partly as a consequence of this ideology, as well as from the bureaucratic and technological features of the hospital itself. Whatever their source, the argument continues, the characteristics of the hospital and of the doctor-patient relationship increase the "powerlessness" of the sick person, "maintain his uncertainty," and systematically "mortify" and "curtail" the "self" with which he enters the sick role and arrives at the hospital door.

This critical perspective links the labeling of illness, the "imperialist" outlook and capitalist behavior of physicians, the "stigmatizing" and "dehumanizing" experiences of patients, and the problems of the health-care system more generally to imperfections and injustices in the society as a whole. Thus, for example, the various forms of social inequality, prejudice, discrimination, and acquisitive self-interest that persist in capitalistic American society are held responsible for causing illness, as well as for contributing to the undesirable attitudes and actions of physicians and other medical professionals. Casting persons in the sick role is regarded as a powerful, latent way for the society to exact conformity and maintain the status quo. For it allows a semi-approved form of deviance to occur which siphons off potential for insurgent protest and which can be controlled through the supervision or, in some cases, the "enforced therapy" of the medical profession. Thus, however permissive and merciful it may be to expand the category of illness, these observers point out, there is always the danger that the society will become a "therapeutic state" that excessively restricts the "right to be different" and the right to dissent. They feel that this danger may already have reached serious proportions in this society through its progressive medicalization.

The criticism of medicalization and the advocacy of demedicalization have not been confined to rhetoric. Concrete steps have been taken to declassify certain conditions as illness. Most notable among these is the American Psychiatric Association's decision to remove homosexuality from its official catalogue ("Nomenclature") of mental disorders. In addition, serious efforts have been made to heighten physicians' awareness of the fact that because they share certain prejudiced, often unconscious assumptions about women, they tend to over-attribute psychological conditions to their female patients. Thus, for example, distinguished medical publications such as the *New England Journal of Medicine* have featured articles and editorials on the excessive readiness with which medical specialists and textbook authors accept the undocumented belief that dysmenorrhea, nausea of pregnancy, pain in labor, and infantile colic are all psychogenic disorders, caused or aggravated by women's emotional problems. Another related development is feminist protest against what is felt to be a too great tendency to define pregnancy as an illness, and childbirth as a "technologized" medical-surgical event, prevailed over by the obstetrician-gynecologist. These sentiments have contributed to the preference that many middle-class couples have shown for natural childbirth in recent years, and to the revival of midwifery. The last example also illustrates an allied movement, namely a growing tendency to shift some responsibility for medical care and authority over it from the physician, the medical team, and hospital to the patient, the family, and the home.

A number of attempts to "destratify" the doctor's relationships with patients and with other medical professionals and to make them more open and egalitarian have developed. "Patients' rights" are being asserted and codified, and, in some states, drafted into law. Greater emphasis is being placed, for example, on the patient's "right to treatment," right to information (relevant to diagnosis, therapy, prognosis, or to the giving of knowledgeable consent for any procedure), right to privacy and confidentiality, and right to be "allowed to die," rather than being "kept alive by artificial means or heroic measures . . . if the situation should arise in which there is reasonable expectation of . . . recovery from physical or mental disability.[15] In some medical milieux (for example, community health centers and health maintenance organizations), and in critical and self-consciously progressive writings about medicine, the term "client" or "consumer" is being substituted for "patient." This change in terminology is intended to underline theimportance of preventing illness while stressing the desirability of a non-supine, non-subordinate relationship for those who seek care to those who provide it. The emergence of nurse-practitioners and physician's assistants on the American scene is perhaps the most significant sign that some blurring of the physician's supremacy vis-a-vis other medical professionals may also be taking place. For some of the responsibilities for diagnosis, treatment, and patient management that were formerly prerogatives of physicians have been incorporated into these new, essentially marginal roles.[16]

Enjoinders to patients to care for themselves rather than to rely so heavily on the services of medical professionals and institutions are more frequently heard. Much attention is being given to studies such as the one conducted by Lester Breslow and his colleagues at the University of California at Los Angeles which suggest that good health and longevity are as much related to a self-enforced regimen of sufficient sleep, regular, well-balanced meals, moderate exercise and weight, no smoking, and little or no drinking, as they are to professionally administered medical care. Groups such as those involved in the Women's Liberation Movement are advocating the social and psychic as well as the medical value of knowing, examining, and caring for one's own body. Self-therapy techniques and programs have been developed for conditions as complicated and grave as terminal renal-disease and hemophilia A and B. Proponents of such regimens affirm that many aspects of managing even serious chronic illnesses can be handled safely at home by the patient and his family, who will, in turn, benefit both financially and emotionally. In addition, they claim that in many cases the biomedical results obtained seem superor to those of the traditional physician-administered health-care-delivery system.

---

15 This particular way of requesting that one be allowed to die is excerpted from the "Living Will" (revised April, 1974, version), prepared and promoted by the Euthanasia Educational Council.

16 See the article by David Rogers, "The Challenge of Primary Care," in J.H. Knowles (Ed.), *Doing better and feeling worse: Health in the United States.* (pp. 81-104). New York: Norton & Company.

The underlying assumption in these instances is that, if self-care is collectivized and reinforced by mutual aid, not only will persons with a medical problem be freed from some of the exigencies of the sick role, but both personal and public health will thereby improve, all with considerable savings in cost. This point of view is based on the moral supposition that greater autonomy from the medical profession coupled with greater responsibility for self and others in the realm of health and illness is an ethically and societally superior state.

> We have the medicine we deserve. We freely choose to live the way we do. We choose to live recklessly, to abuse our bodies with what we consume, to expose ourselves to environmental insults, to rush frantically from place to place, and to sit on our spreading bottoms and watch paid professionals exercise for us. . . . Today few patients have the confidence to care for themselves. The inexorable professionalization of medicine, together with reverence for the scientific method, have invested practitioners with sacrosanct powers, and correspondingly vitiated the responsibility of the rest of us for health. . . . What is tragic is not what has happened to the happened to the revered professions, but what has happened to us as a result of professional dominance. In times of inordinate complexity and stress we have been made a profoundly dependent people. Most of us have lost the ability to care for ourselves. . . . I have tried to demonstrate three propositions. First, medical care has less impact on health than is generally assumed. Second, medical-care has less impact on health than have social and environmental factors. And third, given the way in which society is evolving and the evolutionary imperatives of the medical care system, medical care in the future will have even less impact on health than it has now. . . . We have not understood what health is. . . . But in the next few decades our understanding will deepen. The pursuit of health and of well-being will then be possible, but only if our environment is made safe for us to live in and our social order is transformed to foster health, rather than suppress joy. If not, we shall remain a sick and dependent people. . . . The end of medicine is not the end of health but the beginning. . . .[17]

The foregoing passage (excerpted from Rick Carlson's book, *The End of Medicine)* touches upon many of the demedicalization themes that have been discussed. It proclaims the desirability of demedicalizing American society, predicting that, if we do so, we can overcome the "harm" that excessive medicalization has brought in its wake and progress beyond the "limits" that it has set. Like most critics of medicalization on the American scene, Carlson inveighs against the way that medical care is currently organized and implemented, but he attaches exceptional importance to the health-illness-medical sector of the society. In common with other commentators, he views health, illness, and medicine as inextricably associated with values and beliefs of American tradition that are both critical and desirable. It is primarily for this reason that in spite of the numerous signs that certain *structural* changes in the delivery of care will have occurred by the time we reach the year 2000, American society is not likely to undergo a significant process of *cultural* demedicalization.

Dissatisfaction with the distribution of professional medical care in the United States, its costs, and its accessibility has become sufficiently acute and generalized to make the enactment of a national health-insurance system in the foreseeable future likely. Exactly what form that system should take still evokes heated debate about free enterprise and socialism, public and private regulation, national and local government, tax rates, deductibles and co-insurance, the right to health care, the equality principle, and the principle of distributive justice. But the institutionalization of a national system that will provide more extensive and equitable health-insurance protection

17 Carlson, The End of Medicine, pp. 44, 141, and 203-31.

now seems necessary as well as inevitable even to those who do not approve of it.

There is still another change in the health-illness-medicine area of the society that seems to be forthcoming and that, like national health insurance, would alter the structure within which care is delivered. This is the movement toward effecting greater equality, collegiatity, and accountability in the relationship of physicians to patients and their families, to other medical professionals, and to the lay public. Attempts to reduce the hierarchical dimension in the physician's role, as well as the increased insistence on patient's rights, self-therapy, mutual medical aid, community medical services and care by non-physician health professionals, and the growth of legislative and judicial participation in health and medicine by both federal and local government are all part of this movement. There is reason to believe that, as a consequence of pressure from both outside and inside the medical profession, the doctor will become less "dominant" and "autonomous," and will be subject to more controls.

This evolution in the direction of greater egalitarianism and regulation notwithstanding, it seems unlikely that all elements of hierarchy and autonomy will, or even can, be eliminated from the physician's role. For that to occur, the medical knowledge, skill, experience, and responsibility of patients and paramedical professionals would have to equal, if not replicate, the physician's. In addition, the social and psychic meaning of health and illness would have to become trivial in order to remove all vestiges of institutionalized charisma from the physician's role. Health, illness, and medicine have never been viewed casually in any society and, as indicated, they seem to be gaining rather than losing importance in American society.

It is significant that often the discussions and developments relevant to the destratification and control of the physician's role and to the enactment of national health insurance are accompanied by reaffirmations of traditional American values: equality, independence, self-reliance, universalism, distributive justice, solidarity, reciprocity, and individual and community responsibility. What seems to be involved here is not so much a change in values as the initiation of action intended to modify certain structural features of American medicine, so that it will more fully realize long-standing societal values.

In contrast, the new emphasis on health as a right, along with the emerging perspective on illness as medically and socially engendered, seems to entail major conceptual rather than structural shifts in the health-illness-medical matrix of the society. These shifts are indicative of a less fatalistic and individualistic attitude toward illness, increased personal and communal espousal of health, and a spreading conviction that health is as much a consequence of the good life and the good society as it is of professional medical care. The strongest impetus for demedicalization comes from this altered point of view. It will probably contribute to the decategorization of certain conditions as illness, greater appreciation and utilization of non-physician medical professionals, the institutionalization of more preventive medicine and personal and public health measures, and, perhaps, to the undertaking of non-medical reforms (such as full employment, improved transportation, or adequate recreation) in the name of the ultimate goal of health.

However, none of these trends implies that what we have called *cultural* demedicalization will take place. The shifts in emphasis from illness to health, from therapeutic to preventive medicine, and from the dominance and autonomy of the doctor to patient's rights and greater control of the medical profession do not alter the fact that health, illness, and medicine are central preoccupations in the society which have diffuse symbolic as well as practical meaning. All signs suggest that they will maintain the social, ethical, and existential significance they have acquired, even though by the year 2000 some structural aspects of the way that medicine and care are organized and delivered may have changed. In fact, if the issues now being considered the rubric of bioethics are predictive of what lies ahead, we can expect that in the future, health, illness, and medicine will acquire even greater importance as one of primary symbolic media through which American society will grapple with fundmental questions of value and belief. What social mechanisms we will develop to come to terms with these "collective conscience" issues, and exactly what role physicians, health professionals, biologists, jurists, politicians, philosophers, theologians, social scientists, and the public at large will play in their resolution remains to be seen. But it is a distinctive characteristic of an advanced modern society like our own that scientific, technical, clinical, social, ethical, and religious concerns should be joined in this way.

The Recovery of Health

Ivan Illich

Much suffering has been man-made. The history of man is one long catalogue of enslavement and exploitation, usually told in the epics of conquerors or sung in the elegies of their victims. War is at the heart of this tale, war and the pillage, famine, and pestilence that came in its wake. But it was not until modern times that the unwanted physical, social, and psychological side-effects of so-called peaceful enterprises began to compete with war in destructive power.

Man is the only animal whose evolution has been conditioned by adaptation on more than one front. If he did not succumb to predators and forces of nature, he had to cope with use and abuse by others of his own kind. In his struggle with the elements and with his neighbor, his character and culture were formed, his instincts withered, and his territory was turned into a *home*.

Animals adapt through evolution in response to changes in their natural environment. Only in man does challenge become conscious and the response to difficult and threatening situations take the form of rational action and of conscious habit. Man can design his relations to nature and neighbor, and he is able to survive even when his enterprise has partly failed. He is the animal that can endure trials with patience and learn by understanding them. He is the sole being who can and must resign himself to limits when he becomes aware of them. A conscious response to painful sensations, to impairment, and to eventual death is part of man's coping ability. The capacity for revolt and for perseverance, for stubborn resistance and for resignation, are integral parts of human life and health.

But nature and neighbor are only two of the three frontiers on which man must cope. A third front where doom can threaten has always been recognized. To remain viable, man must also survive the dreams which so far myth has both shaped and controlled. Now society must develop programs to cope with the irrational desires of its most gifted members. To date, myth has fulfilled the function of setting limits to the materialization of greedy, envious, murderous dreams. Myth assured the common man of his safety on this third frontier if he kept within its bounds. Myth guaranteed disaster to those few who tried to outwit the gods. The common man perished from infirmity or from violence; only the rebel against the human condition fell prey to Nemesis, the envy of the gods.

Industrialized Nemesis

Prometheus was hero, not Everyman. Driven by radical greed *(pleonexia),* he trespassed beyond the limits of man (*aitia and mesotes*) and in unbounded presumption (*hubris*) stole fire from heaven.[1] He thus inevitably brought Nemesis on

Illich, I. Medical Nemisis. London: Calder and Boyars, 1975 pp. 251-275.

1 On the political use of divine envy, see Svend Ranulf, *The Jealousy of the Gods and Criminal Law in Athens*, trans. Annie J. Fausboll, 2 vols (Copenhagen: Levin Y Munksgaard, 1933-34). On hubris calling forth nemesis, see David Grene, *Greek Political Theory: The Image of Man in Thucydides and Plato* (Chicago: Univ. of Chicago Press, Phoenix

himself He was put into irons and chained to a Caucasian rock. An eagle preyed all day on his liver, and heartlessly healing gods kept him alive by regrafting his liver each night. Nemesis inflicted on him a kind of pain meant for demigods, not for men. His hopeless and unending suffering turned the hero into an immortal reminder of inescapable cosmic retaliation.

The social nature of nemesis has now changed. With the industrialization of desire and the engineering of corresponding ritual responses, hubris has spread. Unbounded material progress has become Everyman's goal. Industrial hubris has destroyed the mythical framework of limits to irrational fantasies, has made technical answers to mad dreams seem rational, and has turned the pursuit of destructive values into a conspiracy between purveyor and client. Nemesis for the masses is now the inescapable backlash of industrial progress. Modern nemesis is the material monster born from the overarching industrial dream. It has spread as far and as wide as universal schooling, mass transportation, industrial wage labor, and the medicalization of health.

Inherited myths have ceased to provide limits for action. If the species is to survive the loss of its traditional myths, it must learn to cope rationally and politically with its envious, greedy, and lazy dreams. Myth alone can do the job no more. Politically established limits to industrial growth will have to take the place of mythological boundaries. Political exploration and recognition of the necessary material conditions for survival, equity, and effectiveness will have to set limits to the industrial mode of production.

Nemesis has become structural and endemic. Increasingly, man-made misery is the by-product of enterprises that were supposed to protect ordinary people in their struggle with the inclemency of the environment and against the wanton injustice inflicted on them by the elite. The main source of pain, of disability, and of death is now engineered, albeit nonintentional, harassment. Our prevailing ailments, helplessness, and injustice are largely the side-effects of strategies for more and better education, better housing, a better diet, and better health.

A society that values planned teaching above autonomous learning cannot but teach man to keep his engineered place. A society that relies for locomotion on managed transport must do the same. Beyond a certain level, energy used for transportation immobilizes and enslaves the majority of nameless passengers and provides advantages only for the elite. No new fuel, technology, or public controls can keep the rising mobilization and acceleration of society from producing rising harriedness, programmed paralysis, and inequality. The same is true for agriculture. Beyond a certain level of capital investment in the growing and processing of food, malnutrition will become pervasive. The results of the Green Revolution will then rack the livers of consumers more thoroughly than Zeus's eagle. No biological engineering can prevent undernourishment and food poisoning beyond this point. What is happening in the sub-Saharan Sahel is only a dress rehearsal for encroaching world famine. This is but the application of a general law: When more than a certain proportion of value is produced by the industrial mode, subsistence activities are paralyzed, equity declines, and total satisfaction diminishes. It will not be the sporadic famine that formerly came with drought and war, or the occasional food shortage that could be remedied by good will and emergency shipments. The coming hunger is a by-product of the inevitable concentration of industrialized agriculture in rich countries and in the fertile regions of poor countries. Paradoxically, the attempt to counter famine by further increases in industrially efficient agriculture only

Books, 1965; orig. *Man in His Pride*); and E.R. Dodds, *The Greeks and the Irrational* (Berkeley: Univ. of California Press, 1951), especially chap. 2.

widens the scope of the catastrophe by depressing the use of marginal lands. Famine will increase until the trend towards capital-intensive food production by the poor for the rich has been replaced by a new kind of labor-intensive, regional, rural autonomy. Beyond a certain level of industrial hubris, nemesis *must* set in, because progress, like the broom of the sorcerer's apprentice, can no longer be turned off.

Defenders of industrial progress are either blind or corrupt if they pretend that they can calculate the price of progress. The torts resulting from nemesis cannot be compensated, calculated, or liquidated. The down-payment for industrial development might seem reasonable, but the compound-interest installments on expanding production now accrue in suffering beyond any measure or price. When members of a society are regularly asked to pay an even higher price for industrially defined necessities—in spite of evidence that they are purchasing more suffering with each unit—*Homo economics*, driven by the pursuit of marginal benefits, turns into *Home religiosus*; sacrificing himself to industrial ideology. At this point, social behavior begins to resemble that of the drug addict. Expectations become irrational and nightmarish. The self-inflicted portion of suffering outweighs the damage done by nature and all the torts inflicted by neighbors. Hubris motivates self-destructive mass behavior. Classical nemesis was the punishment for the rash abuse of privilege. Industrial nemesis is the retribution for dutiful participation in the technical pursuit of dreams unchecked by traditional mythology or rational self-restraint.

War and hunger, pestilence and natural catastrophes, torture and madness remain man's companions, but they are not shaped into a new *Gestalt* by the nemesis that overtakes them. The greater the economic progress of any community, the greater the part played by industrial nemesis in pain, impairment, discrimination, and death. The more intense the reliance on techniques making for dependence, the higher the rate of waste, degradation, and pathogenesis which must be countered by yet other techniques and the larger the work force active in the removal of garbage, in the management of waste, and in the treatment of people made literally redundant by progress.

Reactions to impending disaster still take the form of better educational curricula, more health-maintenance services, or more efficient and less polluting energy transformers, and solutions are still sought in better engineering of industrial systems. The syndrome corresponding to nemesis is recognized, but its etiology is still sought in bad engineering compounded by self-serving management, whether under the control of Wall Street or of The Party. Nemesis is not yet recognized as the materialization of a social answer to a profoundly mistaken ideology, nor is it yet understood as a rampant delusion fostered by the nontechnical, ritual structure of our major industrial institutions. just as Galilee's contemporaries refused to look through the telescope at Jupiter's moons because they feared that their geocentric world- view would be shaken, so our contemporaries refuse to face nemesis because they feel incapable of putting the autonomous rather than the industrial mode of production at the center of their sociopolitical constructs.

From Inherited Myth to Respectful Procedure

Primitive people have always recognized the power of a symbolic dimension; they have seen themselves as threatened by the tremendous, the awesome, the uncanny. This dimension set boundaries not only to the power of the king and the magician, but also to that of the artisan and the technician. Malinowski claims that only industrial society has allowed the use of available tools to their utmost efficiency; in all other societies, recognizing sacred limits to the use of sword and of plow was a necessary foundation for ethics. Now, after several generations of licentious technology, the finiteness of nature intrudes again upon our consciousness. The limits of the universe are subject to operational probings. Yet at this moment of crisis it would be foolish to found the limits of human actions on some substantive ecological ideology which would modernize the mythic sacredness of nature. The engineering of an eco-religion would be a caricature of traditional hubris. Only a widespread agreement on the procedures through which the autonomy of postindustrial man can be equitably guaranteed will lead to the recognition of the necessary limits to human action.

Common to all ethics is the assumption that the human act is performed within the human condition. Since the various ethical systems assumed, tacitly or explicitly, that this human condition was more or less given, once and for all, the range of human action was narrowly circumscribed.

In our industrialized epoch, however, not only the object but also the very nature of human action is new.[2] Instead of facing gods we confront the blind forces of nature, and instead of facing the dynamic limits of a universe we have now come to know, we act as if these limits did not translate into critical thresholds for human action. Traditionally the categorical imperative could circumscribe and validate action as being truly human. Directly enjoining limits to one's actions, it demanded respect for the equal freedom of others. The loss of a normative "human condition" introduces a newness not only into the human act but also into the human attitude towards the framework in which a person acts. If this action is to remain human after the framework has been deprived of its sacred character, it needs a recognized ethical foundation within a new imperative. This imperative can be summed up only as follows: "Act so that the effect of your action is compatible with the permanence of genuine human life." Very concretely applied, this could mean: "Do not raise radiation levels unless you know that this action will not be visited upon your grandchild." Such an imperative obviously cannot be formulated as long as "genuine human life" is considered an infinitely elastic concept.

Is it possible, without restoring the category of the sacred, to attain the ethics that alone would enable mankind to accept the rigorous discipline of this new imperative? If not, rationalizations could be created for any atrocity: "Why should background radiation not be raised? Our grandchildren will get used to it!" In some instances, fear might help preserve minimal sanity, but only when consequences were fairly imminent. Breeder reactors might not be made operational for fear that they would serve the Mafia for next year's extortions or cause cancer before the operator died. But only the awe of the sacred, with its unqualified veto, has so far proved independent of the computations of mundane self-interest and the solace of uncertainty about remote consequences. This could be reinvoked as an imperative that genuine human life deserves respect both now and in the future. This recourse to the sacred, however, has been blocked in our present crisis. Recourse to faith provides an escape for those who believe, but it cannot be the foundation for an ethical imperative, because faith is either there or not there; if it is absent, the faithful cannot blame the infidel. Recent history has shown that the taboos of traditional cultures are irrelevant in combatting an overextension of industrial production. The taboos were tied to the values of a particular society and its mode of production, and it is precisely those that were irrevocably lost in the process of industrialization.

It is not necessary, probably not feasible, and certainly not desirable to base the limitation of industrial societies on a shared system of substantive beliefs aiming at the common good and enforced by the power of the police. It is possible to find the needed basis for ethical human action

---

2 I have taken this argument, in part, verbatim from Hans Jonas, "Technology and Responsibility: Reflections on the New Task of Ethics," *Social Research* 40 (1972):31-54.

without depending on the shared recognition of any ecological dogmatism now in vogue. This alternative to a new ecological religion or ideology is based on an agreement about basic values and on procedural rules.

It can be demonstrated that beyond a certain point in the expansion of industrial production in any major field of value, marginal utilities cease to be equitably distributed and over-all effectiveness begins, simultaneously, to decline. If the industrial mode of production expands beyond a certain stage and continues to impinge on the autonomous mode, increased personal suffering and social dissolution set in. In the interim-between the point of optimal synergy between industrial and autonomous production and the point of maximum tolerable industrial hegemony-political and juridical procedures become necessary to reverse industrial expansion. If these procedures are conducted in a spirit of enlightened self-interest and a desire for survival, and with equitable distribution of social outputs and equitable access to social control, the outcome ought to be a recognition of the carrying capacity of the environment and of the optimal industrial complement to autonomous action needed for the effective pursuit of personal goals. Political procedures oriented to the value of survival in distributive and participatory equity are the only possible rational answer to increasing total management in the name of ecology.

The recovery of personal autonomy will thus be the result of political action reinforcing an ethical awakening. People will want to limit transportation because they want to move efficiently, freely, and with equity; they will limit schooling because they want to share equally the opportunity, time, and motivation to learn *in* rather than *about* the world; people will limit medical therapies because they want to conserve their opportunity and power to heal. They will recognize that only the disciplined limitation of power can provide equitably shared satisfaction.

The recovery of autonomous action will depend, not on new specific goals people share, but on their use of legal and political procedures that permit individuals and groups to resolve conflicts arising from their pursuit of different goals. Better mobility will depend, not on some new kind of transportation system, but on conditions that make personal mobility under personal control more valuable. Better learning opportunities will depend, not on more information about the world better distributed, but on the limitation of capital-intensive production for the sake of interesting working conditions. Better health care will depend, not on some new therapeutic standard, but on the level of willingness and competence to engage in self-care. The recovery of this power depends on the recognition of our present delusions.

The Right to Health

Increasing and irreparable damage accompanies present industrial expansion in all sectors. In medicine this damage appears as iatrogenesis. Iatrogenesis is clinical when pain, sickness, and death result from medical care; it is social when health policies reinforce an industrial organization that generates ill-health; it is cultural and symbolic when medically sponsored behavior and delusions restrict the vital autonomy of people by undermining their competence in growing up, caring for each other, and aging, or when medical intervention cripples personal responses to pain, disability, impairment, anguish, and death.

Most of the remedies now proposed by the social engineers and economists to reduce iatrogenesis include a further increase of medical controls. These so-called remedies generate second-order iatrogenic ills on each of the three critical levels: they render clinical, social, and cultural iatrogenesis self-reinforcing.

The most profound iatrogenic effects of the medical technostructure are a result of those nontechnical functions which support the increasing institutionalization of values. The technical and the nontechnical consequences of institutional medicine coalesce and generate a new kind of suffering: anesthetized, impotent, and solitary survival in a world turned into a hospital ward. Medical nemesis is the experience of people who are largely deprived of any autonomous ability to cope with nature, neighbors, and dreams, and who are technically maintained within environmental, social, and symbolic systems. Medical nemesis cannot be measured, but its experience can be shared. The intensity with which it is experienced will depend on the independence, vitality, and relatedness of each individual.

The perception of nemesis leads to a choice. Either the natural boundaries of human endeavor are estimated, recognized, and translated into politically determined limits, or compulsory survival in a planned and engineered hell is accepted as the alternative to extinction. Until recently the choice between the politics of voluntary poverty and the hell of the systems engineer did not fit into the language of scientists or politicians. Our increasing confrontation with medical nemesis now lends new significance to the alternative: either society must choose the same stringent limits on the kind of goods produced within which all its members may find a guarantee for equal freedom, or society must accept unprecedented hierarchical controls [3] to provide for each member what welfare bureaucracies diagnose as his or her needs.

In several nations the public is now ready for a review of its health-care system. Although there is a serious danger that the forthcoming debate will reinforce the present frustrating medicalization of life, the debate could still become fruitful if attention were focused on medical nemesis, if the recovery of personal responsibility for health care were made the central issue, and if limitations on professional monopolies were made the major goal of legislation. Instead of limiting the resources of doctors and of the institutions that employ them, such legislation would tax medical technology and professional activity until those means that can be handled by laymen were truly available to anyone wanting access to them. Instead of multiplying the specialists who can grant any one of a variety of sick-roles to people made ill by their work and their life, the new legislation would guarantee the right of people to drop out and to organize for a less destructive way of life in which they have more control of their environment. Instead of restricting access to addictive, dangerous, or useless drugs and procedures, such legislation would shift the full burden of their responsible use onto the sick person and his next of kin. Instead of submitting the physical and mental integrity of citizens to more and more wardens, such legislation would recognize each man's right to define his own health-subject only to limitations imposed by respect for his neighbor's rights. Instead of strengthening the licensing power of specialized peers and government agencies, new legislation would give the public a voice in the election of healers to tax-supported health jobs. Instead of submitting their performance to professional review organizations, new legislation would have them evaluated by the community they serve.

Health as a Virtue

Health designates a process of adaptation. It is not the result of instinct, but of an autonomous yet culturally shaped reaction to socially created reality. It designates the ability to adapt to changing environments, to growing up and to aging, to healing when damaged, to suffering, and to the peaceful expectation of death. Health embraces the future as well, and therefore includes anguish and the inner resources to live with it.

Health designates a process by which each person is responsible, but only in part responsible

3 The Honorable James McRuer, *Ontario Royal Commission Inquiry into Civil Rights* (Toronto: Queen's Printer, 1968, 1969, 1971). On self-governing professions and occupations, see chap. 79. The granting of self-government is a delegation of legislative and judicial functions that can be justified only as a safeguard to public interests.

to others. To be responsible may mean two things. A man is responsible for what he has done, and responsible to another person or group. Only when he feels subjectively responsible or answerable to another person will the consequences of his failure be not criticism, censure, or punishment but regret, remorse, and true repentance.[4] The consequent states of grief and distress are marks of recovery and healing, and are phenomenologically something entirely different from guilt feelings. Health is a task, and as such is not comparable to the physiological balance of beasts. Success in this personal task is in large part the result of the self-awareness, self-discipline, and inner resources by which each person regulates his own daily rhythm and actions, his diet, and his sexual activity. Knowledge encompassing desirable activities, competent performance, the commitment to enhance health in others—these are all learned from the example of peers or elders. These personal activities are shaped and conditioned by the culture in which the individual grows up: patterns of work and leisure, of celebration and sleep, of production and preparation of food and drink, of family relations and politics. long-tested health patterns that fit a geographic area and a certain technical situation depend to a large extent on long-lasting political autonomy. They depend on the spread of responsibility for healthy habits and for the sociobiological environment. That is, they depend on the dynamic stability of a culture.

The level of public health corresponds to the degree to which the means and responsibility for coping with illness are distributed among the total population. This ability to cope can be enhanced but never replaced by medical intervention or by the hygienic characteristics of the environment. That society which can reduce professional intervention to the minimum will provide the best conditions for health. The greater the potential for autonomous adaptation to self, to others, and to the environment, the less management of adaptation will be needed or tolerated.

A world of optimal and widespread health is obviously a world of minimal and only occasional medical intervention. Healthy people are those who live in healthy homes on a healthy diet in an environment equally fit for birth, growth, work, heating, and dying; they are sustained by a culture that enhances the conscious acceptance of limits to population, of aging, of incomplete recovery and ever-imminent death. Healthy people need minimal bureaucratic interference to mate, give birth, share the human condition, and die.

Man's consciously lived fragility, individuality, and relatedness make the experience of pain, of sickness, and of death an integral part of his life. The ability to cope with this trio autonomously is fundamental to his health. As he becomes dependent on the management of his intimacy, he renounces his autonomy and his health must decline. The true miracle of modern medicine is diabolical. It consists in making not only individuals but whole populations survive on inhumanly low levels of personal health. Medical nemesis is the negative feedback of a social organization that set out to improve and equalize the opportunity for each man to cope in autonomy and ended by destroying it.

---

4 Alfred Schutz, "Some Equivocations in the Notion of Responsibility," in *Collected Papers*, vol 2., *Studies in Social Theory* (The Hague: Nijhoff, 1964), pp.274-6.

The Impact of Technology on the Future of Health/Illness Education

Joan E. Watson

Many discussions of future societal trends have suggested that electronic advancements will move the workplace to the home.[1, 2, 3] Toffler labeled this phenomenon the electronic cottage.[4] A ubiquitous information system network will predominate the twenty-first century, the basis of which is the home computer. The possibilities for health services will be infinite.

The use of home computers in health care will evolve from the current status to one where physicians have instant access to patient medical histories via pocket computers. This information plus current signs and symptoms can be input, and the physician can receive the probability of a diagnosis.[5] It is similar to the electronic chess game; the more it plays, the more competent it becomes. The physicians' computer will reflect the consultation of hundreds of colleagues all dealing with like problems.

Early in the twenty-first century, home computers will be as common as the television set is today. These computers will be used by the lay public in the same way doctors use their pocket computers. In addition, the public will receive most primary health care at home. Futurists advocate more efficient and economical systems of preventive medicine, medical testing, and data collection and processing.[6] The home computer can provide a means to this end and the hardware necessary to provide this type of health care currently is available. Wichlein projects remote medical diagnosis is possible by simply adding a camera and microphone to a home two-way cable system and videotex.[7] The following encounter will be typical of twenty-first century health care.

> A man notices abdominal pain in the stomach area. He accesses his already entered medical history on his home computer and adds the new complaint. He answers a series of diagnostic questions and is directed to complete his physical exam. The physical parameters are read directly to the computer by the electronic sensing thermometer, stethoscope, and ECG. The individual merely touches himself with the instruments according to the verbal directions and visual descriptions on the screen. Based on these preliminary data, the computer gives the diagnosis—peptic ulcer, probability 65%—further tests needed. He is directed to the local laboratory where a general battery of tests is completed and input under his identification code.

Watson, J. E. The impact of technology on the future of health/illness education. Health Education Quarterly, 10 (2) pp. 95-104. Copyright 1983. Reprinted by permission of Wiley-Liss, a division of John Wiley & Sons, Inc.

1 Shane HG.: The Silcon Age and Education. *Phi Delta Kappan*, 303-307, January 1982.

2 Pritchard WG.: Instructional Computing in 2001: A Scenario. *Phi Delta Kappan*, 322-25, January 1982.

3 Dickson P: *The Future of the Workplace: The Coming Revolution in Jobs.* New York: Weybright and Talley, 1976.

4 Toffler A: *The Third Wave.* Toronto: Bantam Books, 1981.

5 Ramo S: *America's Technology Slip.* New York: John Wiley & Sons, 1980.

6 Wichlein J: *Electronic Nightmare: New Communications and Freedom.* New York: The Viking Press, 1981.

7 Atkinson RC.: Computerized Instruction and the Learning Process. *American Psychologist* 23:225-39, April 1968.

> If he is unable to go there, the lab on wheels will make a house call. After picking up the diagnostic medications from the "drive-thru" pharmacy, he returns home to complete his tests. He takes his medication and completes his nuclear magnetic resonance image of his stomach by standing in front of his electronic camera. The tests are complete. Final diagnosis—peptic ulcer, probability 95%. The prescriptions for medication and diet print out, or he can access the local pharmacy for delivery. The comparative value, risk, and cost of the medications recommended can be accessed if he desires. Based on learning style, he is directed to access two patient education programs, "How to feed your ulcer" and "Decrease your stress through relaxation and exercise." He also can request other health information if he is interested. In fact, he will be provided the same information his physician receives if he requests.
>
> The local health clinics are staffed with a variety of health professionals who are available for consultation, There he can see specialists to assist him in directing the physiological, psychological, social, and educational components of his health program.

This skeptical patient may desire a second opinion from a specialist. By inputing the code, all his medical data are analyzed by a gastroenterologist at the Mayo Clinic. Diagnosis returned—ulcer, probability 99%—concur with treatment. Had the analyses revealed evidence of bleeding or signs that the patient was in imminent danger, he would have been directed to the local hospital where a specialist would direct his care.

Potential of Home Computer Systems

Primary health care through a personal home computer has the potential to increase the number of people receiving health care. Many people today are hesitant to enter the health care system because of fear associated with the belief their complaints are trivial, unpleasant examination procedures, and inconvenience. Home diagnosis can reduce if not eliminate these fears, Closed circuit diagnosis was tested at Logan Airport in Boston during the late 1960s. This successful program put a sick traveler in touch with a hospital-based physician through a nurse and a two-way television system.[6] A similar experiment was conducted in Canada in 1976 which connected nurses in remote clinics with specialists in an urban hospital. These studies indicated at least initial acceptance by consumers.[6]

Computer Assisted Instruction (CAI) is a viable, effective method of instruction that has developed with increasing momentum in a variety of educational settings. While it is not advocated as a teacher replacement, the utilization and effectiveness of computer assisted instruction has been documented.[7, 8, 9, 10, 11] The use of CAI in the education of health professionals, especially medical students, has gained wide acceptance in recent years.[12] A survey of the North American medical schools in 1975 indicated courses involving CAI had increased from one in 1965 to 351 in 1975.[13, 14] Provisions have been made for institutions to share courseware materials. For

8 Anandam K, Kelly J,: Evaluating technology in education. *Journal of Educational Technology Systems* 1:21-31, 1981.

9 Jamison D, Suppes P, Wells S.: The Effectiveness of Alternate Instructional Media: A Survey. *Review of Educational Research* 44:1-68, 1974.

10 Zinn KL.: Instructional Uses of Computers in Higher Education. *The Fourth Inventory of Computers in Higher Education: An Interpretive Report, EDUCOM*. Princeton, NJ:1979.

11 *More Hands for Teachers*. Report of the Commissioner's Advisory Committee on Instructional Computing. Department of Education, Tallahassee, FL: 1980.

12 Deland E (Ed): *Information Technology in Health Science Education*. New York: Plenum Press, 1978.

13 Lefever RD, Johnson JK: *Survey of the Use of Computers in Instruction*. Washington D.C.: Association of American Medical Colleges, 1976.

14 Tidball CS: *Overview of Survey of the Use of Computers in Instruction*. Washington DC: Association of American Medical Colleges, 1976.

instance, through the Health Education Network, Inc. schools of medicine nationwide can have access to the CAI programs available at the Massachusetts General Hospital and Ohio State University.[15]

CAI has been utilized to produce instructional programs based on simulation. Programmed Logic for Automated Teaching Operations (PLATO) developed at the University of Illinois is one example of such a system.[16] The combination of videodisc with CAI has augmented the power of simulation in instruction.[17] The American Heart Association has developed a totally self-contained instructional unit for teaching CPR which combines a videodisc player, a monitor, a computer, and an audio machine.[18] As the student practices CPR on the manikin, he or she receives feedback on the effectiveness of the skill performance as well as individualized instruction.

The use of home computer systems of health care has significant implications for health/illness education. Increased convenient access to health information will increase the general public health literacy. The American people are demonstrating an increased interest in improving their health. There is a general public concern with exercise, nutrition, occupational safety, and environmental health that attests to a desire to promote health and prevent disease. The Surgeon General's recent report acknowledges and encourages this public interest in health by placing a high national priority on disease prevention.[19] The home computer will assist health professionals to incorporate learning styles in instructional design. However, it will not eliminate the need for professionals to be involved in the learning process. "No matter how many questions the computer answer them.[20] The role of the teacher will demand more creativity and initiative.[21] In addition to adjusting for learning style, the computer can provide a wide variety of direct problem solving experiences through simulations and modeling.[22] Shane implies that by using the computer as a tool and drawing upon the instructional skills of professionals, learning in the next century will increase as a result of a more comprehensive approach to education.[1]

Although many hospitals today have added the computer to the patient care technology and educational institutions include CAI in the instruction of health professionals, there is little evidence in support of the use of computer assisted patient instruction. One hospital in New York has reported using portable Apple computers for in-patient cardiac patient teaching.[23] Wygonik advocates the use of computer generated print-outs to enhance the effectiveness of patient education,[24] but he does not suggest the patient can benefit from in-hospital individual computer

15 Tidball CS: Health Education Network. In E Deland (Ed), *Information Technology in Health Science Education.* New York: Plenum Press, 1978.

16 Hody GL, Avner RA: The PLATO System: An Evaluative Description. In Edward Deland (Ed), *Information Technology in Health Science Education.* New York: Plenum Press, 1978.

17 DeChenne JA, Evans R: Simulating Medical Emergencies. *Instructional Innovator* 27(1):23, January 1982.

18 Hessinger L: Computer and Videodisc: A New Way to Teach CPR. *Biomedical Communications* 8(3):12-13, September 1981.

19 United States Department of Health, Education and Welfare. *Healthy People: The Surgeon General's Report on Health Promotion and Disease Prevention.* Public Health Service. Washington DC: Government Printing Office, 1979. (DHEW publication no. 79-5507).

20 Osborne A: Will your job exist in 2005? *Instructional Innovator* 25(3): 27-30, March 1980.

21 Dede C: Educational technology: the next ten years. *Instructional Innovator* 25(3): 17-24, March 1980.

22 Melmed AS: Information Technology for U.S. schools. *Phi Delta Kappan*, 308-315, January 1982.

23 Lyons C, Krasnowski J, Greenstein A, et al: Interactive Computerized Patient Education. *Heart & Lung* 11:340-41, July-August 1982.

24 Wygonik E: Hospital information systems: the computer comes to patient education. In D Bille (Ed), *Practical*

assisted instruction. Health professionals providing hospital based health education as well as community based health education must incorporate the present and future instructional technologies in their practice if health/illness education is to be in phase with the society of the future. If the practitioners are to accomplish this goal, the utilization and production of computer assisted instruction must be included in the undergraduate and graduate health care educational programs.

Possibly the most significant advantage of home computers in health/illness education is the potential to contribute to the individual's perception of internal control. "Our species will survive neither by totally rejecting nor unconditionally embracing technology—but by humanizing it; why allowing people access to the informational tools they need to shape and reassert control over their lives."[25] Home computers will be an integral part of general instructional technology in the future; and the use of this technology will allow people to control aspects of their lives never before possible. Health professionals who continue to force lack of patient control and submission to health care are not only anachronistic, but also contributing to public despair, The public has a *right to know* as established by the 1973 American Hospital Association Patient Bill of Rights and reiterated in the 1982 American Hospital Association Statement on Patient Education. Recently, with few exceptions, Supreme Court judges have upheld the public's right to see, hear, and read what they please. While censorship of health/illness information by health professionals should not be tolerated today, it certainly will not be tolerated by the more information conscious society of the future.

Problems of Home Computer Health Education Use

Technological advances have made a significant impact on the ability of health professionals to identify and treat diseases in our society, while less can be said of the effect of technology on illness prevention. There is little evidence to suggest instructional technology developments have had a significant influence on the health/illness status of this country. However, the potential for such an influence is great. Health professionals have a habit of letting all forms of technology "happen to them" rather than taking the initiative in projecting and planning for technologies to serve society's needs, If the projected future of health/illness education is to become reality, health professionals and consumers must consider some issues of consequence. Through such an analysis, it is possible and desirable to invent or prevent future developments. The following are some problems commonly identified with this new technology.

Depersonalization

> The computer as a "thinking machine" with its human-like qualities of memory and logic, is challenging our beliefs in human uniqueness. By now doing things that once only people could do, the computer is forcing us to new conceptions of the relationship between man and machine. At one and the same time, the computer provides an opportunity for enhancing human endeavors and gives the humanist a chance to ponder new concepts of uniqueness.[26]

Depersonalization is not a recent development in the health care system; and health professionals frequently are accused of "treating the dis-

Approaches to Patient Teaching. Boston: Little, Brown and Co., 1981.

25 Shamberg M: Television. In L Hickman, A Al-Hibri (Eds): *Technology and Human Affairs*. St. Louis: C.V. Mosby Co, 1981.

26 Slack C, Porter D, Slack W: Some nostalgic reflections on computer assisted instruction. In E Deland (Ed), *Information Technology in Health Science Education*. New York: Plenum Press, 1978.

ease/organ" rather than the individual. While health/illness is viewed as a very personal condition by most lay people, the health care system is seen as having a depersonalization effect.[27] This pervasive lack of individuality in health care led to the development of the following new roles within the system: primary nurse, primary physician, clinical nurse specialist, patient advocate, and patient care managers. Although these people function differently, one common aspect of their roles is assisting the individual to cope with the health care system.

Depersonalization is common in our health care system today. The potential decrease in personal contact associated with home computer diagnosis and treatment can not create that sense of depersonalization; it already exists. In fact, use of home computers may reduce the depersonalization felt by consumers of health care and bring them out of their homes with a feeling of greater personal control. It is possible and probable people may prefer the computer to their doctor.[28] Increased access to health information through use of home computers will serve to demystify medical care for consumers. Greater understanding of medical care can lead to a greater sense of individual control, greater acceptance and adoption of health behavior, and consumers who take an active responsibility for their own health promotion.

Patients at the Salt Lake City Veterans Administration Hospital experience computer psychological assessment and diagnosis. When compared to psychiatrists' assessments and diagnoses, the computer was found to be more accurate, less costly, and require less time. The 132 patients processed both ways indicated 89% preferred the computer, and 56% said they answered the computer's questions more truthfully. Seventy-eight percent agreed that the computer was not too impersonal.[29]

Sagan forecasts an early acceptance of machine intelligence and states "there is nothing inhuman about an intelligent an intelligent machine."[30] The wearers of cardiac pacemakers are not resentful of machine intelligence, but exemplary of this acceptance. Ellis and Raines at the University of Minnesota reported acceptance of microcomputer health education by the 420 volunteers they tested in 1975.[31] Computer Assisted Instructional programs were developed on specific health topics such as coronary risk factor control and weight control. The non-computer oriented volunteers rated the programs positively on patient appeal as well as helpfulness. Personalization can occur by using the computer to implement meta-cognition research. The potential for learner awareness of internal learning processes shifts the instructional technology emphasis from incidental learning to intentional learning.[32]

Cost

The escalating cost of health care is riot a new issue, but one that continues to challenge health care providers and consumers. The question of who will pay for health/illness education is a salient concern of educators. Blue Cross and Blue Shield Association published the White Paper which encouraged programs of community health/illness education,[33] yet with very few exceptions this support has not been realized

27 Wu R: *Behavior and Illness*, Englewood Cliffs, NJ: 1973.

28 Evans C: *The Micro Millennium.* New York: Washington Square Press, 1979.

29 Lesse S: The preventive psychiatry of the future. In E Cornish (Ed), *1999 The World of Tomorrow.* Washington DC: World Future Society, 75-81, 1978.

30 Sagan C: *Broca's Brain.* New York: Ballantine Books, 1979.

31 Ellis L. Raines J: Health education using microcomputers: initial acceptability. *Preventive Medical* 10:77084, 1981.

32 Gagne R: Is educational technology in phase? *Educational Technology* 20(2):7-14, February 1980.

33 *White Paper—Patient Health Education.* Chicago: Blue Cross, Blue Shield Association, 1974.

through direct reimbursement. In-hospital education usually if funded by third party reimbursement by including it in the cost of the room. While it is an admirable ambition, in reality, all patients do not receive the instruction for which they pay!

It is likely that the issue of reimbursement for health/illness education will be resolved in the near future. Health care agencies will have to document clearly the patient education provided. It will not be possible to continue to mask the cost of patient education by categorizing it under a "reimbursable" program such as cardiac rehabilitation or renal dialysis. When education is recognized as an integral part of health care, reimbursement in the same manner as diagnosis and treatment can result. While there are those people who believe no one should profit from providing services essential to people's lives,[6] it is obvious that the cost of health/illness education in the future cannot be hidden. Health care spending will be increasingly scrutinized by consumers and third-party payers. "Those services that can conclusively demonstrate cost savings and cost efficiencies will be more likely to be desired by the market-place, and in turn, supported by Blue Cross and Blue Shield Plans.[34]

The use of home computer for primary health care can assure health/illness education will not be available exclusively to the affluent. The cost of home computers will continue to decrease over the next 20 years and the computer will be as common to the home of the twenty-first century as the television is today. While the cost of designing and producing computer programs to provide this health/illness education may be high initially, it will be minuscule when compared with the amount spent today because of ignorance of appropriate health care. Today's health care system exemplifies the notion that people pay most for things they understand the least; and the increased access to second opinions and health/illness information should reduce drastically the cost of care in the future.

Privacy

Privacy in the age of computers is addressed by most authors who write about the future. A 1979 Harris Poll revealed nearly two-thirds of the citizens queried responded they were concerned about threats to personal privacy in America.[6] We must plan for an individual's right to privacy and give this protection high priority.

> The right to privacy is based on a belief in the essential dignity and worth of the individual. Maintaining one's individuality involves the right to be free from certain types of intrusions and to have personal control over time, conditions, and extent to which one's thoughts, beliefs, attitudes, opinions, and personal history are to be shared or withheld from others. Without privacy, the concept of individuality is meaningless.[35]

Concern for individual privacy is not a computer problem; it is a computer induced societal problem. The true study of technology is a study of its relationships with those who create and use it.[8] Computers are secure until some human being chooses to violate that security. While computers make access to private information easier, people must use the accessed information malevolently if privacy violation is to be a problem. Justice Brandeis warned, long before the privacy issue included computers, "The greatest dangers to liberty lurk in insidious encroachment by men of zeal, well-meaning but without understanding."[36]

---

34 LeBrun P, Gendel T, Rice K, Gerber D, Raichel T: *Blue Cross and Blue Shield Plan Support for Health Education Services: A Discussion of Issues*. Chicago: Blue Cross and Blue Shield Association, 1982.

35 Grayson LP: Education, Technology, and Individual Privacy. *Educational Communication and Technology Journal* 26(3):195-206, Fall 1978.

36 Olmstead v. U.S. In *United States Reports:277*. Washington, D.C.:U.S, Printing Office, 1927.

Following the tradition established in Sweden, Wichlein advocates a non-governmental Privacy Board that would hear complaints and have authority to rectify computer/individual errors.[6]

Protection of privacy related to personal health/illness status may be a minor concern by comparison. Individuals generally are not reticent in discussing details of their health/illness, and therefore less interested in the need for privacy related to health matters. Evans suggests a system of codes and computer generated checks that could easily protect health/illness records from the average inquiry, perhaps more effectively than our present "easily scrutinized, forged and copied paper records."[28] As society deals with the issues of job discrimination based on health, prevention of disease, and insurability of individuals, the concern for protecting health status privacy will be reduced.

Control

Health professionals have been deluged with technological advances to assist with diagnosis, monitoring, and treatment. While the presence and use of this technology indicates an initial acceptance, there is equal evidence of misuse which may be indicative of non-acceptance or ignorance. Empirical data indicate the acceptance level of computer technology in the health professions is ambivalent at best. Bleich reviewed physician use of computers and concluded doctors welcome the challenge of a new device especially if it performs tedious calculations and is under their complete control.[37]

A 1973-74 project evaluated 29 health care computer projects including: administrative services; business services; patient education; history taking; health testing; analysis of physiological measures; medical records, and appointment scheduling. A reluctant response of health professionals, especially physicians, to the use of computers was found.[38] Giebink's survey of computer utilization indicated few physicians expected the system to help them with patient care activities, but they believed computers could help with non-direct patient care functions. Although this same study indicated nurses often were more positive toward computer utilization, too frequently they shared the reservations of the physicians. The Ohio State University College of Medicine has been in the forefront of development and utilization of computer assisted instruction for health professional education.[39] In spite of perhaps the largest single collection of CAI courseware related to health professional education,[40] there exists no provision at The Ohio State University for patient health/illness education via computer.

Underutilization of technology in health/illness education is pervasive in today's health care systems. Health professionals who wish to alter this course must consider the following questions: 1) Does the present instructional technology fail to provide an effective educational opportunity? 2) Are health professionals rigidly clinging to the anachronistic past? 3) Does current and future technology reduce health professionals' feelings of control? 4)Are health professionals frightened by prospects of how easily and accurately their jobs can be computerized? It is time for health professionals to stop reacting to technological developments and address these and other issues of control, because

37 Bleich H: Management of clinical problems by physician computer dialogue. In E Deland (Ed) *Information Technology in Health Science Education*. New York: Plenum Press, 1978.

38 Giebrink G, Hurst L: *Computer Projects in Health Care*. Ann Arbor: Health Administration Press, 1975.

39 Pengov RE.: The Evolution and Use of Computer Assisted Instruction (CAI) in Health Sciences Education at The Ohio State University College of Medicine. In E Deland (Ed), *Information Technology in Health Science Education*. New York: Plenum Press, 1978.

40 Kamp M, Brigham C.: Current Status of Computer Assisted Instruction in the Health Sciences. *Journal of Medical Education* 49(3):279, 1974.

the consumers of the twenty-first century will not tolerate excessive control by the health care system. Health professional influence based on attitudes toward these issues of control will be a determinant of the health care system of the future.

Summary

The direction of future technology and its impact on the health care system will be shaped by economic, social, and political factors. If health professionals are to influence the health care of the future, a sense of involvement in developing technology must be realized immediately. It is time for health professionals and consumers to think about the unthinkable. While not enough is known about what causes individual health/illness behavior, how it might be altered, or how desirable health/illness behavior can be determined, it is projected the technology of the future will evolve a well-informed individual who experiences a sense of control over health related behavior. Rather than letting current and future technology simply happen, health professionals should feel an obligation to participate in designing the health care system of the future.